Pediatric

Edited by

HOWARD BAUCHNER, MD
Professor of Pediatrics and Public Health
Director, Division of General Pediatrics
Department of Pediatrics
Boston Medical Center
Boston University School of Medicine
Boston, MA

ROBERT J. VINCI, MD
Professor of Pediatrics
Program Director
Boston Combined Residency Program
Department of Pediatrics
Boston Medical Center
Boston University School of Medicine
Boston, MA

MELANIE KIM, MD
Associate Professor of Pediatrics
Associate Program Director
Boston Combined Residency Program
Department of Pediatrics
Boston Medical Center
Boston University School of Medicine
Boston, MA

CAMBRIDGE
UNIVERSITY PRESS

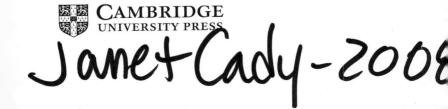

Janet Cady - 2008

CAMBRIDGE UNIVERSITY PRESS
Cambridge, New York, Melbourne, Madrid, Cape Town, Singapore,
São Paulo, Delhi

Cambridge University Press
32 Avenue of the Americas, New York, NY 10013-2473, USA

www.cambridge.org
Information on this title: www.cambridge.org/9780521709361

© 2007, 2003, Pocket Pediatrics by PocketMedicine.com, Inc.

This publication is in copyright. Subject to statutory exception
and to the provisions of relevant collective licensing agreements,
no reproduction of any part may take place without
the written permission of Cambridge University Press.

First published 2007

Printed in the United States of America

A catalog record for this publication is available from the British Library.

Library of Congress Cataloging in Publication Data

Pediatrics / [edited by] Howard Bauchner, Robert Vinci, Melanie Kim.
  p.   cm.
ISBN-13: 978-0-521-70936-1 (pbk.)
ISBN-10: 0-521-70936-9 (pbk.)
1. Pediatrics – Handbooks, manuals, etc.   I. Bauchner, Howard, 1951–
II. Vinci, Robert J.   III. Kim, Melanie, 1952–
[DNLM: 1. Pediatrics – Handbooks. WS 39 P37191 2007]
RJ48.P428   2007
618.92–dc22   2007016912

ISBN   978-0-521-70936-1 paperback

Cambridge University Press has no responsibility for
the persistence or accuracy of URLs for external or
third-party Internet Web sites referred to in this publication
and does not guarantee that any content on such
Web sites is, or will remain, accurate or appropriate.

Every effort has been made in preparing this book to provide accurate and
up-to-date information that is in accord with accepted standards and practice at
the time of publication. Nevertheless, the authors, editors, and publisher can
make no warranties that the information contained herein is totally free from
error, not least because clinical standards are constantly changing through
research and regulation. The authors, editors, and publisher therefore disclaim
all liability for direct or consequential damages resulting from the use of
material contained in this book. Readers are strongly advised to pay careful
attention to information provided by the manufacturer of any drugs or
equipment that they plan to use.

NOTICE

Because of the dynamic nature of medical practice and drug selection and dosage, users are advised that decisions regarding drug therapy must be based on the independent judgment of the clinician, changing information about a drug (e.g., as reflected in the literature and manufacturer's most current product information), and changing medical practices.

While great care has been taken to ensure the accuracy of the information presented, users are advised that the authors, editors, contributors, and publisher make no warranty, express or implied, with respect to, and are not responsible for, the currency, completeness, or accuracy of the information contained in this publication, nor for any errors, omissions, or the application of this information, nor for any consequences arising therefrom. Users are encouraged to confirm the information contained herein with other sources deemed authoritative. Ultimately, it is the responsibility of the treating physician, relying on experience and knowledge of the patient, to determine dosages and the best treatment for the patient. Therefore, the author(s), editors, contributors, and the publisher make no warranty, express or implied, and shall have no liability to any person or entity with regard to claims, loss, or damage caused, or alleged to be caused, directly or indirectly, by the use of information contained in this publication.

Further, the author(s), editors, contributors, and the publisher are not responsible for misuse of any of the information provided in this publication, for negligence by the user, or for any typographical errors.

Contents

Preface

The way that physicians care for patients is changing. The time spent with patients has become shorter, so that busy clinicians both need and want authoritative information in a quick, easy-to-use format.

Pediatrics has been designed to provide a comprehensive review of clinical pediatrics, with advice for appropriate diagnostic and therapeutic interventions for the most common pediatric problems encountered in the clinical setting. The topics are organized under headings on differential diagnosis, evaluation, treatment, complications and prognosis so that the user will find the desired information quickly and easily.

It is our hope that *Pediatrics* will provide clinicians in any setting with a text that will help them feel comfortable managing both the most common and clinically challenging presentations of acutely ill children.

Howard Bauchner, Robert J. Vinci, and Melanie Kim

ACETAMINOPHEN POISONING

HENAN SEDIK, M.D., F.A.A.P.

HISTORY AND PHYSICAL
- History of ingestion:
  - Tylenol® preparations
  - Over-the-counter analgesics/cold remedies
- Toxic dose >150 mg/kg in acute ingestion
  - Stage I (0.5–24 h):
    - Nausea
    - Vomiting
    - Diaphoresis
    - Pallor
    - Malaise
  - Stage II (24–72 h): latent period: initial symptoms resolve; hepatic dysfunction develops
  - Stage III (3–7 d):
    - Progressive hepatic encephalopathy: jaundice, confusion, hyperammonemia, & bleeding diathesis

TESTS
- Acetaminophen level: 4 h after ingestion
- Plot level on Rumack and Matthew's semilogarithmic nomogram
- Liver function tests
- Serum toxicology screen for co-ingestions

DIFFERENTIAL DIAGNOSIS
- Accidental vs. intentional
- Chronic ingestions
- Other hepatotoxins
- Viral hepatitis/hepatic disease
- Reye's

MANAGEMENT
- GI decontamination
- Antidote: N-acetylcysteine (NAC)

SPECIFIC THERAPY
- Decontamination:
  - Gastric lavage: within first hour after ingestion.
  - Avoid ipecac unless toxic co-ingestion

- ➤ Activated charcoal:
  - All patients w/in 4 h of ingestion
  - Consider beyond 4 h for co-ingestions or delayed absorption of acetaminophen (e.g., ingestion of sustained-release preparations or agent that slows gut motility)
- ■ *N*-acetylcysteine (NAC):
  - ➤ Antidote
  - ➤ Most efficacious if administered w/in 8 h of ingestion
  - ➤ Use if:
    - 4-hour level >150 mcq/mL
    - Patient presents 6–8 h after ingestion: give initial dose while level pending
  - ➤ Oral dose: loading dose 140 mg/kg, then 70 mg/kg q4h for 17 doses, diluted 1:4 in a carbonated beverage, PO or NG
  - ➤ Side effects: nausea, vomiting
  - ➤ Repeat dose if patient vomits within 1 h; use antiemetics
  - ➤ IV NAC (not FDA approved in U.S.) recommended for:
    - Pts who cannot tolerate oral NAC due to intractable vomiting & for whom further delay will result in decreased efficacy
    - Pts whose medical condition precludes enteral use of NAC (e.g., corrosive ingestion, GI bleeding or obstruction)
    - Fulminant hepatic failure
    - Pregnancy

FOLLOW-UP

- ■ Serum acetaminophen level in "minimal risk of hepatic toxicity" range on nomogram (or ingestion <140 mg/kg): sent home
- ■ Potential hepatotoxicity: admitted for antidote therapy
- ■ Repeat monitoring of acetaminophen levels at 4 h intervals
- ■ NAC should not be discontinued if subsequent levels fall below possible hepatic toxic zone
- ■ Monitor liver function and coagulation profile

COMPLICATIONS AND PROGNOSIS

Complications

- ■ Fulminant hepatic failure
- ■ Renal failure
- ■ Anaphylaxis with IV NAC

Prognosis

- ■ No toxicity with ingestion of single dose <150 mg/kg

- Hepatocellular necrosis: may resolve with ICU care
- Fulminant hepatic failure: may require transplant

ACNE VULGARIS

PAULINE SHEEHAN, M.D.

HISTORY AND PHYSICAL
- 85% teenagers & young adults affected

History
- Risk factors: relative with severe disease, hyperandrogenism

Physical signs
- Disorder of pilosebaceous unit; prominent on face, chest & back
- Noninflammatory lesions:
    - Microcomedones
    - Open comedones (blackheads)
    - Closed comedones (whiteheads)
- Inflammatory lesions:
    - Papules
    - Pustules
    - Cysts
    - Nodules

TESTS
- Free & total testosterone & DHEA-S, LH, FSH, prolactin in females who:
    - Fail traditional therapy
    - Evidence of hyperandrogenism

DIFFERENTIAL DIAGNOSIS
- Rash caused by systemic or topical steroids, anticonvulsants, isoniazid
- Folliculitis
- Acne rosacea

MANAGEMENT
- Goal: to prevent scarring and emotional sequelae
- Noticeable improvement: 6–8 wk
- Proper usage & dosage of medications important

- Avoid creams, lotions, cosmetics, hair care products containing oil (use oil-free, non-comedogenic, water-based products)
- Picking & excessive scrubbing can lead to scarring

SPECIFIC THERAPY

- Depending on type, severity & distribution of lesions
- Generally begin w/ topical therapy with keratolytic agent alone or w/ topical antibiotic; then progress to systemic therapy w/ oral antibiotics, OCPs, antiandrogens
- Non-inflammatory:
  - ➤ Benzoyl peroxide:
    - gels, creams, lotions, soaps, shaving creams, washes
    - Start w/ water-based gel or cream
    - Lower concentrations less irritant
  - ➤ Tretinoin:
    - Creams, gels, solutions
    - Start with lowest concentrations; work up as tolerated
    - Apply thin layer every other night, wash off in am
  - ➤ May add azelaic acid:
    - Anti-inflammatory, comedolytic; fades hyperpigmentation
    - Less potent than tretinoin but tolerated better
  - ➤ May add adapalene gel: similar effect as tretinoin but less local irritation
  - ➤ Tazarotene gel: for acne & psoriasis
- Moderate inflammatory:
  - ➤ As for non-inflammatory; then consider:
    - Topical clindamycin, tetracycline, or erythromycin
    - Add oral therapy PRN: tetracycline, doxycycline, minocycline
    - Second-line oral therapy: erythromycin, amoxicillin, cephalexin
- Severe inflammatory:
  - ➤ As for moderate inflammatory; then consider:
    - Increase frequency & dosage of oral antibiotics
    - Consider intralesional steroids, isotretinoin (only for severe recalcitrant acne)
    - Oral contraceptives, hormonal therapy (spironolactone)

FOLLOW-UP

- Re-evaluate in 6–8 wk
- Adjust therapy accordingly
- Continue antibiotics for 3 mo & reconsider therapy
- Judicious use of antibiotics important

COMPLICATIONS AND PROGNOSIS

- Scarring
- Hyper- or hypopigmentation
- Beware psychological impact

ACUTE ABDOMINAL PAIN

JAIME BELKIND-GERSON, M.D.

HISTORY AND PHYSICAL

History

- Type, character, & radiation of pain
- Previous abdominal pain
- Vomiting, diarrhea, bowel function
- ? GI bleeding
- Cough, fever
- Precipitating events, diet
- Intake of drugs or toxins
- Trauma
- Past surgical history

Physical signs

- Fever
- Pharyngitis
- Evidence of pneumonia, costovertebral angle tenderness
- Location & character of pain
- Presence or absence of bowel sounds
- Liver, spleen size
- Peritoneal signs
- Rectal exam (test for blood)
- Pelvic exam/testicular exam

TESTS

- CBC
- Urinalysis
- Abdominal flat plate and upright films
- Amylase, lipase, ALT/AST, bilirubins, glucose
- Stool culture and tests for ova and parasites
- BUN/creatinine
- Pregnancy test

- Toxicology screen
- Chest x-ray
- Abdominal ultrasound
- In selected cases, GI contrast studies and/or CT

DIFFERENTIAL DIAGNOSIS
- Trauma:
  - Duodenal hematoma
  - Pancreatitis
  - Liver or spleen laceration
- Intra-abdominal medical disorders:
  - Constipation
  - Gastroenteritis
  - Peptic ulcer disease
  - UTI
  - Pelvic inflammatory disease (PID)
  - Pancreatitis
- Intra-abdominal surgical disorders:
  - Appendicitis
  - Intussusception
  - Complicated pancreatitis
  - Obstruction from previous surgery
- Extra-abdominal disorders:
  - Pneumonia
  - Psychogenic pain
  - Testicular or ovarian torsion
  - Pregnancy
  - PID
- Systemic disorders:
  - Lead poisoning
  - Sickle cell anemia
  - Diabetic ketoacidosis
  - Porphyria
- Surgical disorder suggested by:
  - Pain that wakes child at night
  - Severe pain
  - Fever, vomiting (particularly bilious or feculent)
  - Rebound tenderness
  - Lack of bowel sounds
  - Abdominal distention
  - Failure to pass flatus

MANAGEMENT

General measures
- Avoid analgesics
- NPO with IV fluid & electrolyte replacement
- NG tube for relief of GI obstruction
- Consider surgical and/or gastroenterologist consult

SPECIFIC THERAPY
- Varies according to etiology
- Prompt attention to potential surgical cases is high priority

FOLLOW-UP
- Frequent contact w/ pt discharged with diagnosis of abdominal pain

COMPLICATIONS AND PROGNOSIS
- Varies according to etiology:
  - Dehydration
  - Electrolyte imbalances
  - Sepsis
  - Intestinal perforation, intestinal obstruction, & hemorrhage

Prognosis
- Very good for most medical disorders (e.g., infectious diarrhea, gastroenteritis, constipation)
- Excellent for surgical disorders treated in a timely manner (e.g., appendicitis, intussusception, testicular torsion, obstruction due to adhesions, ectopic pregnancy)

ACUTE ASTHMA

SUZANNE F. STEINBACH, M.D.

HISTORY AND PHYSICAL

History
- Presence/duration: cough, wheeze, shortness/labored/rapid breathing
- Home therapy: # & frequency of steroids, bronchodilator doses
- Previous attacks:
  - Use of steroids
  - ER/hospital/ICU care
  - Intubation

- Best baseline peak expiratory flow (PEF)
- Trigger exposures

Physical signs

- Respiratory rate
- Oxygen sat
- Ability to speak
- Retractions
- Trachea midline, crepitus
- Air entry, inspiratory to expiratory ratio (I:E), wheeze, asymmetries
- Mental status

TESTS

- PEF
- CXR:
  - ➤ Asymmetric exam
  - ➤ Poor response to therapy
- ABG: poor response to therapy

DIFFERENTIAL DIAGNOSIS

- Bronchiolitis
- Laryngotracheobronchitis (croup)
- Foreign body aspiration
- Vocal cord dysfunction
- Airway compression
- Anaphylaxis

MANAGEMENT

What to do first

- Assess severity:
  - ➤ Mild:
    - Mild tachypnea
    - Normal mental status and color
    - Speaks in sentences
    - ± mild retractions
    - PEF >80%
    - O_2 sat >95%
    - $PaCO_2$ <35
    - ± end-expiratory wheeze (E)
    - Good response
  - ➤ Moderate:
    - Moderate tachypnea & retractions

- Normal mental status
- Speaks in phrases
- Pale
- PEF: 50–80%
- O_2 sat: 91–95%, $PaCO_2$ <42
- E or inspiratory (I) & E wheeze
- Incomplete response to therapy
➤ Severe:
  - Severe tachypnea or apnea
  - Depressed or agitated mental status
  - ± severe retractions
  - Single word or short phrases
  - ± cyanotic
  - Decreased aeration
  - PEF <50
  - O_2 sat <91, $PaCO_2$ >41
  - Poor response to therapy

General measures
■ Reassure
■ Educate
■ Hydrate; avoid overhydration
■ O_2: O_2 sat >90%
■ Bronchodilators:
  ➤ Inhaled albuterol
  ➤ Ipratropium bromide
  ➤ SQ epinephrine/terbutaline
  ➤ IV terbutaline
■ Corticosteroids

SPECIFIC THERAPY
■ Mild:
  ➤ Albuterol 0.02 mL/kg (max, 1.0 mL) in NS nebulized or 2–4 puffs w/ spacer q20 min up to 3×, then q4 h at home, taper
  ➤ Consider oral steroids: 1–2 mg/kg (max, 60 mg/d) divided bid for 3–10 d
■ Moderate/severe:
  ➤ O_2 to keep O_2 sat >90%
  ➤ Albuterol 0.03 mL/kg (max, 1.0) in NS nebulized w/ ipratropium q20 min up to 3× or 4–8 puffs with spacer q20 min up to 4 h

➤ Steroids PO or IV: 2–4 mg/kg/day: in extremis or no response to
   1st dose or incomplete response to 2nd dose of albuterol
■ In extremis, can't do PEF, deteriorates suddenly:
➤ Epinephrine 1:1,000, 0.01 mg = mL/kg sq (max, 0.3–0.5 mL),
   repeat q15 min × 3
➤ Terbutaline 1:1,000, 0.01 mg = mL/kg sq (max, 0.25 mL)

Side effects and complications of treatment
■ O_2: hypoventilation in chronic CO_2 retainers
■ Beta-2 agonists: tachycardia, anxiety, tremor, head/abdominal pain,
  arrhythmias
■ Ipratropium: migratory anisocoria, tremor
■ Steroids: GI upset, acne, hyperglycemia, hypertension, weight gain,
  hypokalemia, psychosis

Contraindications:

Absolute
■ Sedation, mucolytic drugs

Relative
■ Chest physiotherapy; antibiotics (OK for pneumonia, sinusitis)

FOLLOW-UP
■ Assess after bronchodilator therapy & 1 h later
■ Poor response (persistent severe asthma): transfer to ER or ICU with
  O_2, albuterol, steroids:
➤ SQ epinephrine/terbutaline
➤ Continuous albuterol nebs, 0.5 mg/kg/h
➤ $MgSO_4$ 25 mg/kg (max, 2.0 g) q6h
➤ Heliox 70/30
➤ Terbutaline IV: 10 mcg/kg over 10 min then 0.2 mcg/kg/min,
   titrate up to max 8 mcg/kg/min; monitor EKG, cardiac enzymes
■ Incomplete response (persistent moderate asthma):
➤ Repeat albuterol q20 min × 3 or space to qh × 3–4 h
➤ Corticosteroids
➤ ER or hospital >3 h
■ Good response (mild asthma):
➤ Space albuterol q2 h
➤ Consider steroids
■ Discharge: <2 signs in moderate category, PEF >80%
■ Follow-up 2–3 days

- Persistent asthma (see "Chronic Asthma" entry): begin or step up preventive therapy

COMPLICATIONS AND PROGNOSIS
- Pneumomediastinum: 5–15% hospitalized pts, rarely symptomatic, supportive care
- Pneumothorax: rare, if large or tension; chest tube
- Atelectasis: common, mistaken for pneumonia, Rx longer steroid course
- Pneumonia: uncommon, likely viral or *Mycoplasma*
- Respiratory failure: rare

Prognosis
- Short-term: good
- Long-term: good if anti-inflammatory preventive therapy used

ACUTE LYMPHOBLASTIC LEUKEMIA (ALL)

KIMBERLY STEGMAIER, M.D.

HISTORY AND PHYSICAL
- Fever
- Anorexia/weight loss
- Fatigue
- Bone pain/limp
- Bleeding/bruising
- Arthralgias
- Lymphadenopathy
- Hepatosplenomegaly
- Petechiae/purpura
- Pallor

TESTS
- CBC
  - Elevated WBC
  - Neutropenia
  - Anemia
  - Thrombocytopenia
  - Blasts
- Bone marrow aspirate & biopsy:
  - >25% lymphoblasts

- Histochemical stain:
  - Periodic acid-Schiff (PAS) +
  - Terminal deoxynucleotidyl transferase (TdT) +
  - Myeloperoxidase
- Cytogenetic analysis: translocations (prognosis)
- Immunophenotype analysis:
  - Cell surface markers (3 classes):
    - B-progenitor
    - Mature B-cell
    - T-cell
- Ca, Phos, LDH, uric acid, K
- If febrile, blood & urine cultures
- CXR
- Coagulation studies
- Lumbar puncture: CSF cytocentrifugation: blasts
- Echocardiogram, ECG

DIFFERENTIAL DIAGNOSIS
- Nonmalignant:
  - Juvenile rheumatoid arthritis
  - Immune thrombocytopenia purpura
  - Infectious mononucleosis
  - Pertussis
  - Aplastic anemia
  - Acute infectious lymphocytosis
  - Osteomyelitis
- Malignant:
  - Acute myelogenous leukemia
  - Neuroblastoma
  - Lymphoma
  - Myelodysplastic syndrome
  - Rhabdomyosarcoma

MANAGEMENT
- Prevent uric acid nephropathy:
  - IV hydration
  - Alkalinization
  - Allopurinol
- Fever and neutropenia:
  - Identify infection

➤ Broad-spectrum antibiotics
- Transfusion support
- Correct coagulopathy
- Nutritional support
- Central access for chemotherapy
- Psychosocial support

SPECIFIC THERAPY
- Pts classified high or standard risk
- Therapy depends on classification
- High-risk criteria:
    ➤ Age <1 or >10 y
    ➤ WBC >50,000/mcL
    ➤ T-cell phenotype
    ➤ Anterior mediastinal mass
    ➤ CNS disease
    ➤ Translocation: t(4;11) or t(9;22)
    ➤ Slow response to induction therapy
    ➤ Four phases of therapy
- Induction: intensive chemotherapy for 1 mo
    ➤ Induction agents: prednisone, vincristine, methotrexate, asparaginase, anthracyclines
    ➤ >95% complete remission
- CNS therapy: prevent relapse
    ➤ Intrathecal agents: hydrocortisone, methotrexate, cytarabine
    ➤ Some high-risk pts: cranial irradiation
- Intensification:
    ➤ Cytoreduce & suppress leukemic growth
    ➤ Multiple drugs: prevent resistant clone
- Continuation:
    ➤ Less intensive: eliminate minimal residual disease
    ➤ Maximally tolerated doses used outpatient for >=2 y
- Exceptions: high-risk pts with t(9;12), Philadelphia chromosome: bone marrow transplant after induction

FOLLOW-UP
- After induction outpatient q1–3 wk
- Monitor for side effects: exam, CBC, LFTs, renal function
- Evaluate: febrile episodes
- Monitor long-term complications

COMPLICATIONS AND PROGNOSIS
- Infection:
  - ➤ Major cause morbidity/mortality
  - ➤ Risk factors:
    - Mucosal barrier breakdown
    - Neutropenia
    - Central venous catheters
  - ➤ Bacteria
  - ➤ Fungal
  - ➤ Viral: herpes zoster/simplex
  - ➤ Other opportunistic infections: *Pneumocystis carinii* (Bactrim for prophylaxis)
- Tumor lysis syndrome:
  - ➤ Elevated K, Phos, uric acid, LDH
  - ➤ Hyper- or hypocalcemia
  - ➤ Uric acid nephropathy: possible acute renal failure
- Bleeding
- Anemia: severe can lead to cardiac failure

Prognosis
- Event-free survival (EFS) for standard-risk pts: 75–85%
- EFS for high-risk pts: 60–80%
- Late complications:
  - ➤ Neuropsychological abnormalities
  - ➤ Neuroendocrine insufficiencies
  - ➤ Cardiac dysfunction
  - ➤ Cataracts
  - ➤ Short stature
  - ➤ Obesity

ACUTE OTITIS MEDIA

HOWARD BAUCHNER, M.D.

HISTORY AND PHYSICAL
- Often URI ± fever
- Older children: ear pain
- Examine ear, head, neck
- Middle ear effusion: w/out signs & symptoms of acute illness, does not indicate AOM

- Key to Dx: particularly in younger children, assess tympanic membrane (TM) mobility using pneumatic otoscopy
- Red, bulging, distinct fullness, immobile TM

TESTS
- Tympanometry or other test of mobility
  - Assess TM mobility
  - Confirm presence of middle ear fluid

DIFFERENTIAL DIAGNOSIS
- External otitis
- Middle ear effusion w/out acute disease
- Mastoiditis
- Infections of oropharynx, teeth, scalp

MANAGEMENT
- Antibiotics
- Pain relief

SPECIFIC THERAPY

Treatment
- First-line Rx: amoxicillin
- Drug-resistant *S. pneumoniae* (DRSP):
  - Risk factors:
    - Young age
    - Community with high rates of DRSP
    - Recent antibiotic therapy
    - Exposure to large numbers of children
  - Treatment
    - High-dose amoxicillin or amoxicillin-clavulanate
    - Other antibiotics: cefuroxime axetil, ceftriaxone
    - CDC recommendation: daily IM ceftriaxone for 3 d, however can give 1 injection and see if patient improves
    - Other cephalosporins & macrolides do not treat DRSP
    - Some antibiotics, e.g., azithromycin, not reliably effective against other bacteria such as *H. influenzae*
- Penicillin allergy:
  - Oral cephalosporins, macrolides, co-trimoxazole
  - High rates of resistance to co-trimoxazole
- Length of Rx:
  - Infants/young children: 10 d

➤ Older children: 7 d <u>or</u> consider no antibiotic Rx reasonable with close contact maintained
■ Pain relief:
  ➤ Acetaminophen
  ➤ NSAIDs
  ➤ Otic drops

FOLLOW-UP
■ 48–72 hr: if no clinical improvement, contact provider
■ Next visit: examine young infants for middle ear effusion
■ 3–4 mo follow-up: necessary if child has recurrent AOM, middle ear effusion or child is not hearing well

COMPLICATIONS AND PROGNOSIS
■ Complications rare
■ In infants, may be associated with bacteremia
■ Older children do well
■ Mastoiditis can occur in children treated with antibiotics
■ Prognosis:
  ➤ Effusions resolve
    • 60% by 1 mo
    • 80% by 2 mo
    • 90% by 3 mo
  ➤ Hearing loss associated with recurrent episodes

ACUTE RENAL FAILURE (ARF)

MICHAEL J. G. SOMERS, M.D.

HISTORY AND PHYSICAL

History
■ Change in urine output, color, stream
■ Volume depletion
■ Nephrotoxin exposure
■ Recent pharyngitis, impetigo, diarrhea
■ Previous UTIs
■ Abdominal surgery or tumor
■ Family history:
  ➤ Renal disease
  ➤ Dialysis or renal transplant

Physical signs
- Vital signs, esp. BP
- Hydration/perfusion status
- Pericardial effusion
- Pulmonary edema
- Abdominal mass
- Palpable bladder
- Rashes or purpura
- Peripheral edema
- Joint swelling or anomalies
- Bony anomalies/rickets
- Mental status or DTR changes

TESTS
- CBC
- Plasma and urine osmolality, electrolytes, Cr
- BUN, Ca, phos
- Albumin
- Microscopic urinalysis
- If clinically indicated:
    - Complement levels
    - ANA or dsDNA
    - ASLO titers or streptozyme
    - Urine protein/Cr ratio
- Renal US: bladder; Doppler assessment of renal blood flow

DIFFERENTIAL DIAGNOSIS
- Prerenal:
    - Hypovolemia:
        - Vomiting, diarrhea
        - Hemorrhage
        - Shock
    - Hypoperfusion:
        - Cardiac dysfunction
        - Hypoxia
    - Redistribution of intravascular fluid:
        - Leak (sepsis, burns)
        - Hypoalbuminemia (nephrosis)
- Postrenal (obstruction):
    - Urinary tract anomalies
    - Stones

- ➤ Blood clots
- ➤ Foreign bodies
- ➤ Surgical adhesions
- ➤ Malignancy
- ■ Renal:
  - ➤ Vascular occlusion: bilateral renal artery or vein thrombosis
  - ➤ Glomerular: HUS, nephritis
  - ➤ Tubular: ATN, nephrotoxins
- ■ Differentiating tests:
  - ➤ Fractional excretion of sodium: urine (U) and plasma (P) samples: $(UNa \times PCr/UCr \times PNa) \times 100$
  - ➤ Prerenal:
    - • U Osm >350
    - • U Na <20
    - • U/P Osm >1.5
    - • U/P Cr >40
    - • FENa <1
  - ➤ Postrenal:
    - • U Osm <350
    - • U Na >40
    - • U/P Osm <0.5
    - • U/P Cr <15
    - • FENa variable
  - ➤ Renal (acute nephritis):
    - • U Osm >350
    - • U Na <30
    - • U/P Osm >1.5
    - • U/P Cr >40
    - • FENa <1
  - ➤ Renal (ATN):
    - • U Osm <350
    - • U Na >40
    - • U/P Osm <1
    - • U/P Cr <20
    - • FENa >1

MANAGEMENT
- ■ Weights bid
- ■ Strict I/O
- ■ Renal diet (low K & phos)
- ■ Avoid nephrotoxin

- Adjust medications for GFR
- Assess volume:
  - Depleted: restore volume, IV normal saline (NS)
  - Replete: limit insensible losses (300 mL/M^2/d D_5W or $\frac{1}{4}$ NS) + mL/mL replacement of output
  - Overloaded: limit fluids to output alone
- Correct abnormal electrolytes
  - Hyperkalemia
    - K^+ <6.5 mEq/L: dietary restriction
    - K^+ >6.5 mEq/L: Kayexalate 1 g/kg po or pr; ECG changes: 10% Ca gluconate 0.5–1.0 mL/kg IV, dextrose 0.5 g/kg IV, insulin 0.1 units/kg IV; or bicarb 0.5–1.0 mEq/kg IV; or 0.5% albuterol nebulization
  - Acidosis:
    - Rx w/ bicarb IV or sodium citrate po 1–2 mEq/kg/d
    - Correct ionized Ca before alkali therapy
- Hypertension:
  - Na & fluid restriction
  - Vasodilators or diuretics
  - Avoid ACE inhibitors

SPECIFIC THERAPY
- Dialysis:
  - Uncontrollable fluid overload
  - Uncontrollable hyperkalemia
  - Intractable acidosis
  - Progressive severe uremia
  - Dialyzable toxin
- Low-phosphate diet, Ca carbonate phosphate binders (hyperphosphatemia)
- Activated vitamin D po, or if cardiac effects, IV 10% Ca gluconate (hypocalcemia)
- Treat underlying cause

FOLLOW-UP
- Frequent blood chemistries
- Quantify urine output closely
- Reassess volume status

COMPLICATIONS AND PROGNOSIS
- Depends on underlying cause
- Stroke

- Seizures
- CHF
- Pulmonary edema
- Death
- Recovery by 2 mo if healthy & underlying cause abates or is effectively treated
- Possible irreversible cortical necrosis & chronic renal insufficiency if:
  - Prolonged anuria
  - Significant ischemia or hypoxia

ACUTE RHEUMATIC FEVER (ARF)

STEVE SESLAR, M.D.
SHARON E. O'BRIEN, M.D.

HISTORY AND PHYSICAL
Diagnosis by modified Jones criteria
- Evidence of preceding group A streptococcal (GAS) infection
- 2 major or 1 major + 2 minor criteria

History
- Rare age <4 y
- GAS infection: pharyngitis, impetigo
- Decreased activity, easily fatigued
- Pallor
- Rarely abdominal pain or epistaxis
- Family Hx of ARF

Physical signs
- Major criteria:
  1. Arthritis: migratory polyarthritis, larger joints (knees, ankles, elbows, wrists)
  2. Carditis: tachycardia, heart murmur of valvulitis (mitral or aortic regurgitation), friction rub, severe CHF
  3. Rash: erythema marginatum (nonpruritic evanescent rash on trunk or extremities)
  4. Subcutaneous nodules: firm painless, freely mobile nodules (diameter 0.2–2 cm), extensor surfaces of large joints
  5. Sydenham chorea: movement disorder of fast, clonic, involuntary movements, esp face & limbs, muscular hypotonus & emotional lability

- Minor criteria:
  1. Arthralgias
  2. Fever
- Exceptions to Jones criteria
  - Chorea or indolent carditis may occur as only manifestions
  - Recurrence may not fulfill Jones criteria

TESTS
- Throat culture
- Antistreptolysin-O titers:
  - Children: >320 Todd units
  - Adults: >240 Todd units or 2-fold increase over baseline
- Antibodies to other streptococcal antigens (confirm GAS infection in unclear cases):
  - Antideoxyribonuclease B (anti-DNAase B)
  - Antihyaluronidase
  - Antistreptokinase
  - Antinicotinamide adenine-dinucleotidase (anti-NADase)
- C-reactive protein, ESR: minor criteria if elevated
- ECG: minor criteria if P-R interval prolonged
- Echocardiogram: signs of valvulitis w/o accompanying auscultatory findings; not enough as only criteria of carditis

DIFFERENTIAL DIAGNOSIS
- Juvenile rheumatoid arthritis
- SLE or other connective tissue disease
- Infective or reactive arthritis
- Seronegative spondyloarthropathies
- Infections (Hansen disease, Lyme disease, *Yersinia*)
- Familial Mediterranean fever
- Antiphospholipid syndrome
- Leukemias
- Sickle cell anemia
- Sarcoidosis

MANAGEMENT
- Treat GAS infection
- American Heart Association recommends antibiotic prophylaxis for at least 10 y to prevent recurrence if no residual valvular disease after last episode of ARF or until "well into adulthood." Residual heart disease may require life-long prophylaxis.

SPECIFIC THERAPY
- Severe carditis: prednisone 2 mg/kg/d in 4 divided doses, 2–6 wks
- Mild to moderate carditis: high-dose aspirin (90–100 mg/kg/d) in 4–6 divided doses; ESR guide for Rx length
- Symptomatic arthritis: salisalicylates or other NSAIDs, do not start until definitive diagnosis is made as may mask joint manifestions
- Bedrest

FOLLOW-UP
- Severe carditis:
  - Admit for IV steroids
  - Monitor cardiac status & treat as indicated
- Milder carditis:
  - Outpatient
  - Anti-GAS Rx, high-dose aspirin & NSAIDs for symptomatic arthritis
- Symptoms & ESR determine length of treatment

COMPLICATIONS AND PROGNOSIS

Complications
- Valve deformities
- Thromboembolism
- Cardiac hemolytic anemia

Prognosis
- Depends on whether permanent cardiac damage
- More severe disease at presentation: greater likelihood of residual heart disease
- Risk of permanent cardiac damage higher after recurrence of rheumatic fever
- Arthritis self-limited:
  - Few days to several wks
  - No permanent damage
- Chorea gradually subsides over weeks to months, usually does not cause permanent neurologic sequelae

ADOLESCENT CONTRACEPTION

LINDA GRANT, M.D.

HISTORY AND PHYSICAL
- Match to pt needs:
  - Estrogen sensitivity

> Chronic disease
> Frequency of coitus

History
- Contraindications to hormonal methods:
  > Thromboembolism
  > Liver disease
  > Estrogen-sensitive neoplasm
  > CVA

Physical signs
- Pelvic exam if already sexually active
- May delay pelvic until coital initiation if protected

TESTS
- Gonorrhea, chlamydia, Pap
- RPR
- CBC
- Pregnancy testing
- Offer HIV, hepatitis C testing

DIFFERENTIAL DIAGNOSIS
- Methods for pts w/ chronic illness:
  > Sickle cell: medroxyprogesterone decreases sickling
  > Seizure disorder:
    - No Norplant if on anticonvulsants (except valproic acid)
    - Increase OCP estrogen (ethinyl estradiol) to 50 mcg; increased metabolism

MANAGEMENT
- Confidentiality essential; review state laws on adolescent confidentiality rights
- Ask about sexual activity
- Explain risks, benefits of all methods
- Abstinence & condoms only methods that protect from STDs
- Test for gonorrhea & chlamydia q6 mo
- Annual Pap, pelvic exam
- OCP: monitor BP
- Begin hormonal methods while on or completing menses
- OCP:
  > May need to try several formulations
  > <= 35 mcg ethinyl estradiol
- Injectable: medroxyprogesterone:

- ➤ <14 wks since last injection or >14 wks & no unprotected sex in last 2 wk: urine HCG & give injection
- ➤ >14 wk & unprotected sex: return after 2 wks of protected sex for HCG & injection
- ■ Injectable: medroxyprogesterone acetate/estradiol cypionate
  - ➤ Every 28–30 days; not longer than 33 days
- ■ Emergency contraception:
  - ➤ Within 72 hours of coitus
  - ➤ 100 mcg of ethinyl estradiol + 1 mg norgestrel *or* 0.5 mg levonorgestrel, repeated in 12 h or 0.75 mg levonorgestrel (Plan B) repeated in 12 h
  - ➤ Nausea management
- ■ Condoms: adequate water-based lubrication to prevent breakage

SPECIFIC THERAPY
- ■ OCP:
  - ➤ Advantages:
    - • Low failure rates
    - • Decreases dysmenorrhea, acne, menstrual flow
    - • Protects against ovarian/uterine cancer
    - • Side effects reversible
  - ➤ Disadvantages:
    - • Medical visits
    - • Daily use
- ■ Injectable: medroxyprogesterone:
  - ➤ Advantages:
    - • Little effort
    - • No estrogen
    - • Can be used while breastfeeding
    - • No drug interactions
    - • Decreases sickling episodes
  - ➤ Disadvantage: medical visit
    - • Side effects take months to resolve
    - • Fertility may take up to 30 months to return
- ■ Injectable: medroxyprogesterone/estradiol cypionate:
  - ➤ Advantages:
    - • Little effort
    - • Contains both estrogen and progesterone so cycles more regular than with progesterone alone
    - • Fertility returns within several cycles of discontinuation
  - ➤ Disadvantages; frequency of injections

- Emergency contraception:
  - Advantage: easy to use
  - Disadvantage: must be aware of contraceptive failure to use
- Condoms:
  - Advantages:
    - Easily available
    - Low cost
    - STD protection
  - Disadvantages:
    - Intermittent use
    - Breakage
    - Latex allergy (polyurethane alternative)
- Norplant: more commonly used by older/parenting adolescent
- Diaphragm, female condom: require body touching; often unacceptable, particularly w/ younger teen
- Withdrawal: still practiced by many teens
- IUDs: high rate of STDs; good for older, parenting teen
- Abstinence: should always be discussed as an option, particularly with young teens

FOLLOW-UP
- Return q3 mo, increasing to q6 mo when reliable pattern established
- Ask about contraceptive use at every visit

COMPLICATIONS AND PROGNOSIS
- OCP:
  - Nausea
  - Menstrual changes
  - Headaches
  - Libido changes
  - Drug interactions
- Medroxyprogesterone:
  - Menstrual irregularities
  - Weight gain
  - May decrease bone density
  - Hair thinning
- Emergency: nausea
- Condom: latex, spermicide allergies
- Adolescents who have sex before age 18 have $5\times$ greater chance of cervical cancer than those beginning sex after age 22
- Best contraceptive: one the pt will use

ADRENAL INSUFFCIENCY

SULEIMAN NJELAWUNI MUSTAFA-KUTANA, M.D.

HISTORY AND PHYSICAL
- Often history of steroid use
- Often history of antecedent stress: trauma, infection
- Glucocorticoid deficiency:
  - Fasting hypoglycemia
  - Nausea, vomiting
  - Fatigue
- Mineralocorticoid deficiency:
  - Muscle weakness
  - Weight loss
  - Fatigue
  - Nausea, vomiting, anorexia
  - Salt craving
  - Hypotension
  - Shock
- Adrenal androgen deficiency:
  - Decreased pubic and axillary hair
  - Decreased libido
  - Hyperpigmentation

TESTS
- ACTH stimulation test (diagnostic)
- AM cortisol:
  - Primary adrenal insufficiency: low; fails to respond to ACTH stimulation
  - Secondary adrenal insufficiency: low to normal, won't increase with stress or ACTH stimulation
- ACTH: elevated
- Serum electrolytes, glucose:
  - Hyponatremia
  - Hyperkalemia in primary adrenal insufficiency
  - Hypoglycemia

DIFFERENTIAL DIAGNOSIS
- Primary cause
  - Autoimmune polyglandular syndrome
  - Bilateral adrenal hemorrhage

➤ Congenital adrenal hypoplasia
➤ X-linked adrenal hypoplasia; seen with Duchenne muscular dystrophy or glycerol kinase deficiency
➤ Deficient ACTH receptor
➤ Infection:
  • Bacterial
  • Fungal
  • HIV
  • Tuberculosis
➤ Adrenoleukodystrophy
■ Secondary cause:
  ➤ Central: suppression or deficient ACTH or CRH:
    • Hypopituitarism
    • Stop prolonged course of steroid therapy
    • Infants born to mothers on steroid therapy
  ➤ End-organ unresponsiveness:
    • Cortisol resistance
    • Aldosterone resistance

MANAGEMENT
■ Adrenal insufficiency crisis:
  ➤ Rapid volume expansion w/ IV NS
  ➤ IV hydrocortisone 50–100 mg
  ➤ Subsequent hormonal therapy:
    • IV hydrocortisone 50 mg/m^2 q24h
    • OR IV Solumedrol 2.5 mg/m^2 q8h
  ➤ No K until serum K normal

SPECIFIC THERAPY
■ Glucocorticoid maintenance therapy:
  ➤ Replace w/ minimum effective dose, avoid long-acting glucocorticoid
  ➤ Cortisol 3 mg/m^2 q8h po
  ➤ Cortisone acetate 10 mg/m^2 q8h po
  ➤ Prednisone 5 mg/m^2/d divided bid po
  ➤ IM cortisone (Solu-Cortef)
  ➤ Stress situation: triple dose
■ Mineralocorticoid maintenance therapy: oral fludrocortisone acetate 0.1 mg/d

FOLLOW-UP
■ If temporary, weaning of treatment possible

- Most causes: lifelong therapy & follow-up with endocrine
- Dosing adjusted for growth

COMPLICATIONS AND PROGNOSIS
- Depends on underlying cause
- Side effect of replacement therapy: suppressed growth, osteoporosis
- Adrenal insufficiency crisis: shock, possible death if not treated in timely manner

---

ALOPECIA

ALBERT C. YAN, M.D., F.A.A.P.

HISTORY AND PHYSICAL

History
- Antecedent event (illness, fever, surgery, trauma, psychosocial)
- Medication use
- Assoc. skin rashes or lesions
- Assoc. systemic diseases, esp. thyroid, diabetes
- Recent hair treatments or braiding

Physical signs
- Generalized or localized pattern
- Morphologic pattern: round or irregular
- Scarring: shiny areas w/ no visible hair follicles
- Non-scarring: normal presence of hair follicles but assoc. hair loss
- Erythema or pustules: inflammation

TESTS
- Alopecia areata:
  - CBC (R/O pernicious anemia)
  - TFTs (R/O thyroiditis)
  - Glucose screening (R/O diabetes)
- Tinea capitis: fungal culture
- Microscopic exam of hair shaft & bulb
- Biopsy (uncertain Dx)

DIFFERENTIAL DIAGNOSIS

Non-scarring
- Tinea capitis:
  - Scaling
  - Pruritus

> Lymphadenopathy
> Alopecia.
- Telogen effluvium:
  > Generalized hair shedding
  > Antecedent traumatic event 2–4 mo before
- Alopecia areata:
  > Localized, round areas of hair loss; nail pitting
  > Vitiligo
  > Pernicious anemia
  > Atopic disease
  > Myasthenia gravis
  > Endocrine disorders
- Trichotillomania:
  > Often bizarre patterns; hairs of several different lengths
  > Child may not admit to manipulating hair, parents often unaware
  > Usually scalp, eyebrows, eyelashes
- Androgenetic alopecia: pattern of hair loss on vertex & family Hx
- Anagen effluvium: generalized hair loss from chemotherapy
- Developmental hair problems: Hx of difficulty growing long hair & seldom needing haircuts

Scarring

- Tinea capitis w/ kerion formation
- Trichotillomania
- Traction & other traumatic alopecias:
  > Typically seen in braided or chemically treated hair
  > Folliculitis may be present
- Acne keloidalis:
  > Small follicular papules on back of neck & posterior scalp
  > Healing w/ small keloidal papules leading to progressive hair loss
- Lichen planopilaris: inflammatory hair loss w/ multifocal scarring alopecia
- Scalp cellulitis
- Folliculitis decalvans: rare disorder; multifocal round areas of hair loss surrounded by pustules
- Keratosis pilaris atrophicans: may be assoc w/ atrophic scarring of lateral eyebrows

MANAGEMENT

General measures
- Directed toward specific Dx
- Antibiotics:

- ➤ Tinea capitis: griseofulvin
- ➤ Folliculitis decalvans, folliculitis keloidalis, or dissecting cellulitis of scalp:
  - Erythromycin
  - Cephalexin
  - Tetracycline
- ■ Removal of offending agent:
  - ➤ Telogen & anagen effluvium
  - ➤ Trichotillomania
  - ➤ Traumatic or traction alopecia
- ■ Pediatric dermatology consult

SPECIFIC THERAPY
- ■ Tinea capitis: griseofulvin 20 mg/kg divided bid
- ■ Topical or injected steroids:
  - ➤ Alopecia areata
  - ➤ Lichen planopilaris
- ■ Trial of topical steroids:
  - ➤ Fluocinonide bid × 2 wks, stop for 1 wk, & repeat
  - ➤ If no improvement w/in 2–3 mo, abandon treatment
- ■ Androgenetic alopecia: minoxidil

FOLLOW-UP
- ■ depends on etiology

COMPLICATIONS AND PROGNOSIS
- ■ Depends on disease process
- ■ Non-scarring (telogen or anagen effluvium): excellent
- ■ Others: chronic processes or chronic sequelae

ALTERED MENTAL STATUS

SCOT BATEMAN, M.D.

HISTORY AND PHYSICAL

History
- ■ Immediate prior events:
  - ➤ Trauma
  - ➤ Fever, infection
  - ➤ Ingestion, drugs in the home
  - ➤ CNS symptoms:
    - Headache

- Ataxia
- Vomiting
- Seizure

➤ Environmental exposures:
- Carbon monoxide
- Lead

Physical signs

- Glasgow Coma Scale
- Hyperthermia or hypothermia
- Increased ICP:
    - ➤ Hypertension
    - ➤ Bradycardia
    - ➤ Slow, irregular respirations
- Pupil size and reactivity
- Meningeal irritation
- Fruity breath aroma (diabetic ketoacidosis [DKA])

TESTS

- ABG
- Dextrose
- CBC
- Electrolytes:
    - ➤ Calcium
    - ➤ Magnesium
    - ➤ Ammonia
- Liver function tests
- Blood and urine toxicology screen
- Serum osmolarity
- CSF studies
- Cervical spine and head CT for suspected trauma
- Lumbar puncture
- ECG

DIFFERENTIAL DIAGNOSIS

- CNS infection
- Head trauma
- Ingestions
    - ➤ Dilated pupils (anticholinergics, sympathomimetics)
    - ➤ Constricted pupils (narcotics, cholinergics, benzodiazepines)
    - ➤ Nystagmus (barbiturates, alcohol, phenytoin, carbamazepine, PCP)
- Metabolic disturbance, hypoglycemia, DKA, hyponatremia

■ Seizures
■ Increased ICP from intracranial hemorrhage or brain tumor

MANAGEMENT

What to do first
■ Assess airway, breathing, & circulation
■ Stabilize cervical spine
■ Rapid neurologic assessment

General measures
■ NPO with IV fluids; avoid excess fluid if suspected CNS process
■ Antibiotics for suspected infections

SPECIFIC THERAPY
■ IV glucose for hypoglycemia
■ Naloxone for opioid overdose
■ Gastric lavage & activated charcoal, if indicated, for suspected toxin ingestion
■ Give specific toxin antidote; contact regional Poison Control Center

FOLLOW-UP
■ Depends on etiology
■ Most require hospitalization for observation for 24–48 h

COMPLICATIONS AND PROGNOSIS

Complications
■ Aspiration pneumonia
■ Persistent vegetative state
■ Brain death

Prognosis
■ Depends on etiology & prevention of secondary events such as hypoxia

---

AMENORRHEA

LIANA R. CLARK, M.D.

HISTORY AND PHYSICAL
■ Primary amenorrhea
  ➤ No uterine bleeding by age 14 without breast/pubic hair development

➤ By age 16 with breast/pubic hair development
■ Secondary amenorrhea: absence of menses for length of 3 cycles after menarche

History
■ Sexual activity
■ Pregnancy symptoms
■ Weight loss
■ Weight gain

Physical
■ Hirsutism
■ Tanner stage
■ Virilization
■ Acne
■ Nutritional status
■ Height, weight

TESTS
■ Pregnancy test: first
■ Thyroid function, ESR, LH, FSH, free & total testosterone if indicated by history and physical
■ Consider chromosomes in primary amenorrhea
■ Consider pelvic ultrasound

DIFFERENTIAL DIAGNOSIS
■ Pregnancy
■ Rheumatologic condition
■ Thyroid disease
■ Tumor

MANAGEMENT
■ Provera challenge
  ➤ 10 mg qhs for 10 nights
  ➤ Withdrawal bleed establishes anovulation & normal endometrium
■ Labs:
  ➤ Hypergonadotropic hypogonadism
    • High LH & FSH
    • Low LH and/or FSH
  ➤ Polycystic ovary syndrome (PCOS): LH/FSH ratio >=3:1

SPECIFIC THERAPY
- Hypergonadotropic hypogonadism:
  - ➤ Supplement estrogen/progesterone with combined OCP
  - ➤ May also use Premarin/Provera regimen but more difficult to follow
- Hypogonadotropic hypogonadism
  - ➤ Correct underlying condition if possible
  - ➤ Supplement estrogen/progesterone as above
- PPCOS
  - ➤ Suppress androgen production with combined OCP or Premarin/Provera as above
  - ➤ Add spironolactone for significant hirsutism

FOLLOW-UP
- Monitor q3–6 mo
- PCOS: recheck androgens after 6 mo on hormonal suppression and annually after that
- If amenorrhea due to anorexia nervosa or other weight loss may stop OCP when gains weight

COMPLICATIONS AND PROGNOSIS
- Hormonal replacement: hyperlipidemia and blood clots
- Unopposed estrogen in anovulatory states predisposes to endometrial cancer
- Hypergonadotropic hypogonadism
  - ➤ Generally permanent
  - ➤ Improves with weight gain or treatment of illness
- PCOS: protection of ovary by androgen suppression improves later fertility outcomes

ANAPHYLAXIS

ANDREW MACGINNITE, M.D., PH.D.

HISTORY AND PHYSICAL
- Onset minutes after exposure to allergen: nuts, seafood, eggs, medication, insect sting, latex
- Urticaria & angioedema, esp. eyelids, lips, glottis; described as tingling sensation
- Difficulty swallowing
- Inspiratory stridor

- Bronchospasm
- Hypotension
- Lacrimation, conjunctivitis, rhinorrhea
- Abdominal symptoms: nausea, vomiting, cramps, diarrhea
- Rarely, arrhythmias

TESTS
- Usually not necessary
- Equivocal cases: serum tryptase level elevated

DIFFERENTIAL DIAGNOSIS
- Vasovagal syncope or near-syncope
- Asthma exacerbation
- Not IgE-mediated anaphylactoid reaction: clinically indistinguishable
- Isolated urticaria and/or angioedema

MANAGEMENT
- Stabilize respiratory status:
  - Epinephrine 0.01 mL/kg (max, 0.3 mL) 1:1,000 solution IM or SQ; can repeat
  - Albuterol 0.03 mL/kg (max, 1 mL) nebulized in 2–3 cc normal saline
  - Oxygen
- Stabilize blood pressure:
  - IV fluids: 20 mL/kg normal saline bolus
  - Epinephrine and/or dopamine drips

General measures
- Corticosteroids (prevent biphasic reaction)
- Antihistamine:
  - H1 blocker: diphenhydramine
  - H2 blocker: ranitidine
- Consider admission to monitor for biphasic reaction w/ hypotension or significant respiratory distress
- Discharge w/ prescription for Epi-pen (>30 kg) or Epi-pen Jr (<30 kg) & instructions for use

SPECIFIC THERAPY
- Avoidance of allergen:
  - Food allergen or drug: may develop tolerance if complete elimination for 1–3 y
  - Foods w/ lifelong allergies: peanut, tree nuts, fish, shellfish

- Immunotherapy:
  - ➤ May be effective for insect allergy
  - ➤ Not shown to be effective for food allergy

FOLLOW-UP
- If cause unclear, skin testing by allergist to identify precipitant

COMPLICATIONS AND PROGNOSIS
- Death
- Vascular collapse
- Respiratory arrest
- High risk:
  - ➤ Asthmatics
  - ➤ Peanut or tree nut allergy
  - ➤ Family or personal Hx of atopy
  - ➤ Away from home
  - ➤ Accidental ingestion
  - ➤ Lack of recognition
  - ➤ Delayed administration of epinephrine
  - ➤ Worsening after initial improvement

Prognosis
- Food allergy percipitant: 30% tolerant after complete elimination for 1–3 y except for peanut, tree nuts, fish, shellfish
- Immunotherapy for insect allergy: good results for clinical protection

ANEMIA

SHARON SPACE, M.D.

HISTORY AND PHYSICAL
- Often detected by screening & comparing results to established norms based on age

History
- Activity level

Physical
- Pallor in skin, mucous membranes, nailbeds
- Jaundice/scleral icterus suggests hemolysis
- Skeletal abnormalities (frontal bossing, maxillary prominence due to extramedullary hematopoiesis) associated with congenital anemias

- Severe anemia or rapid fall in Hgb – signs of CHF – murmur, gallop, tachycardia
- Lymphadenopathy, splenomegaly suggest underlying infection, malignancy

TESTS
- CBC with differential and platelet count
  - RBC indices: particularly MCV (mean cellular volume)
- Reticulocyte count
- To diagnose microcytic anemia: Mentzer index = MCV/RBCM
  - <11.5 suggests iron deficiency
  - >13.5 suggests thalassemia trait
- Iron studies (order of changes):
  - Decreased ferritin (loss of storage Fe)
  - Decreased Fe and elevated TIBC (loss of circulating iron)
  - Decreased Hb, MCV (loss of functional Fe)
- Hemoglobin electrophoresis: elevated Hb A2 with B-thal trait
- Hypochromic microcytic RBC on peripheral smear
- Normocytic anemia
  - Hemolysis
    - Increased bilirubin, decreased haptoglobin indicates hemolysis
    - Direct Coombs (for IgG and IgM/complement antibody)
    - Urinalysis: Free hemoglobin in urine with intravascular hemolysis
    - RBC agglutination, spherocytes on peripheral smear
  - Anemia of chronic disease
    - Decreased Fe, TIBC, elevated ferritin and ESR associated with anemia of chronic disease
  - Appropriate workup for chronic disease (BUN, creatine, ANA)

DIFFERENTIAL DIAGNOSIS
- Based on various categorization schemes
- Microcytic anemia: low MCV
  - Iron deficiency (see Iron deficiency entry)
  - Thalassemia trait (see separate chapter)
  - Lead
- Normocytic anemia: normal MCV
  - Hemolysis
  - Chronic disease
  - Drug exposure
  - Recent illness

- Macrocytic anemia: high MCV
  - Folate/vitamin B_{12} deficiency
- Decreased production: low reticulocyte count
  - Blackfan-Diamond anemia
  - Transient erythroblastemia of childhood
  - Infection
  - Drugs
  - Aplastic anemia
  - Marrow infiltration
- Increased destruction: evidence of hemolysis, high reticulocyte count
  - Hemoglobinopathy (sickle cell anemia)
  - Membrane disorders (hereditary spherocytosis)
  - Enzyme deficiencies (G6PD, pyruvate kinase deficiency)
- Hemolysis (autoimmune, transfusion reaction, drug-induced)
- Hypothyroidism: normocytic, normochromic anemia
- Myelodysplasia: anemia ± neutropenia, thrombocytopenia, macrocytosis

MANAGEMENT
- Determine severity; compare to baseline Hgb/Hct if available
- If severe, with evidence of CHF, draw labs, including type and cross, and transfuse PRBC

SPECIFIC THERAPY
- Iron deficiency: see specific chapter
- Anemia of chronic disease
  - Treat underlying disease
  - Consider epoetin alfa: dosing varies
    - Peak effect seen in 2–3 wk
    - Give Fe supplement with epoetin alfa for 4–6 wk
- Hemolytic anemia
  - Supportive care
  - Prednisone helpful in some cases

FOLLOW-UP
- Iron deficiency: see specific chapter
- Anemia of chronic disease: monitor Hb/Hct; epoetin alfa as indicated

COMPLICATIONS AND PROGNOSIS
- Evidence that iron deficiency anemia may affect cognitive development in young children

- Autoimmune hemolytic anemia
  - IgM antibody: self-limited disease, does not recur
  - IgG: may have underlying autoimmune disease, can be chronic
- Severe anemia affects work capacity

ANIMAL BITES

FRANZ E. BABL, M.D., M.P.H.

HISTORY AND PHYSICAL

History
- Identification of animal
- Assess force of bite (large or small animal)
- Provoked or unprovoked
- Animal behavior at time of bite
- Animal vaccination status
- Location of bite
- Bleeding
- Associated symptoms or injury
- Pt tetanus status

Physical signs
- Signs of local infection
- Location of bite: hand injuries, cat bites at high risk for infection
- Associated injuries to muscles, nerves, tendons, & vessels

TESTS
- Radiographs:
  - Deep injuries
  - Possible fracture or joint involvement
- Other tests as indicated by physical exam (e.g., CT for possible dural puncture)
- Wound culture, if infected or presenting >8 h after injury

DIFFERENTIAL DIAGNOSIS
- Preschoolers with no history of bites:
  - Ringworm
  - Granuloma annulare
  - Other superficial ovoid skin eruptions
- Human bites

MANAGEMENT

What to do first

- Wound cleansing; sponge away visible dirt
- Irrigation with copious sterile saline by high-pressure syringe
- Debridement:
  - ➤ Remove devitalized tissue
  - ➤ Surgical debridement for extensive wounds
- Elevation
- Wound closure:
  - ➤ Nonpuncture wound <8 h of injury
  - ➤ No sutures >8 h after injury or for puncture wound
  - ➤ Steri-strips for small wounds
  - ➤ Bite on face (cosmetic considerations): suture when possible

SPECIFIC THERAPY

- Consider rabies post-exposure prophylaxis (contact Public Health Dept.)
- Tetanus immunization
- Antimicrobial therapy
  - ➤ Prophylaxis (Rx for 2–3 d)
    - Moderate to severe wounds, esp. w/ edema or crush injury or deep puncture wound
    - Facial bites
    - Hand & foot bites
    - Genital bites
    - Immunocompromised pt
  - ➤ No antimicrobial agents for superficial abrasions
- Consider inpatient care for:
  - ➤ Infected wounds
  - ➤ Serious hand bites
  - ➤ Extensive soft-tissue injury or wound involving joint, tendon, cartilage, or bone
  - ➤ Potential poor pt compliance

Treatment options

- Antibiotics for dog & cat bites
  - ➤ Oral
    - Amoxicillin-clavulanate
    - Co-trimoxazole + clindamycin, if penicillin-allergic
  - ➤ IV
    - Ampicillin-sulbactam

- For penicillin-allergic pts: extended-spectrum cephalosporin or co-trimoxazole + clindamycin

FOLLOW-UP
- Return if redness, discharge, swelling, fever, or chills
- Follow-up wound inspection within 48 h
- Social service evaluation of home
- Public Health Dept. reporting

COMPLICATIONS AND PROGNOSIS
- Infection: 5% of dog bites and as many as 80% of cat bites
- Transmission of disease
  - Cat-scratch disease
  - Tularemia
  - Rabies

Prognosis
- Usually excellent with local wound care, post-exposure prophylaxis, & prompt identification of infection

ANKLE INJURIES

ELIZABETH CALMAR, M.D.

HISTORY AND PHYSICAL

History
- Mechanism of injury:
  - Inversion (lateral ligaments) vs. eversion (medial ligaments)
  - Motor vehicle accident:
    - High energy
    - Talar neck or Lisfranc fractures
  - Fall from height: calcaneus fractures
  - Repetitive sprains: tarsal coalition
  - Chronic overuse with pain: stress fracture
- Ambulation after injury
- When did swelling occur?
- Previous ankle injury

Physical signs
- Signs of associated injuries
- Examine uninjured ankle

- Obvious deformity to injured ankle
- Palpate to identify area of tenderness:
  - Anterolateral: anterior talofibular ligament; most common injury
  - Lateral: calcaneofibular ligament
  - Medial: deltoid ligament
  - Posterolateral: posterior talofibular ligament
- Fifth metatarsal tenderness (fracture)
- Anterior drawer test: most sensitive for joint instability

TESTS
- True AP, lateral, & mortise films of ankle
- Foot films for metatarsal fracture
- CT: displaced Salter or triplanarfracture

DIFFERENTIAL DIAGNOSIS
- Ankle sprains/strains:
  - 75–80% of ankle injuries in children & adolescents
  - Grade I: mild strain
  - Grade II: partial tear
  - Grade III: complete tear
- Fractures:
  - Lateral malleolus: fibula
  - Medial malleolus: tibia
  - Bimalleolar
  - Trimalleolar
  - Fracture dislocations
  - Fracture of 5th metatarsal w/ inversion injuries
- Dislocations:
  - Tibiotalar
  - Talonavicular
  - Talocalcaneal

MANAGEMENT
What to do first
- Non-weight bearing (NWB)
- Immobilize & splint

General measures
- Minimize swelling
- Control pain

- Prevent further injury
- RICE: rest, ice, compression (splint w/ Ace or Air cast), elevation
- Analgesics & anti-inflammatory drugs

SPECIFIC THERAPY
- Sprains:
  - ➤ Grade I:
    - Air cast
    - Weight bearing as tolerated
  - ➤ Grade II & III:
    - Posterior plaster splint
    - NWB
- Fractures:
  - ➤ Nondisplaced:
    - Posterior splint
    - NWB
    - Crutches
  - ➤ Displaced: emergency ortho evaluation
  - ➤ Open fractures and dislocations:
    - Immediate ortho consult
    - Possible operative debridement (open fractures)

FOLLOW-UP
- Acute sprains: initial NWB, followed by physical therapy to restore full mobility
- Fracture/dislocation: depends on extent of initial injury
- Close F/U for pts w/ compromised tissue healing (i.e., diabetics)
- Growth plate injuries: close F/U in 1–2 d, even if nondisplaced

COMPLICATIONS AND PROGNOSIS
Complications
- Leg length discrepancy (crush injuries to growth plate)
- Infections (open fractures)
- Arthritis with significant joint involvement or disruption

Prognosis
- Sprains: usually do well w/ optimal initial care
- Growth plate fractures: depend on extent of injury:
  - ➤ Salter I, II, III: >90% excellent long-term
  - ➤ Salter IV: proper realignment at articular surface needed
  - ➤ Salter V: significant potential for growth disruption

ANOREXIA

LIANA R. CLARK, M.D.

HISTORY AND PHYSICAL

- Mild:
  - Mild body image distortion
  - Weight >=90% average weight/height
  - No symptoms/signs of weight loss
  - Healthy weight loss methods (>1,000 cal/d, moderate exercise, no purging)
- Moderate:
  - Moderate body image distortion
  - Weight <=90% average weight/height
  - Refusal to stop losing weight
  - Symptoms/signs of weight loss
  - Unhealthy weight loss methods (<1,000 cal/d, excessive exercise, purging)
- Severe:
  - Severe body image distortion
  - Weight <=85% average weight/height
  - Refusal to stop losing weight
  - Symptoms/signs of extreme malnutrition
  - Unhealthy weight loss methods (<1,000 cal/d, excessive exercise, purging)
  - Denial

History

- Eating behaviors:
  - Restricting, binging, or purging
  - Calories eaten/day
  - Laxative/purgative use
- Weight:
  - Maximum/minimum weights
  - Why dieting
  - Goal weight
- Symptoms:
  - Fatigue
  - Cold intolerance
  - Presyncope/syncope
  - Abdominal pain

➤ Constipation
➤ Weakness
■ Mood:
    ➤ Depression
    ➤ Suicidal ideation

Physical signs
■ Hypotension
■ Bradycardia
■ Hypothermia
■ % ideal body weight
■ Degree of emaciation
■ Lanugo
■ Livedo reticularis

TESTS
■ CBC, ESR
■ Electrolytes, calcium, magnesium, phosphate
■ BUN, creatine
■ LFTs
■ Cholesterol, total protein, albumin
■ T4, TSH
■ LH, FSH
■ ECG, DEXA scan

DIFFERENTIAL DIAGNOSIS
■ Tuberculosis
■ Cerebral neoplasm
■ Hyperthyroidism/hypothyroidism
■ Addison
■ Diabetes mellitus
■ Depression
■ Malabsorptive states
■ Gastroesophageal obstruction
■ Sarcoidosis

MANAGEMENT
■ Mild:
    ➤ Monitor diet & weight plan
    ➤ Refer to nutritionist
    ➤ Establish weight loss limit

- Moderate:
  - ➤ Establish weight gain goal
  - ➤ Collaborate w/ psychologist & nutritionist
  - ➤ Guidelines for daily activities
  - ➤ Weekly follow-up
  - ➤ Establish criteria for hospitalization
- Severe:
  - ➤ Facilitate hospitalization
  - ➤ Refer to eating disorder specialist
  - ➤ Treat as for moderate after discharge
- Criteria for hospitalization:
  - ➤ Hypovolemia & hypotension
  - ➤ Hypothermia
  - ➤ Electrolyte imbalance/dehydration
  - ➤ Heart rate <55 beats/min
  - ➤ Presyncope or syncope
  - ➤ Uncontrolled binging & purging
  - ➤ Acute food refusal
  - ➤ Persistent weight loss

SPECIFIC THERAPY
- Amenorrhea (hypogonadotropic hypogonadism): estrogen (combined OCP, Premarin, patch) replacement w/ progesterone
- Osteopenia: calcium supplement
- Diet:
  - ➤ Initially 800–1,000 Kcal/d
  - ➤ Increase calories by 200–300 q2–3 d
  - ➤ May need supranormal calories for weight gain

FOLLOW-UP
- Long-term, weekly to monthly, as condition warrants

COMPLICATIONS AND PROGNOSIS
- Cardiac rhythm abnormalities
- Decreased intestinal motility
- Amenorrhea
- Osteopenia
- Mortality: 5.9%

Prognosis
- 50% good, 25% intermediate, 25% poor

AORTIC STENOSIS (AS)

SHARON E. O'BRIEN, M.D.

HISTORY AND PHYSICAL

History
- Depends on age & severity of obstruction to left ventricular (LV) outflow:
  - Neonate:
    - "Critical AS"
    - Low cardiac output & LV failure
  - Older children:
    - Rare
    - Exertional chest pain, easily fatigued, dizziness or syncope
- Mild or moderate: asymptomatic or mild exercise intolerance
- Severe: sudden cardiac death

Physical signs
- Neonatal critical AS:
  - Cool extremities
  - Thready pulse
  - Increased work of breathing
  - Murmur may be absent or faint
  - CHF
- Blood pressure:
  - Usually normal
  - Significant AS may have narrow pulse pressure
- Systolic thrill: R upper sternal border or suprasternal notch
- Harsh systolic ejection murmur, loudest at R upper sternal border; radiates to neck
- Diastolic murmur if aortic regurgitation (AR) present
- Mild to moderate:
  - Early systolic ejection click, best heard at apex & L sternal edge
  - Unlike pulmonic stenosis, click intensity doesn't vary w/ respirations

TESTS
- ECG:
  - Usually normal
  - Severe AS may see LVH strain

- CXR:
  - Dilated ascending aorta
  - Cardiomegaly (neonatal critical AS or AR)
- Echocardiogram:
  - Abnormal valve
  - Assess systolic pressure gradient & LV function
  - Assess for AR
  - Detect anomalies of mitral valve or aortic arch
  - VSD or PDA: up to 20% of cases
- Exercise stress test: ECG changes or symptoms not seen at rest

DIFFERENTIAL DIAGNOSIS
- Pulmonary stenosis
- Subaortic stenosis
- Coarctation of aorta

MANAGEMENT
- Neonatal critical AS: admit to ICU for stabilization, urgent cardiac catheterization for balloon dilation or surgery
- Mild to moderate: serial echocardiograms q1–2 y to assess for progression; more frequent for higher degrees of obstruction
- Activities:
  - Mild: no restriction
  - Moderate: restrict strenuous activities & competitive sports
  - Severe or symptomatic disease: refer for treatment
- Maintain oral hygiene & antibiotic prophylaxis for bacterial endocarditis

SPECIFIC THERAPY
- Indications for intervention are peak-to-peak systolic pressure:
  1. >=70 mmHg regardless of symptoms
  2. 50–70 mmHg with symptoms and ST-T wave changes on ECG, indicating myocardial ischemia at rest or w/ exercise
  3. <50 mmHg & asymptomatic: no intervention; follow for progression
- Intervention:
  - Cardiac cath & balloon valvuloplasty unless significant aortic valve regurgitation
  - Surgical valvotomy or valve replacement

FOLLOW-UP
- Aortic insufficiency or calcification w/ restenosis likely to occur years or decades later; requires reoperation & often aortic valve replacement

■ Annual exam & ECG: detect restenosis or progressive aortic insufficiency

COMPLICATIONS AND PROGNOSIS

Complications
■ Severe disease: LV dysfunction
■ Endocardial fibroelastosis (neonatal critical AS)
■ Rarely, sudden cardiac death
■ Aortic insufficiency from progressive valve degeneration over time or balloon valvuloplasty

Prognosis
■ Neonatal critical AS: guarded; may have LV dysfunction even after successful balloon dilation or surgical valvotomy
■ Older infants & children w/ mild to moderate AS: good, although disease progression over 5–10 y common

APLASTIC ANEMIA

SHARON SPACE, M.D., AND HALLIE KASPER, R.N.

HISTORY AND PHYSICAL
■ Acquired bone marrow failure
■ Majority idiopathic
■ Other etiologies:
  ➤ Drug/chemical exposure
  ➤ Radiation
  ➤ Infection (EBV, HIV, hepatitis)
  ➤ Pregnancy
  ➤ Leukemia

History
■ Most common in adolescents age 13–18

Physical signs
■ Signs and symptoms of bone marrow failure:
  ➤ Anemia:
    • Fatigue
    • Headache
    • Pallor
    • Flow murmur

- ➤ Thrombocytopenia:
  - Bleeding
  - Bruising
- ➤ Neutropenia:
  - Mouth ulcers
  - Fever
  - Infections

TESTS

- CBC with differential and platelet count: pancytopenia
- Reticulocyte count: <0.1%
- Bone marrow biopsy (not aspirate): hypocellular marrow without blasts

DIFFERENTIAL DIAGNOSIS

- Leukemia
- Idiopathic thrombocytic purpura
- Fanconi anemia
- Myelodysplasia

MANAGEMENT

- Packed red cells and platelet transfusions PRN; patients with fewer transfusions have better outcome with stem cell transplant
- Fever and neutropenia:
  - ➤ Blood and other appropriate cultures
  - ➤ Broad-spectrum antibiotics

SPECIFIC THERAPY

- Allogeneic stem cell transplant:
  - ➤ HLA-matched sibling first choice
  - ➤ Matched unrelated donor if no sibling match & no response to immunosuppression
- Immunosuppression:
  - ➤ Antithymocyte globulin (ATG), steroids, cyclosporine
  - ➤ May not see response for 2–3 mo
- Hematopoietic growth factors:
  - ➤ GM-CSF, G-CSF, erythropoietin, thrombopoietin
  - ➤ Supportive care before definitive treatment

FOLLOW-UP

- Frequent (>= weekly) follow-up to monitor blood counts, assess needs for transfusion
- Immediate evaluation and treatment for fever and neutropenia

COMPLICATIONS AND PROGNOSIS
- Depends on residual marrow function: decreased cellularity = worse prognosis
- 50% mortality in first 6 mo
- 90% survival with matched sibling stem cell transplant; 20% develop moderate-severe graft-versus-host disease (GVHD)
- 30% survival with unrelated matched stem cell transplant:
  - High risk of graft failure (50%)
  - High incidence of GVHD
  - Better prognosis in younger children
- 40–70% survival with immunosuppression; 60% develop serum sickness
- 10–30% risk of relapse
- 10% risk of myelodysplasia or acute leukemia
- Often persistent thrombocytopenia after marrow recovery
- Many cases: underlying clonal bone marrow disorder; worst outcome (myelodysplasia, hematologic malignancy, Fanconi anemia)

APPARENT LIFE-THREATENING EVENTS (ALTE)

MICHAEL J. CORWIN, M.D.

HISTORY AND PHYSICAL
Syndrome defined as:
- Frightening to observer
- Characterized by:
  - Apnea
  - Color change
  - Marked change in muscle tone
  - Choking or gagging

History
- Review of key event:
  - Sleep/wake state
  - Presence of breathing efforts
  - Duration
  - Color change
  - Crying or other sounds
  - Body movements
  - Muscle tone
  - Association w/ feeding or emesis

- Current health status:
  - Acute illness (eg, URI)
  - Chronic illness:
    - Respiratory
    - Neurologic
    - Gastroesophageal reflux (GER)
    - Cardiac
    - Metabolic
    - Congenital anomalies
  - Environmental conditions:
    - Bedding
    - Position
    - Overheating
- Past Hx:
  - Prematurity
  - ALTE
- Family Hx:
  - SIDS
  - ALTE
  - Metabolic problem

TESTS
- CBC
- Serum bicarbonate
- Cardiorespiratory monitoring
- As indicated:
  - Neurologic:
    - EEG
    - Brain imaging
  - Cardiac:
    - ECG
    - Echocardiogram
  - Serum electrolytes
  - Esophageal pH monitoring (GER)
  - Polysomnography: simultaneous recordings of multiple physiologic signals for 8 h w/ channels selected based on symptoms

DIFFERENTIAL DIAGNOSIS
- Normal child
- Infection:
  - Respiratory

➤ Systemic
■ Neurologic:
  ➤ Seizures
  ➤ CNS tumor
■ Cardiac arrhythmias
■ GER
■ Upper airway obstruction
■ Drugs:
  ➤ Poisoning
  ➤ Iatrogenic
  ➤ Post-anesthesia
■ Metabolic disease
■ Child abuse (Munchausen by proxy)
■ Control of breathing disorder

MANAGEMENT
■ If attributable to factors not requiring further evaluation (eg, normal behavior, minor coughing or gagging):
  ➤ Reassure family
  ➤ Advice to assess & avoid future episodes
■ If convincing & sufficiently severe to warrant further investigation:
  ➤ Hospitalize for evaluation based on Hx/physical
  ➤ Manage based on underlying cause
  ➤ No cause identified in term infant, no persistent symptoms or sequelae, & no concerning family issues:
    • Reassure family
    • Advice to assess & avoid future episodes

SPECIFIC THERAPY
■ No cause identified in preterm infant or term infant w/ persistent symptoms or sequelae, or concerning family issues: consider home cardiorespiratory monitor for 2 mos

FOLLOW-UP
Follow-up dependent on whether underlying cause is identified

COMPLICATIONS AND PROGNOSIS
■ Idiopathic:
  ➤ Recurrence rate low unless:
    • Premature infant
    • ALTE symptoms persistent (hours) or associated w/ sequelae

➤ Multiple episodes: worse prognosis mandates systematic search for underlying cause, incl. child abuse

APPENDICITIS

HAROON PATEL, M.D.

HISTORY AND PHYSICAL

History
- Most common abdominal surgical condition in children
- Ages 4–15 y
- Periumbilical abdominal pain often initial symptom, followed by anorexia, vomiting
- Pain moves to RLQ over ~12 h
- Low-grade temperature (if > 39°C, consider perforation or other diagnosis)

Physical signs
- Focal RLQ tenderness with guarding
- Rovsing's sign (referred tenderness)
- Psoas & obturator signs
- Percussion tenderness: better (kinder) than eliciting rebound tenderness
- Diffuse tenderness = perforation, esp. in very young
- Relatively nontender despite other findings (possible retrocecal appendix)
- Rectal exam crucial, especially for pelvic appendix and other diagnoses

TESTS
- CBC: in 90%, WBC elevated to 10–15,000/cu mm
- Urinalysis:
  - ➤ To R/O stone/UTI
  - ➤ May be positive (few WBCs, RBCs) if appendix on/near ureter or bladder
- Other studies not needed if examined by experienced surgeon
- Plain film: useful in 15%; may show fecalith, but usually nonspecific
- Ultrasound
- CT (with contrast)

DIFFERENTIAL DIAGNOSIS

- Varies by age
- Classic history may be absent in 50%
- 30–50% of perforated appendicitis have been seen by MD before
- Gastroenteritis:
  - More vomiting (before pain), diarrhea
  - Higher fever
  - Sick contacts
- Mesenteric adenitis: often preceded by URI
- Gynecologic:
  - Ovarian torsion
  - Mittelschmerz
- Urinary:
  - UTI
  - Stone
- Other:
  - Pneumonia
  - HSP
  - DKA
  - Cholelithiasis
  - Peptic ulcer
  - Sickle cell disease
  - Severe constipation (diagnosis of exclusion)

MANAGEMENT

What to do first

- IV fluids
- NPO pending evaluation

General measures

- Pain medication after surgeon evaluation
- Antibiotics:
  - Aerobic + anaerobic coverage
  - More extensive if perforated
- Surgical consult

SPECIFIC THERAPY

- Appendectomy (open or laparoscopic)
- Delayed appendectomy in "appendiceal mass/abscess":

- ➤ IV antibiotics
- ➤ Percutaneous imaging-guided drainage
- ➤ Appendectomy in 6–8 wks

FOLLOW-UP
- Standard postop care
- Nonperforated appendix: begin oral fluids 6–8 h after surgery
- Perforated appendix:
    - ➤ Delay oral fluids until postop ileus resolves (3–4 d)
    - ➤ Prolonged antibiotics (until ~48 h of normal temp & WBC)

COMPLICATIONS AND PROGNOSIS
- ~100 deaths/year from perforated appendicitis in the very young
- Wound infection (~2% nonperforated vs. ~20% perforated)
- Intraabdominal abscess (5%)
- Postoperative adhesive bowel obstruction (3–5%)

APPROACH TO INGESTIONS

ROBERT VINCI, M.D.

HISTORY AND PHYSICAL

History
- Characteristics of ingestion:
    - ➤ Time elapsed since ingestion
    - ➤ Products ingested
    - ➤ Amount ingested & potential for toxicity
    - ➤ Sustained-release preparation
    - ➤ Symptoms since ingestion
- List of medications in home
- Missing pills
- Administration of home remedies
- Underlying medical conditions
- Assess for suicidal ideation

Physical signs
- Assess ABCs
- Baseline heart rate, temperature
- Examine breath for odors

- Pupil size, nystagmus
- Careful neurologic exam, incl. mental status
- Specific toxidromes:
  - Narcotics:
    - Coma
    - Respiratory depression
    - Pinpoint pupils
  - TCAs:
    - Seizures
    - Coma
    - Arrhythmias
  - Sympathomimetics:
    - Seizures
    - Dilated pupils
    - Hyperpyrexia
    - Tachycardia

TESTS
- Dextrose stick
- ABG & serum electrolytes: metabolic acidosis (salicylates, iron, ibuprofen, ethylene glycol, methylene glycol)
- Compare measured serum & calculated osmolarity
- Serum & urine toxicology screen
- Specific drug levels, if available
- ECG
- KUB for pill fragments

DIFFERENTIAL DIAGNOSIS
- Acute head injury
- Suicide
- CNS infection

MANAGEMENT

What to do first
- Establish ABCs

General measures
- Identify toxin
- Contact Poison Control Center
- Consider gastric emptying
- Decrease GI absorption
- Antidote therapy, if available

SPECIFIC THERAPY

- Syrup of ipecac no longer recommended for ED use
- Gastric lavage controversial; may increase risk of aspiration
- Activated charcoal:
  - Decreases GI absorption
  - Ineffective for:
    - Heavy metals
    - Hydrocarbons
    - Alcohols
    - Solvents
  - Repeat q4–6h
  - Do not give as sorbitol-based preparation more than q12–24h
  - Indications:
    - Theophylline
    - Drugs metabolized by liver with enterohepatic recirculation (i.e., barbiturates, phenytoin)
- IV fluids for drugs excreted primarily by kidney
- Urinary alkalinization to promote excretion of some drugs (salicylates)
- Specific antidotes:
  - Narcotics: naloxone
  - Iron: deferoxamine
  - Methemoglobinemia: methylene blue
  - Acetaminophen: *N*-acetylcysteine
  - TCAs: sodium bicarbonate
  - Digitalis: Fab antibodies
  - Methanol or ethylene glycol: fomepizole
- Whole-bowel irrigation (iron ingestion)
- Consider dialysis or hemoperfusion

FOLLOW-UP

- Depends on agent ingested & clinical manifestations

COMPLICATIONS AND PROGNOSIS

- CNS dysfunction if hypoxic with initial presentation
- Depends on agent ingested

Prognosis

- Depends on agent ingested & clinical manifestations

ASPIRIN OVERDOSE

LISE NIGROVIC, M.D.

HISTORY AND PHYSICAL

History
- Contained in many OTC products
- History of ingestion of aspirin product
- Symptoms w/in 3–6 h:
  - Vomiting
  - Tinnitus
  - Change in mental status
- Toxic dose: 15 mg/kg
- Suicide attempt vs. ingestion

Physical signs
- Acute toxicity:
  - Tachypnea and respiratory alkalosis
  - Fever, lethargy, coma, and seizures
  - Metabolic acidosis
  - Hyperglycemia
  - Coagulopathy
- Chronic ingestion/toxicity:
  - Hepatitis and elevated liver enzymes
  - Severe metabolic acidosis and seizures

TESTS
- Dextrose stick/serum glucose
- Electrolytes
- ABG
- Liver function tests
- Coagulation studies
- CBC
- Aspirin level:
  - Peaks 60–90 min after ingestion
  - Enteric-coated tablets absorbed more slowly; delays peak level
- KUB: may show enteric-coated tablets

DIFFERENTIAL DIAGNOSIS
- Infection: viral or bacterial
- DKA

- Iron overdose
- Ethylene glycol poisoning

MANAGEMENT
- Supportive care
- Cardiovascular monitoring
- Gastric decontamination to prevent absorption
- Consider gastric lavage w/in 6 h or w/ aspirin bezoar
- Multidose activated charcoal (1 g/kg): in first 12–24 h due to delayed absorption & gastric dialysis
- Monitor labs closely
- Fluid resuscitation:
  - Correct deficit aggressively
  - Glucose-containing fluid
  - Limit intake (demonstrated cerebral edema)
  - Add potassium once urine output begins
- Hospitalization: children w/ toxic levels (>30–50 mg/dL)

SPECIFIC THERAPY
- Treatment needed for >100 mg/kg
- Alkalinize urine:
  - Keep pH >8.0
  - Enhances excretion by trapping ionized drug in renal tubules
  - Contraindications: cerebral or pulmonary edema
- Reverse metabolic acidosis to protect brain:
  - Correct PT w/ vitamin K
  - Consider hemodialysis:
    - Progressive CNS deterioration
    - Acute renal failure
    - Profound metabolic derangement
    - Pulmonary or cerebral edema

FOLLOW-UP
- Check aspirin level at 2 and 6 h after ingestion
- Discharge when level in therapeutic range & social service evaluation completed

COMPLICATIONS AND PROGNOSIS
- Aspirin nomogram accurately predicts toxicity risk
- Risk of overdose depends on drug level:
  - Therapeutic: 20–30 mg/dL
  - Mild symptoms: 30–50 mg/dL

- ➤ Moderate syndrome: 50–70 mg/dL
- ➤ Neurologic symptoms: 70 mg/dL
- ➤ Poor prognosis: >100 mg/dL
- ■ Chronic salicylate poisoning: symptoms at lower levels

ATAXIA

JANET SOUL, M.D., F.R.C.P.C.

HISTORY AND PHYSICAL

History
- ■ Acute, recurrent, or chronic
- ■ Truncal or appendicular
- ■ Sensory abnormalities, weakness
- ■ Impairment of mental status or consciousness, vertigo
- ■ Recent illness, trauma, ingestion, medications, environmental exposures, travel
- ■ Past history of migraine, seizures, tumor, other neurologic or systemic disease
- ■ Chronic/recurrent: family history of ataxia, other neurologic disorders

Physical signs
- ■ Careful neurologic exam to distinguish between cerebellar ataxia, sensory ataxia, weakness, or encephalopathy
- ■ Acute-onset:
    - ➤ Vital signs
    - ➤ Mental status/LOC
    - ➤ Brain stem reflexes
    - ➤ Deep tendon reflexes (DTR)
    - ➤ Power

TESTS
- ■ Head CT (&/or MRI brain ± spine)
- ■ CBC, electrolytes, BUN/Cr
- ■ Liver function tests
- ■ Toxicology screen
- ■ CSF exam
- ■ EEG
- ■ Recurrent/chronic:
    - ➤ Head CT &/or MRI

➤ CSF exam
➤ NCV/EMG (if sensory deficits, depressed DTR, weakness)
➤ Amino & organic acids
➤ Lactate & pyruvate
➤ Specific genetic tests for inherited ataxia

DIFFERENTIAL DIAGNOSIS

■ Acute/recurrent:
➤ Brain tumor
➤ Toxic ingestion
➤ Intracranial hemorrhage
➤ Blunt head trauma
➤ Migraine
➤ Acute postinfectious cerebellitis
➤ Miller Fisher syndrome (ataxia, areflexia, ophthalmoplegia)
➤ Pseudoataxia (epileptic)
➤ Opsoclonus/myoclonus syndrome
➤ Conversion disorder
■ Chronic/recurrent:
➤ Brain tumor
➤ Cerebellar malformation (e.g., Dandy-Walker, Chiari)
➤ Spinocerebellar ataxia (inherited, many types)
➤ Episodic ataxia (type 1 & 2)
➤ Friedrich ataxia, abetalipoproteinemia (sensory neuropathy)
➤ Metabolic (e.g., Hartnup, mitochondrial, peroxisomal leukodys-
trophies)
➤ Ataxia-telangiectasia

MANAGEMENT

General measures

■ Acute:
➤ Diagnose & treat emergent causes:
• Trauma
• Hemorrhage
• Tumor (may have hydrocephalus and/or increased ICP)
• Ingestion
• Meningoencephalitis
■ Protect patient from self-injury, esp. falls

SPECIFIC THERAPY

■ Physical therapy for chronic or recurrent ataxia
■ Vitamin E for abetalipoproteinemia

- Acetazolamide for episodic ataxia
- Treatment based on underlying metabolic disorder

FOLLOW-UP
- In 1–2 mo after acute ataxia to ensure resolution vs. progression
- Long-term follow-up (chronic/recurrent):
  - Establish diagnosis
  - Provide genetic counseling for family
  - Determine response to therapy

COMPLICATIONS AND PROGNOSIS

Prognosis
- Determined by underlying etiology and severity
- Postinfectious ataxia: complete recovery, but resolution may take weeks to months

ATOPIC DERMATITIS

SEAN PALFREY, M.D.
JOSH SHARFSTEIN, M.D.

HISTORY AND PHYSICAL

History
- Onset usually early in life
- Chronically relapsing course
- Usually very pruritic
- Exposure to allergens, infection, stress
- Family history of asthma, allergic disease

Physical signs
- Small, dry, itchy papules and patches of skin
- Identify area of body affected:
  - In infancy: face, scalp, extensor surfaces of extremities
  - In older children: usually popliteal & antecubital fossa, backs of upper arms, back of neck, behind ears, and on cheeks & forehead
- Skin usually rough, dry
- Skin thickened, excoriated from scratching

TESTS
- Clinical diagnosis
- Pts who do not respond to therapy may benefit from:
  - Fungal scraping

➤ CBC (Wiskott-Aldrich)
➤ Skin biopsy (rarely indicated)

DIFFERENTIAL DIAGNOSIS
■ Contact dermatitis (usually can identify offending agent)
■ Nummular eczema: no central clearing as in tinea
■ Scabies: underlying skin usually normal in appearance
■ Tinea infections:
  ➤ Usually circular
  ➤ Few in number
  ➤ Located on face, trunk
■ Psoriasis
■ Seborrhea
■ Lupus

MANAGEMENT
General measures
■ Limit exposure to allergens.
■ Minimize repetitive wetting & drying of skin.
■ Unscented soaps w/ moisturizers
■ Emollients to moisturize skin
■ Anti-inflammatory drugs
■ Antihistamine to control itching

SPECIFIC THERAPY
■ Emollients (hydrolated petrolatum or Eucerin):
  ➤ Important: apply to wet skin after bathing
  ➤ May also apply tid to qid
■ Topical steroids:
  ➤ Use weakest effective strength, beginning w/ 1% hydrocortisone.
  ➤ Avoid steroids on face, if possible.
■ Ointments more effective than creams of equal potency

FOLLOW-UP
■ Response to treatment should occur within days.

COMPLICATIONS AND PROGNOSIS
■ Most cases manageable w/ elimination of allergens, use of unscented soaps, emollients, topical steroids
■ Secondary infection w/ staph (bullous lesions) or strep (impetigo)
■ Eczema herpeticum
■ Systemic absorption of steroids
■ Skin atrophy from chronic steroid use

ATRIAL SEPTAL DEFECT (ASD)

SHARON O'BRIEN, M.D.

HISTORY AND PHYSICAL
- Usually asymptomatic
- Thin for age
- Active precordium w/ prominent right ventricular heave
- Wide, fixed-split S2
- No click as w/ pulmonary stenosis
- Systolic ejection murmur at upper LSB
- Large or long-standing shunt:
  - Easy fatigability
  - Asymmetric chest wall
  - Diastolic rumble at lower sternal border

TESTS
- ECG:
  - R axis deviation
  - Right atrial (RA) enlargement
  - Right ventricular (RV) conduction delay (RSR in V1)
  - RV hypertrophy
- CXR:
  - Cardiomegaly
  - Enlarged RA & RV
  - Increased pulmonary vascular markings
  - Prominent main pulmonary artery
- Echocardiogram:
  - RA & RV volume overload, RV hypertension, & any associated defects (partial anomalous pulmonary venous return or mitral valve prolapse)
  - Defect size & location:
    - Most defects: secundum type (middle of septum)
    - 30% primum defects (lower septum)
    - 10% sinus venosus type (entrance to IVC or SVC)

DIFFERENTIAL DIAGNOSIS
- Pulmonary stenosis
- Other left-to-right shunts:
  - Total anomalous pulmonary venous return
  - Arteriovenous malformation

MANAGEMENT
- Follow-up q yr
- May become smaller or spontaneously close within first 5 y of life
- SBE prophylaxis not needed for isolated ASD

SPECIFIC THERAPY
- Closure indications:
  - RA & RV volume overload
  - ASD associated w/ stroke (including PFO)
  - Transcatheter closure: small or moderate-sized secundum defects
  - Surgical closure:
    - Large defects
    - Defects w/ deficient septal rims
    - Defects assoc. w/ anomalies such as partial anomalous pulmonary venous return or sinus venosus defects

FOLLOW-UP
- Every 1–2 y pre- and postoperatively

COMPLICATIONS AND PROGNOSIS
- RA & RV volume overload
- Untreated large defects: pulmonary hypertension & CHF
- Atrial arrhythmias w/ dilated RA pre- or postoperatively secondary to scar in atrium
- Paradoxical emboli & CVA: most typically seen after the 3rd or 4th decades of life

Prognosis
- Excellent in most w/ recognized ASDs

ATTENTION-DEFCIT HYPERACTIVITY DISORDER (ADHD)

HOWARD BAUCHNER, M.D.

HISTORY AND PHYSICAL
- ADHD consists of 3 behaviors:
  - Hyperactivity
  - Impulsivity
  - Inattention

History
- Types:
  - Predominantly inattentive
  - Predominantly hyperactive-impulsive
  - Combined
- Onset age <7 yrs
- Symptoms in 2 or more settings (home, work, school)
- Behaviors do not occur exclusively during the course of pervasive developmental disorder, schizophrenia, or other psychotic disorders

Physical signs
- Findings consistent with assoc conditions:
  - Fragile X syndrome
  - Neurofibromatosis
  - Fetal alcohol syndrome

TESTS
- Behavior reports from 2 sources (parents, teachers, self) necessary for diagnosis
- Connors Rating Scales (narrow-band checklists)
- Consider psychological/educational testing for co-morbid conditions
- Lead, thyroid function tests, EEG, neuroimaging: not required unless indicated by history

DIFFERENTIAL DIAGNOSIS
- Pervasive developmental disorder
- Major affective disorder
- Reaction to stress
- Hyperthyroidism
- Hearing loss
- Common co-morbid conditions:
  - Learning disabilities
  - Depression
  - Oppositional defiant disorder
  - Conduct disorder
  - Mild mental retardation
  - Anxiety disorders

MANAGEMENT
- Assemble & interpret data from various sources
- If significant co-morbid conditions: specialist referral

■ Referral to CHADD (Children and Adults with Attention Deficit/ Hyperactivity Disorder); may be helpful (954-587-3700, www. chadd.org)

SPECIFIC THERAPY
■ First-line:
➤ Methylphenidate
➤ Methylphenidate extended-release
➤ Dextroamphetamine
➤ Adderall
■ Families may stop therapy on weekends, holidays & summer
■ If adolescent wants to stop drug therapy, consider as trial & negotiate w/ adolescent & family
■ Second-line:
➤ Clonidine
➤ Antidepressants
■ Complementary & alternative medicine: unproven
■ Behavioral and/or psychotherapy

FOLLOW-UP
■ Frequent contact, by telephone or in person, when pharmacologic therapy is started
■ After stable regimen established: follow up q3–6 mo

COMPLICATIONS AND PROGNOSIS
■ Drug side effects:
➤ Loss of appetite: monitor weight
➤ Inability to fall asleep
➤ Manipulate dose & timing of drug therapy to minimize effects
■ Children w/ conduct disorder & oppositional defiant disorder difficult to manage; prognosis guarded in terms of school achievement/ employment
■ Most have ADHD as adolescents (70%) & adults (60%)

BACK PAIN

IRENE TIEN, M.D.

HISTORY AND PHYSICAL

History
■ Onset, duration, history of trauma or recent illness
■ Frequency & intensity of pain

- Neurologic symptoms
- General medical condition
- Nighttime pain
- Pathologic process most likely in children age <4 y; less likely in adolescents

Physical signs
- Spinal exam:
  - ➤ Posture, alignment
  - ➤ Overlying skin condition
  - ➤ Bony tenderness
- Forward bending test: thoracic & lumbar asymmetry and flexibility
- Careful neurologic exam, esp. weakness, abnormal tone, or asymmetric reflexes

TESTS
- Radiographs:
  - ➤ AP & lateral spinal x-rays in all children, esp. with uncertain diagnosis or high suspicion of:
    - Abuse
    - Chronic pain
    - Bony tenderness after trauma
  - ➤ Oblique films (spondylolysis)
  - ➤ Technetium bone scan if normal x-ray and neurologic exam
  - ➤ MRI if normal x-ray and abnormal neurologic exam
  - ➤ CT if bony lesion on x-ray or bone scan
  - ➤ PPD and/or chest x-ray (tuberculosis)
- Lab studies:
  - ➤ CBC, ESR
  - ➤ Rheumatoid factor, ANA, HLA-B27 (suspected rheumatologic disorder)
  - ➤ Consider blood culture

DIFFERENTIAL DIAGNOSIS
- Developmental: Scheuermann's kyphosis
- Infection:
  - ➤ Diskitis
  - ➤ Vertebral osteomyelitis
  - ➤ Tuberculous spondylitis
  - ➤ Epidural abscess
- Traumatic:
  - ➤ Spondylolysis, spondylolisthesis

- ➤ Herniated disk
- ➤ Slipped vertebral apophysis
- ➤ Fractures
- ➤ Muscle strain
- Neoplasms
- Visceral:
  - ➤ Abdominal neoplasms
  - ➤ Pyelonephritis
  - ➤ Appendicitis
  - ➤ Retroperitoneal abscess
- Psychosomatic (diagnosis of exclusion)

MANAGEMENT
- Generally not emergent problem
- Emergent MRI and neurosurgical evaluation (pts w/ abnormal neurologic exam)

SPECIFIC THERAPY
- Hospitalization:
  - ➤ Diskitis
  - ➤ Vertebral osteomyelitis
  - ➤ Tuberculous spondylitis
  - ➤ Selected spinal fractures
  - ➤ Back pain associated w/ neurologic deficits
  - ➤ Neoplasm-related back pain
  - ➤ Pyelonephritis, appendicitis, retroperitoneal abscess, abdominal neoplasms
  - ➤ Uncontrolled back pain requiring parenteral analgesics
  - ➤ Suspected child abuse or neglect
- Orthopedic evaluation (require follow-up and/or nonsurgical management):
  - ➤ Scheuermann's kyphosis
  - ➤ Painful scoliosis
  - ➤ Spondylolysis, spondylolisthesis
  - ➤ Herniated disk
- Reduction in activity
- NSAIDs

FOLLOW-UP
- Orthopedic follow-up
- Primary care follow-up for adolescents with muscle overuse or strain

COMPLICATIONS AND PROGNOSIS
- At least 50% have identifiable physical cause for back pain, but few require surgical intervention
- No neurologic deficits: generally do well
- Spinal cord lesions: possible serious neurologic sequelae

BELL'S PALSY/FACIAL PALSY

LAURIE DOUGLAS, M.D.

HISTORY AND PHYSICAL
Originally referred to as acute idiopathic facial nerve dysfunction; some evidence linking to HSV 1 infection

History
- Often preceded by URI
- Sometimes heralded by pain or tingling in ear canal or over mastoid
- Rapid onset, few hours to few days
- Weakness of upper & lower face
- Usually unilateral

Physical
- Ability to furrow forehead, close eyes, turn up corners of mouth, puff out cheeks
- Examine for flatter nasolabial fold on affected side
- May affect taste (sugar & salt), lacrimation, salivation
- May cause hyperacusis

TESTS
- For isolated unilateral facial palsy, which appears to be idiopathic or related to HSV 1, no specific tests indicated

DIFFERENTIAL DIAGNOSIS
- Upper motor neuron lesion: spares brow elevation; perform MRI of brain
- Trauma: due to fractures of the temporal bone; perform CT
- Lyme disease
- *Mycoplasma pneumoniae*, Epstein-Barr virus, varicella zoster
- Ramsay Hunt: see vesicles in external ear canal or oropharynx; may affect CN VIII causing vertigo & deafness, presumably due to herpes zoster
- HIV

- Sarcoid: usually causes bilateral facial weakness
- Melkersson-Rosenthal:
  - Recurrent facial paralysis
  - Facial edema
  - +/− lingual plication
  - May be familial
- Mobius: congenital facial diplegia with abducens palsies
- Guillain-Barre: usually bilateral, diminished reflexes
- Brain stem tumor: look for other signs of brain stem involvement

MANAGEMENT
Patch & lubricate eye regularly if unable to close eye fully

SPECIFIC THERAPY
- Value of steroids & acyclovir controversial
- Some evidence that oral prednisone given in first week of symptoms helpful in adults
- Oral acyclovir for 5–10 d in combination with prednisone possibly improves outcome in adults
- Do not use steroids with CSF pleocytosis, immune compromise, hypertension, or suspected infection other than HSV 1

FOLLOW-UP
- Follow every 2–3 wk

COMPLICATIONS AND PROGNOSIS
- Most recover in 4–6 wk
- Nearly all recover in 6 mo

BETA-BLOCKER OVERDOSE

SOPHIA DYER, M.D.

HISTORY AND PHYSICAL
- Initially may be asymptomatic
- Weakness, lethargy
- Bradycardia, hypotension, exacerbation of underlying asthma
- Sinus arrest, high degree AV block, QRS prolongation; in severe overdose, asystole
- Respiratory depression and apnea in life-threatening overdoses
- Seizures and coma, esp. w/ propranolol

TESTS
- Dextrose stick or blood sugar
- ECG
- Serum electrolytes
- Urine and serum toxicology screen
- Pregnancy test (adolescent females)

DIFFERENTIAL DIAGNOSIS
- Calcium channel blocker overdose
- Overdose of clonidine or other alpha-2 agonists
- Digitalis glycoside overdose
- Opiate overdose

MANAGEMENT
What to do first
- Airway control if necessary
- IV access
- Correct hypoglycemia if present
- Fluid bolus for hypotension
- No gastric lavage or emesis (ipecac)

SPECIFIC THERAPY
- Atropine for bradycardia
- Activated charcoal
- Multiple-dose activated charcoal: for sustained-release beta-blockers
- IV glucagon bolus:
  - Continuous glucagon infusions for pts who respond to initial bolus
  - Catecholamine infusions for pts who do not respond to glucagon
- Transcutaneous or transvenous pacing: may aid with heart rate but not blood pressure
- Seizures responsive to benzodiazepines
- Insulin and glucose infusions (experimental); contact local Poison Control Center
- Hemodialysis rarely indicated; only for water-soluble beta-blockers
- Intra-aortic balloon pump or extracorporeal membrane oxygenation in extreme hypotension not responsive to other measures

FOLLOW-UP

- After recovery from overdose, long-term concerns limited to sequelae of initial overdose (i.e., intercurrent renal failure from hypotension)

COMPLICATIONS AND PROGNOSIS

- Prognosis excellent if patient survives cardiovascular effects of overdose

BRAIN TUMORS

JANE E. MINTURN, M.D., PH.D.

HISTORY AND PHYSICAL

History

- 60% infratentorial (cerebellum, brain stem)
- 40% supratentorial (cerebral hemispheres, thalamus)
- Associated:
  - Neurofibromatosis Types I & II
  - Tuberous sclerosis
  - Von Hippel-Lindau
  - Ataxia-telangectasia
  - Gorlin
  - Li-Fraumeni
  - Astrocytoma, medulloblastema associated w/ p53 mutation
- Increased ICP:
  - Headache
  - AM vomiting
  - Impaired vision:
    - Blurriness (papilledema)
    - Diplopia (CN VI palsy)
  - Lethargy
  - School performance & personality changes
  - Ataxia
  - Focal seizures
- Infants:
  - Anorexia
  - Irritability
  - Increasing head circumference
  - Failure to thrive
  - Loss of milestones (developmental delay)

Physical signs
- Papilledema
- Visual field defects
- Cranial nerves:
  - Impaired eye abduction
  - Facial droop
  - Absent gag
  - Limited upward gaze
- Motor defects:
  - Gait
  - Muscle strength
- Ataxia

TESTS
- Head CT:
  - Hydrocephalus
  - Intracranial hemorrhage
- Brain MRI:
  - T1 (anatomic detail)
  - T2 (edema)
  - Gadolinium (blood-brain barrier breakdown)
- Spine MRI: determine dissemination
- CSF (10 d post-op):
  - Cell count
  - Cytology
  - Chemistry

DIFFERENTIAL DIAGNOSIS
Depends on location
- Cerebral hemisphere:
  - Astrocytoma
  - Ependymoma
  - Glioblastoma
  - Meningioma
- Sella/chiasm:
  - Craniopharyngioma
  - Pituitary adenoma
  - Optic nerve glioma
- Cerebellum:
  - Medulloblastoma
  - Astrocytoma
  - Meningioma

- Brain stem:
  - ➤ Astrocytoma
  - ➤ Ependymoma
  - ➤ Glioblastoma
- Cerebral hemorrhage
- Head trauma: cerebral contusion

MANAGEMENT
- ICP w/ impending herniation: emergent ventriculostomy/VP shunt placement
- Reduce edema & decrease ICP: dexamethasone/mannitol/acetazolamide

SPECIFIC THERAPY
- Surgery:
  - ➤ Biopsy, total or partial resection
  - ➤ Relieve increased ICP/CSF obstruction
- Radiation (RT):
  - ➤ Total resection often impossible
  - ➤ Many tumors radiation-sensitive
  - ➤ Avoid/delay if age <3 y
- Chemotherapy (CRx):
  - ➤ Systemic/intrathecal, multiagent regimens; depend on tumor type
  - ➤ Often w/ surgery, RT
  - ➤ High-dose CRx w/ stem cell rescue in young children to avoid RT
- Rehabilitation:
  - ➤ Physical
  - ➤ Occupational
  - ➤ Speech

FOLLOW-UP
- MRI:
  - ➤ Determine extent of resection
  - ➤ Response to treatment
  - ➤ Monitor for recurrence/relapse
- Laboratory eval:
  - ➤ CBC/hepatic/renal function during CRx
  - ➤ Endocrine/electrolytes (hypothalamic & pituitary tumors)
- Off-therapy:
  - ➤ MRI
  - ➤ Endocrine:

- GH levels
- Thyroid function
- Gonadal function
➤ Intellectual/school function

COMPLICATIONS AND PROGNOSIS
■ Depends on tumor type, size & location, extent of disease (metastatic or localized), age, treatment modality
■ Neurologic deficits (depend on tumor location, extent of resection):
  ➤ Blindness
  ➤ Mutism
  ➤ Paralysis
  ➤ Motor deficits
  ➤ Seizures
■ Post-op meningitis, shunt infections
■ Treatment-related complications:
  ➤ CRx:
    - Nausea/vomiting
    - Cytopenia
    - Infection
    - Nephrotoxicity
    - Ototoxicity
    - Encephalopathy
  ➤ RT:
    - Intellectual impairment
    - Growth failure
    - Second malignancies

Prognosis
■ Depends on tumor type, location, & age

BREAST DISORDERS

LINDA M. GRANT, M.D., M.P.H.

HISTORY AND PHYSICAL
■ Asymmetry, gynecomastia common in adolescent
■ Development:
  ➤ Sexual maturity or Tanner stages B1–B5 (ie, when breast budding began, progression)

- Gynecomastia:
  - ➤ 2/3 of all boys
  - ➤ Peak occurrence age 14
  - ➤ Usually bilateral
  - ➤ Upper/lower body segment ratio (Kleinfelter's)
  - ➤ Testicular size

History
- Family Hx of breast disorders
- Gynecologic Hx:
  - ➤ Pregnancy
  - ➤ Irregular menses
- Mass:
  - ➤ Vary w/ cycle vs. increasing in size
  - ➤ Duration clearly delineated
  - ➤ Presence of increased vasculature
  - ➤ Discharge
- Abnormal size:
  - ➤ Rapidity of growth
  - ➤ Unilateral vs. bilateral
  - ➤ Developmental level
  - ➤ History of radiation
  - ➤ Other developmental delay
  - ➤ Systemic illness
  - ➤ Poland syndrome (absence of pectoralis muscle)
- Pain (mastalgia/mastodynia):
  - ➤ Vs. cervical root pain, costochondritis, caffeine, drugs (phenothiazines)
  - ➤ Infection
  - ➤ Erythema
  - ➤ Cracked nipples
  - ➤ Abscess or hematoma
- Discharge:
  - ➤ Milky (common)
  - ➤ Bloody
  - ➤ Hx of headaches or vision changes: more detailed eval.
  - ➤ From nipple or periareolar gland

Physical signs
- Teach self-exam while palpating breast; performed week after menses every month

TESTS
- Mass: ultrasound, may do needle aspiration if cystic
- Mammogram not useful in adolescents; tissue density differences compared w/ adults
- Galactorrhea:
  - ➤ Prolactin level; if elevated (100 ng/mL suggests pituitary adenoma): MRI
  - ➤ TFTs

DIFFERENTIAL DIAGNOSIS
- Mass:
  - ➤ Observe for monthly fluctuations suggesting cyst
  - ➤ Contusions painful, fibroadenomas not
  - ➤ Most masses are fibroadenomas even if hx of recent chest trauma
  - ➤ Cystosarcoma phylloides less common
  - ➤ Intraductal papilloma less common
- Abnormal size:
  - ➤ Enlarged:
    - Virginal hypertrophy
    - Giant fibroadenoma
  - ➤ Small or absent:
    - Turner
    - CAH
    - Previous irradiation
  - ➤ Asymmetric:
    - Normal development vs. unilateral fibroadenoma
    - Virginal hypertrophy
    - Poland syndrome
- Gynecomastia:
  - ➤ Normal puberty
  - ➤ Kleinfelter:
    - Decreased upper/lower body segment ratio
    - Testes <5 mL, firm
- Pain:
  - ➤ Pregnancy
  - ➤ Mastitis
  - ➤ Caffeine use
  - ➤ Idiopathic
- Discharge:
  - ➤ Prolactin-secreting pituitary adenoma

➤ Drug use (illicit, prescription drug, OCP)
➤ Idiopathic

MANAGEMENT
■ Depends on adolescent's development level, duration, & nature of disorder
■ Masses: observed for 2–4 mo if considered cystic or fibroadenoma

SPECIFIC THERAPY
■ Mass:
  ➤ Ultrasound
  ➤ Cystic: needle aspiration
  ➤ Fibroadenoma: consider resection
■ Abnormal size:
  ➤ Enlarged: US for mass
  ➤ Hypertrophy: consider reduction mammoplasty
  ➤ Small or absent: supportive; implants in older teen if debilitating
■ Gynecomastia:
  ➤ Karyotype
  ➤ May do reduction mammoplasty if very enlarged, socially debilitating, & Tanner V for >2 yr
■ Pain:
  ➤ Mastitis: antibiotics
  ➤ Idiopathic:
    • Decrease caffeine
    • Good bra support
    • Possibly vitamin E (unproven)
■ Discharge:
  ➤ Pituitary adenoma: bromocriptine
  ➤ Decrease drug use/breast stimulation

FOLLOW-UP
■ Regular checkups & self-exam

COMPLICATIONS AND PROGNOSIS
■ Usually none
■ Depend on disorder & management strategies:
  ➤ Mass:
    • Most not cancerous
    • Fibroadenomas can recur
    • Family Hx warrants closer follow-up

- Gynecomastia: usually resolves w/in 2 yr
- Discharge: galactorrhea w/ amenorrhea & normal prolactin common, but warrants close follow-up

BREASTFEEDING BASICS

BARBARA L. PHILIPP, M.D., I.B.C.L.C.

HISTORY AND PHYSICAL

- American Academy of Pediatrics (AAP): human milk is the "optimal form of nutrition for infants"
- AAP: exclusive breastfeeding for ~6 mo, continue for at least 12 months, or for as long as mother/baby wish
  - Add complementary foods at about 6 mo
  - Note: WHO recommends breastfeed to 2 years or more
- Anticipatory guidance:
  - Initiate breastfeeding as soon as possible after birth, usually w/in 1st hour of life
  - Advise continuous rooming-in while in hospital
  - Newborns should be nursed whenever they show signs of hunger — 8-12x in 24 hours, usually 10–15 min per breast
  - All babies lose weight 1st few days (up to 7% considered normal)
  - Breast milk production:
    - Day 1: 3 tablespoons (~50 mL)
    - Day 2: 13 tablespoons (~ 200 mL)
    - Day 2–4: lactogenesis stage II (copious production)
  - Stools:
    - Meconium: thick, black, tarry
    - Transition: sludgy, brown
    - Milk stools: loose, yellow with chunks
- Going home:
  - Infant to breast ~8–12× in 24 h
  - 3–4 bowel movements in 24 h
  - At least 6 wet diapers in 24 h
  - Clinician contact 48–72 h after going home
  - Give information regarding management of engorgement
  - Telephone support line/contact person
  - Beware the sleepy baby!
  - Back to birthweight by 10–14 d

- Breastfeeding contraindications
  - HIV+ mother (in U.S.)
  - Few medications such as
    - Chemotherapy
    - Radioactive isotopes
  - Illegal street drugs
  - Galactosemia (lactose = glucose + galactose)
  - Untreated active tuberculosis

History
- Most common reason for stopping in hospital setting: "not enough milk"
- Need to prime the pump (breasts) to tell system (brain) to make breast milk (discourage pacifiers, bottles of infant formula, other supplements)
- Pacifiers, if used at all, should be used once mother and baby breastfeeding well

Physical signs
- Feeding cues:
  - Any signs of hunger
  - Rooting, lipsmacking, fist sucking
- The latch (the way the infant attaches to the breast to ensure production and transfer of adequate milk supply)
  - Tummy to tummy, nipple to nose (cradle hold)
  - Touch middle of infant's face w/ nipple
  - Patiently wait for baby to open mouth widely
  - Bring baby to breast (NOT mom to baby); help baby grab onto breast like grabbing onto "Big Mac sandwich"
  - Good latch:
    - Lips flanged out
    - Wide angle at corner of baby's mouth
    - More of lower than upper areola in baby's mouth
    - No audible clicks or indents in cheeks
    - Jaw movement
    - Audible gulps when milk in w/ rhythmic suck/suck/swallow

TESTS
- Accurate weight important
- Clinical assessment of jaundice

DIFFERENTIAL DIAGNOSIS

■ Breastfeeding problems:
- ➣ Excessive weight loss
- ➣ Engorgement
- ➣ Sore nipples
- ➣ Inverted nipples

MANAGEMENT

■ See w/in 48–72 hours of going home
■ Ensure mother can contact healthcare provider

SPECIFIC THERAPY

■ Causes of excessive weight loss (SAILBOAT):
- ➣ Surgery of breast (reduction > augmentation)
- ➣ Agenesis of mammary tissue
- ➣ Inverted nipples
- ➣ Latch, latch, latch
- ➣ Baby issue: prematurity, poor suck
- ➣ OB issue: retained placental fragments, Sheehan's syndrome
- ➣ Ankyloglossia
- ➣ Time for a change to baby-friendly (The Ten Steps to Successful Breastfeeding)

■ Breast engorgement:
- ➣ Warm water on breasts
- ➣ Bend over (use gravity to drain off milk)
- ➣ Hand expression to soften nipple so baby can attach
- ➣ Baby to breast frequently
- ➣ Cool compresses (bags of frozen vegetables)
- ➣ Pain medication (ibuprofen, acetaminophen)
- ➣ Emotional support

■ Sore nipples:
- ➣ First week:
  - • Correct poor latch
  - • Air-dry nipples
  - • Apply breast milk/lanolin cream onto nipple
- ➣ After first few weeks (causes):
  - • Poor latch
  - • Candidal infection
  - • Secondary bacterial infection

■ Inverted nipples:
- ➣ Pinch test or observe nipple as baby comes off breast

➤ Pull out nipple w/ pump; then have baby latch
➤ Stimulate supply with pumping
➤ Cup-feed expressed milk
➤ Close follow-up
■ Sleepy baby:
  ➤ Office evaluation & weight check
  ➤ Assess latch
  ➤ Assess frequency of breastfeeds & amount of formula supplementation, pacifier sucking
  ➤ Infant to breast frequently
  ➤ Stimulate supply w/ pump, if necessary
  ➤ Offer supplements by a method other than the bottle
    • Cup-feed
    • Finger feed
    • Syringe feed
    • Supplemental nursing system

FOLLOW-UP
■ Close contact (phone, home visits, in-office)
■ Weight checks
■ Peer, lactation consultant support

COMPLICATIONS AND PROGNOSIS
■ Most women can breastfeed
■ Knowledgeable, supportive clinician is key
■ AAP Statement on Breastfeeding and the Use of Human Milk. Pediatrics 1997;100:1035
■ HHS Blueprint for Action on Breastfeeding. US Dept of HHS, Office on Women's Health, 2000
■ Support:
  ➤ La Leche League
  ➤ Academy of Breastfeeding Medicine (www.bfmed.org)
  ➤ American Academy of Pediatrics

BRONCHIOLITIS

SUZANNE F. STEINBACH, M.D.

HISTORY AND PHYSICAL
■ Age <2 y
■ URI with cough

- Low-grade fever
- Tachypnea
- Grunting, flaring, retraction
- Crackles
- Wheeze, prolonged expiration
- Severe cases: apnea/cyanosis

TESTS
- Oxygen saturation
- CXR:
  - Hyperinflation
  - Atelectasis
  - Peribronchial cuffing
- RSV fluorescent antibody screen
- CBC
- ABG: hospitalized pts if poor response to therapy, concern for respiratory failure:
  - Mean PaO_2: 51 (range 31–63)
  - $PaCO_2$ >45+

DIFFERENTIAL DIAGNOSIS
- Asthma
- Cystic fibrosis
- Foreign body aspiration
- Chronic aspiration:
  - Tracheoesophageal fistula
  - Gastroesophageal reflux
- Airway compression
- Airway anomalies:
  - Tracheal stenosis, webs
  - Tracheobronchomalacia

MANAGEMENT
What to do first
- Assess oxygenation/ventilation
- Oxygen if needed

General measures
- Maintain hydration/nutrition
- Cardiorespiratory monitor
- Isolation/contact precaution

SPECIFIC THERAPY

Indications
- Respiratory distress
- Hypoxia

Treatment options
- Oxygen
- Nebulized beta-2-agonist bronchodilators (in 3 mL NS)
  - L-epinephrine 1:1,000, 0.5 mg/kg, max 5 mg
  - Racemic epinephrine 2.25%, 0.05–0.1 mL/kg
  - Albuterol 0.03 mL/kg
  - Albuterol MDI 2 puffs w/ spacer
- Prednisone 2 mg/kg/d IV/PO
- Heliox 70/30
- Ribavirin (controversial)
- Nasal CPAP 6–7 cm H_2O
- Intubation/assisted ventilation

Side effects and complications
- Beta-agonists:
  - Tachycardia
  - Irritability
- Ribavirin: deposits block ventilator tubing

Contraindications to treatment

Absolute
- Mist:
  - No benefit
  - May worsen bronchospasm
- Sedation: suppresses respiratory drive

Relative
- Antibiotics:
  - No benefit unless bacterial infection
  - May increase secondary infection
- Ipratropium bromide: no benefit

FOLLOW-UP
- Monitor respiratory rate, retractions, wheeze, oxygen sat
- Assess response to therapy

COMPLICATIONS AND PROGNOSIS
- Atelectasis: resolves spontaneously
- Aspiration

- Hospitalized pts:
  - 20%: apnea
  - <7%: respiratory failure
  - 1%: death; higher risk in congenital heart disease
- Secondary bacterial infection
- Pneumothorax/pneumomediastinum (rare)

Prognosis
- May recur
- Prevent w/ palivizumab or RSV-IGIV:
  - Age <2 y w/ chronic lung disease (CLD) requiring treatment in past 6 mo
  - Premature infant (no CLD):
    - 29–32 wks gestation to age 6 mo
    - <28 wks gestation to age 12 mo
- Increased risk of recurrent wheezing:
- $^3/_4$ children age 1–2 y
- $^1/_2$ children age 2–3 y

BULIMIA

LIANA R. CLARK, M.D.

HISTORY AND PHYSICAL
- Binge eating
- Average two binge-eating episodes/week for 3 mo
- Binge: rapid consumption of high-calorie food in frenzied manner; usually done alone
- Patient aware of abnormal eating behavior

History
- Vomiting, laxatives, or excessive exercise may be used to counteract binging
- Symptoms
  - Fatigue
  - Heartburn
  - Abdominal pain
- Mood
  - Depressed
  - Substance use
  - Suicidal

Physical
- Hypotension
- Edema
- Calluses on hands
- Muscle cramps
- Normal weight

TESTS
- Basic:
  - CBC
  - Electrolytes
  - BUN
  - Creatinine
  - Glucose
  - Cholesterol
  - Lipids
  - Amylase
  - Total protein
  - Albumin
  - LFTs
- Other test: ECG
- Consider:
  - Urine drug screen
  - UGI with SBFT to rule out GE obstruction

DIFFERENTIAL DIAGNOSIS
- Psychogenic vomiting
- Gastrointestinal obstruction
- Bilateral hernia

MANAGEMENT
- Outpatient management: emphasize breaking binge-purge cycle
- Use nutritionist for healthy meal planning

SPECIFIC THERAPY
- Criteria for hospitalization
  - Hypovolemia
  - Severe electrolyte disturbance
  - Intractable vomiting
  - Medical complications
    - Mallory-Weiss tears

- Aspiration pneumonia
- Pancreatitis

➤ Psychological: behavior therapy
- Medications (SSRIs): may decrease preoccupation with food and weight

FOLLOW-UP
- Needs long-term follow-up, weekly to monthly, as condition warrants

COMPLICATIONS AND PROGNOSIS
- Aspiration pneumonia
- Pneumomediastinum
- Pancreatitis
- Mallory-Weiss tears
- Paralytic ileus
- Cathartic colon
- Tooth enamel erosion with caries and periodontal disease
- Low mortality: 0.3%

CAMPYLOBACTER INFECTIONS

FRANZ BABL, M.D., M.P.H.

HISTORY AND PHYSICAL

History
- Diarrhea, abdominal pain, & fever
- Reservoir domestic & wild birds, animals
- Improperly cooked poultry, untreated water, & unpasteurized milk
- Farmworker or field trip to farm
- Child care centers
- Travel to developing countries

Physical signs
- Signs/symptoms of dehydration (10% of children)
- Intense abdominal pain, malaise, myalgia, & headache (precedes diarrhea in 30–50%)
- Periumbilical, crampy pain; can mimic appendicitis
- Severe cases: tenesmus, malaise, fever; mimic acute inflammatory bowel disease

TESTS

- CBC:
  - ➤ Peripheral WBC count usually normal
  - ➤ Left shift common
- Serum ALT, ALP, ESR: mild elevation in up to 25% of pts
- Stool smears examined w/ dark field microscopy, indirect fluorescent antibody test, or special stains: make presumptive diagnosis possible
- Stool culture
- Blood culture (septic, malnourished, chronically ill, or immunocompromised)
- CSF or joint culture: as clinically indicated

DIFFERENTIAL DIAGNOSIS

- Gastroenteritis: viral, bacterial, & parasitic infections
- Inflammatory diarrhea:
  - ➤ Ulcerative colitis
  - ➤ Crohn's
  - ➤ Pseudomembranous colitis
- Appendicitis

MANAGEMENT

- Assess hydration status & rehydration
- Bacteremia:
  - ➤ Assess & stabilize cardiovascular status
  - ➤ Assess for local infections
- Antibiotics

SPECIFIC THERAPY

- Erythromycin & azithromycin:
  - ➤ Shorten duration of illness & prevent relapse
  - ➤ Eradicate organism within 2–3 d
- Tetracycline: alternative for children $>=8$ y
- Fluoroquinolone (ciprofloxacin): effective but not approved for pts <18 y
- Rx for 5–7 d
- For resistant or bacteremic strains: therapy based on susceptibility tests
- Antimotility drugs: prolong symptoms; contraindicated

FOLLOW-UP

- Review hydration status in first 24 h

■ Follow-up visit w/in 24 h in pts with more than mild dehydration or additional complaints such as abdominal pain & fever
■ Control measures: contact precautions & hand washing

COMPLICATIONS AND PROGNOSIS
■ Guillain-Barre:
  ➤ More common young male adults & during summer
  ➤ Within 10 d of diarrhea (range 6–21 d)
  ➤ Cranial nerve involvement: 1/3 of pts
  ➤ Complete recovery in most
■ Reactive arthritis:
  ➤ More common in young male adults
  ➤ Within 3–40 d of diarrhea (mean 11 d)
  ➤ Oligoarticular, asymmetric, mainly large joints
■ Erythema nodosum
■ Acute idiopathic polyneuritis
■ Reiter

Prognosis
■ Enteritis:
  ➤ 60–70% subside w/in 1 wk
  ➤ 20–30% subside w/in 2 wks
  ➤ 5–10% persist for several wks
  ➤ Can be severe, prolonged, & recurrent in immunocompromised pts
■ Septicemia in immunocompromised host or neonate assoc w/ high mortality rate

CARBON MONOXIDE POISONING

ROBERT VINCI, M.D.

HISTORY AND PHYSICAL

History
■ Fire victims
■ Exposure to smoke or other sources of carbon-containing fuel:
  ➤ Car exhaust, other engines using combustible fuels
  ➤ Wood or coal-burning stoves
  ➤ Kerosene space heaters
  ➤ Faulty home furnace systems
  ➤ Solvents, paint removers

- Headache
- Nausea
- Dizziness
- Visual disturbances
- Fatigue
- Confusion
- Coma
- Family members w/ similar symptoms

Physical signs
- May not correlate with carboxyhemoglobin (COHgb) level
- Vital signs
- Tachycardia
- May appear cyanotic despite normal pulse oximetry (most oximeters can't measure COHgb)
- "Cherry red" skin in minority of patients
- Neuropsychiatric exam
- Assess for suicidal ideation

TESTS
- Co-oximetry if available
- ABG or VBG with CO level
- ECG, cardiac enzymes (to assess myocardial ischemia)
- Serum electrolytes with glucose
- Renal function tests
- CBC
- Chest x-ray (fire victim)
- Pregnancy test (CO transported across placenta)
- Toxicology screen
- Cyanide levels (industrial fire and unexplained metabolic acidosis)
- CT/MRI (CNS involvement)

DIFFERENTIAL DIAGNOSIS
- Smoke inhalation
- Methemoglobinemia
- Lactic acidosis
- Drug ingestion
- Anemia

MANAGEMENT

What to do first
- Remove patient from CO source

- 100% oxygen via non-rebreather system or intubation
- Fire victim:
  - Assess airway
  - Prophylactic intubation for airway thermal injury (i.e., soot, stridor)
- IV access

SPECIFIC THERAPY
- Decrease COHgb half-life:
  - Room air 4–6 h
  - 100% oxygen 30–90 min
  - Hyperbaric oxygen 15–30 min
- Hyperbaric oxygen:
  - Coma & CNS involvement
  - Cardiovascular impairment
  - Levels >25–40% even w/o symptoms
  - Pregnant mother (fetus and newborn at higher risk)
  - Location of nearest chamber: call 1-919-684-2948
- Sodium bicarbonate:
  - Avoid unless severe acidosis (<7.15)
  - Acidosis shifts Hgb dissociation curve to right & promotes tissue oxygen delivery
  - Bicarbonate shifts curve to left & may impair oxygen delivery to tissues
- Treat increased ICP as clinically indicated

FOLLOW-UP
- Discharge if levels <10% & no symptoms
- Monitor COHgb & acid-base status during therapy
- Formal neuropsychiatric testing
- Follow-up CNS imaging
- CO detector for home

COMPLICATIONS AND PROGNOSIS
- Fetal demise
- Rhabdomyolysis
- Impaired cognitive functioning

Prognosis
- Depends on COHgb level and degree of tissue hypoxia
- Delayed neuropsychiatric sequelae, esp if:
  - Coma

➤ Cardiac arrest
➤ Metabolic acidosis
➤ High COHgb level

CARDIAC ARRHYTHMIAS

ALEJANDRO ITHURALDE, M.D.
SHARON E. O'BRIEN, M.D.

HISTORY AND PHYSICAL

■ Lyme disease
■ Collagen vascular disease
■ Drugs: caffeine, stimulants
■ May be asymptomatic
■ Palpitations
■ Chest pain
■ Dizziness
■ Syncope
■ Respiratory distress
■ Exam may be normal
■ CHF
    ➤ Poor perfusion
    ➤ Hypotension
    ➤ Tachycardia, tachypnea
    ➤ Low oxygen saturation
    ➤ Hepatomegaly
    ➤ Rales

TESTS

■ ECG
■ 24-h Holter
■ Event monitor
■ Exercise stress test
■ Electrolytes
■ Toxicology screen
■ Echo

DIFFERENTIAL DIAGNOSIS

■ Sinus arrhythmia:
    ➤ Normal slowing during expiration
    ➤ Exaggerated:

- Acute illness
- Increased vagal tone (drugs)
  ➤ Benign
■ Premature atrial complexes:
  ➤ Common
  ➤ P wave earlier than anticipated; different morphology
  ➤ Narrow QRS
  ➤ Incomplete compensatory pause
  ➤ Benign
■ Premature ventricular complexes (PVC):
  ➤ Wide QRS not preceded by P wave
  ➤ T wave points in opposite direction
  ➤ Unifocal or multifocal
  ➤ Generally full compensatory pause
  ➤ In general, unifocal PVCs benign
  ➤ Red flags:
    - Suspected heart disease
    - Multifocal PVCs/runs of PVCs
    - Symptoms (syncope, chest pain)
    - Family history: sudden death
    - Increased frequency w/ exercise

Narrow complex tachycardia

■ Sinus tachycardia:
  ➤ P wave + in leads I, II, AVF
  ➤ Rate varies
  ➤ Associated: fever, anemia, anxiety, pain, hyperthyroidism, sepsis, CHF
  ➤ Treat underlying cause
■ Atrial flutter:
  ➤ Reentrant mechanism
  ➤ Atrial rate 300 bpm
  ➤ Sawtooth configuration common
  ➤ Variable ventricular response depends on degree of AV block
  ➤ Treatment:
    - Digoxin
    - Diltiazem
    - Type 1C agents
    - Amiodarone
    - Electrical cardioversion
    - Anticoagulation

- Atrial fibrillation:
  - ➤ Atrial rate 350–600
  - ➤ Irregularly irregular ventricular response
  - ➤ Treatment as above

Wide complex tachycardia

- Ventricular tachycardia:
  - ➤ 3 or more PVCs in a row, rate of 120–200 bpm
  - ➤ Treatment:
    - Correct electrolytes
    - Lidocaine (if stable)
    - Synchronized cardioversion (if unstable)
    - Antiarrhythmic therapy
    - EP study/ICD implantation
- Ventricular fibrillation:
  - ➤ Bizarre QRS complexes of varying configuration
  - ➤ Treatment: CPR with defibrillation

Disturbance AV conduction

- First-degree AV block:
  - ➤ PR interval > normal for age
  - ➤ Every P wave followed by QRS
  - ➤ Consider Lyme disease, rheumatic heart disease, collagen vascular disorder, drug toxicity
  - ➤ Benign
  - ➤ Treat underlying cause
- Second-degree AV block:
  - ➤ Mobitz I or Wenckebach
    - Progressive lengthening of PR until QRS complex dropped
    - Consider myocarditis, CHD, drug toxicity, can occur normally in healthy children
  - ➤ Mobitz II: QRS complex dropped w/o lengthening of PR interval
- Third-degree AV block:
  - ➤ Complete AV dissociation
  - ➤ P & QRS complexes regular intervals but ventricular rate slower than atrial rate
  - ➤ May be acquired: surgery, collagen vascular disease, myocarditis
  - ➤ If congenital: consider CHD, maternal lupus
  - ➤ Treatment:
    - Isoproterenol
    - Cardiac pacing

MANAGEMENT
- Assess cardiopulmonary status & treat appropriately
- Supportive care
- Determine cardiac arrhythmias

SPECIFIC THERAPY
- See "Differential diagnosis" section

FOLLOW-UP
- Depends on underlying arrhythmia

COMPLICATIONS AND PROGNOSIS
- Depends on underlying arrhythmia
- CHF
- Cardiogenic shock
- Cardiac arrest and death

CAT-SCRATCH DISEASE

KATHERINE HSU, M.D.

HISTORY AND PHYSICAL
- Hallmark of disease: regional "hot" lymphadenopathy in immuno-competent person
  - Inoculation site papule in 60%, then 1–3 wk later develop lymphadenopathy, with suppuration in 30%
  - Axillary, cervical, inguinal, femoral, or epitrochlear nodes
  - Parinaud oculoglandular syndrome: eye inoculation & unilateral conjunctivitis, then later preauricular adenopathy
- Rare disseminated bone involvement with granulomatous lytic lesions

History
- Feline contact in >90%; rare transmission via other animals or inanimate objects
- Fever, mild systemic symptoms (malaise, headache, anorexia, transient maculopapular rash) in 30%

Physical
- 1% have disseminated illness:
  - High fever
  - Abdominal pain

➤ Weight loss
➤ Liver & spleen involvement with granulomatous lesions (but little hepatic dysfunction)

TESTS

- Culturing *Bartonella henselae* impractical (difficult & slow to grow)
- Indirect fluorescent antibody (IFA) test for *Bartonella* species antibodies available from CDC
- Other IFA & enzyme immunoassay (EIA) tests commercially available, but little comparison data
- If tissue available, histologic findings characteristic but not diagnostic
  ➤ *Bartonella* PCR may detect DNA of organism in tissue sample (available in research settings)

DIFFERENTIAL DIAGNOSIS

- Mycobacterial disease
- Malignancy
- Pyogenic lymphadenitis
- Tularemia
- Brucellosis
- Sporotrichosis
- Mononucleosis syndrome (EBV or CMV)
- Toxoplasmosis

MANAGEMENT

- In immunocompetent patients, use symptomatic care & observation
  ➤ Needle aspirate tense, painful suppurative lymph nodes
  ➤ Avoid I&D of nonsuppurative nodes; may develop chronic draining sinuses
  ➤ Antibiotic uncertain effectiveness in hastening resolution

SPECIFIC THERAPY

- Consider antibiotics for severely ill pts with systemic symptoms & for immunocompromised pts
- Organism probably sensitive to standard doses of co-trimoxazole, azithromycin, rifampin, ciprofloxacin, doxycycline, tetracycline, or gentamicin

FOLLOW-UP

- Spontaneous resolution over weeks to months (usually 2–4 mo)
- Counsel pts to:
  ➤ Avoid contact with cats that scratch or bite
  ➤ Wash sites of cat scratches or bites immediately

> Not permit cats to lick open cuts or wounds
> Control cat flea outbreaks (thought to transmit *B. henselae* from cat to cat)

COMPLICATIONS AND PROGNOSIS

- Neurologic complications can appear 1–3 wk after onset of lymphadenopathy
  > Encephalopathy in up to 5% of pts
  > Sudden-onset seizures, combative or bizarre behavior, lethargy, or coma
  > Neuroimaging usually normal
  > LP results may be normal or show slight pleocytosis or elevated protein
  > Fever absent or low-grade; minimal associated systemic symptoms
  > Recovery over days to weeks
- Optic neuritis, neuroretinitis
  > Sudden-onset painless unilateral visual loss
  > Recovery over months
- Peripheral & cranial nerve neuralgia & paresthesia
- Reports of associated pneumonia, thrombotic thrombocytopenic purpura, hemolytic anemia, erythema nodosum, glomerulonephritis, & endocarditis (mostly in adults)
- Prognosis benign for all forms of illness in immunocompetent patients

CELLULITIS

ERIC FLEEGLER, M.D.

HISTORY AND PHYSICAL

History
- Local trauma, laceration, puncture wound, or foreign body
- Fever, pain, erythema, lymphangitis
- Recent varicella infection
- Chronic disease, chronic steroid use
- Tetanus and vaccination status

Physical signs
- Warmth, erythema, edema, tenderness
- Margin of cellulitis indistinct
- Regional lymphadenopathy (occasional)

- Fever uncommon
- Red streaking proximal: ascending lymphangitis
- Predilection: lower extremity > upper extremity > face

TESTS
- No work-up if small area, minimal pain, no systemic signs
- Consider CBC (usually normal), blood culture if febrile
- Aspiration of wound at leading edge: can instill sterile saline (culture and Gram stain 10–50% greater sensitivity if abscess or bullae)
- Radiographs: if crepitus may show gas in tissues (surgical emergency if fasciitis or gangrene)

DIFFERENTIAL DIAGNOSIS
- Angioedema
- Burns (thermal, radiation, chemical)
- Dermatitis (atopic, contact, exfoliative)
- Erythema multiforme, Stevens-Johnson
- Gas gangrene
- Arthropod envenomation
- Septic or inflammatory joints
- Impetigo, erythema, erysipelas
- Toxic epidermal necrolysis

MANAGEMENT
General measures
- Warm compresses
- Elevation of area
- Consider analgesics
- Antibiotics (most important)

SPECIFIC THERAPY
- Etiology often bacterial: *S. aureus* and group A streptococcus
- Outpatient treatment: dicloxacillin (liquid tastes terrible), cephalexin, or erythromycin
- Parenteral: nafcillin, cefazolin
- Immunocompromised: consider Rx for gram-negative rods or fungi (rare)
- Fresh water exposure: *Aeromonas hydrophila* (GNR)
- *Pneumococcus*:
  - ➤ Typically immunocompromised host
  - ➤ Tissue necrosis, suppuration, bacteremia
- Ludwig angina:
  - ➤ Cellulitis of submandibular space

> Respiratory distress
> Oral flora
- Perineum:
  > Anaerobes or fecal flora
  > May lead to necrotizing fasciitis

FOLLOW-UP
- Re-evaluate at 24–48 h; if worse consider parenteral antibiotics

COMPLICATIONS AND PROGNOSIS

Complications
- Severe infection:
  > Fever
  > Hypotension
  > Dehydration
  > Crepitus
  > Bullae formation
- Facial cellulitis with extension into retro-orbital space
- Bacteremia
- Toxic shock syndrome
- Abscess formation
- Lymphangitis
- Thrombophlebitis
- Gas-forming cellulitis (gangrene): may require amputation, 25% mortality rate

Prognosis
- Excellent; >90% cure rate on initial treatment

CHEST PAIN

PATRICIA R. LAWRENCE, P.N.P.
SHARON E. O'BRIEN, M.D.

HISTORY AND PHYSICAL

History
- Family Hx:
  > Arrhythmia
  > Heart disease
  > Seizure
  > Syncope or sudden death

- Recent surgery/trauma
- Kawasaki
- Medications/street drugs
- Description of pain:
  - Acute or chronic
  - Mode of onset
  - Location, radiation
  - Nature: sharp or dull (sharp usually musculoskeletal)
  - Duration, frequency
  - Aggravating factors:
    - Exercise (of concern)
    - Deep breathing
    - Chest wall movement
    - Palpation (musculoskeletal or pleural)
  - Alleviating factors:
    - Rest
    - Position
- Assoc. symptoms (of concern):
  - Fever
  - Dizziness
  - Nausea
  - Diaphoresis
  - Palpitations
  - Shortness of breath
  - Syncope
- Infants (Sx of concern):
  - Inconsolable irritability
  - Feeding intolerance
  - Pallor
  - Diaphoresis

Physical signs
- Heart rate
- Blood pressure in R arm & leg
- Syndromic appearance (Marfan's syndrome)
- Palpation of chest wall to elicit tenderness
- Auscultation for murmur while supine, sitting
- Assess change in murmur from standing to squatting

TESTS
- 12-lead ECG/rhythm strip:

- ➤ Pre-excitation
- ➤ Abnormal Q waves
- ➤ Hypertrophy
- ➤ ST-segment & T-wave abnormalities
- ■ CXR:
  - ➤ Bony abnormalities
  - ➤ Parenchymal disease
  - ➤ Fluid
  - ➤ Cardiac silhouette
- ■ Echocardiogram:
  - ➤ Coronary arteries
  - ➤ Hypertrophy
  - ➤ Outflow obstruction
  - ➤ Pericardial fluid
  - ➤ Left ventricular function
- ■ 24-h Holter monitor (suspected arrhythmia)
- ■ Exercise stress test

DIFFERENTIAL DIAGNOSIS

- ■ Cardiac:
  - ➤ Pericarditis/myocarditis
  - ➤ Postpericardiotomy syndrome
  - ➤ Arrhythmia
  - ➤ Trauma
  - ➤ Ischemia:
    - • Cocaine
    - • Obstructive lesions
    - • Coronary artery anomalies
    - • Pulmonary hypertension
    - • Hypertrophic cardiomyopathy
  - ➤ Mitral valve prolapse
  - ➤ Aortic dissection
- ■ Pulmonary:
  - ➤ Pneumonia
  - ➤ Pneumothorax
  - ➤ Pleurodynia
- ■ Esophageal:
  - ➤ Esophagitis w/ GER
  - ➤ Foreign body
- ■ Miscellaneous:
  - ➤ Costochondritis

- Asthma
- Sickle cell disease
- Bony abnormality: fracture
- Idiopathic/psychogenic

MANAGEMENT
- Depends on underlying etiology
- Rest/medication
- Reassurance
- Restriction from strenuous activity
- Pediatric cardiology referral

SPECIFIC THERAPY
- Treat cause
- Suspected costochondritis: rest, ibuprofen
- Pericarditis: NSAIDs/steroids
- Pneumonia: antibiotics
- Intervention for pneumothorax, obstructive lesions
- Antiarrhythmics

FOLLOW-UP
- Depends on underlying cause
- Worsening symptoms or changing exam may warrant escalated workup
- Pediatric cardiology referral (cardiac causes)

COMPLICATIONS AND PROGNOSIS
- In general, chest pain in children is noncardiac, prognosis excellent
- Varies w/ etiology
- Cardiac causes:
  - Arrhythmia
  - Sudden death

CHILD ABUSE

MEGAN SANDEL, M.D.

HISTORY AND PHYSICAL
- Physical abuse:
  - Unexplained injuries
  - Delay in seeking medical attention
  - Age inconsistent w/ injury

- Sexual abuse:
  - Sexualized behavior
  - Psychosomatic complaints
  - New behavioral or other psychological problems

History
- Obtained separately from child & parent, if possible
- Detail injury, who involved, where occurred
- Review Hx of previous injuries
- Family Hx (bone or bleeding disorders)
- Social Hx:
  - Domestic violence
  - Previous allegations of abuse
  - Previous or current involvement of social agencies or law enforcement

Physical signs
- Exam for suspected physical abuse:
  - Document location, size, shape, color of bruises
  - Suspicious bruises: symmetric, on central body or back, may resemble objects
  - Consider photographing suspicious bruises
- Exam for suspected sexual abuse:
  - If cooperative, inspect vaginal area, incl. hymen; document findings
  - Note demeanor during exam
  - Normal exam does not mean child was not abused

TESTS
- Suspected physical abuse:
  - CBC, PT/PTT, toxicology screen, U/A
  - LFTs, amylase (GI symptoms)
  - Suspicious bruises: consider skeletal survey in children age <2 or bone scan in age >2
  - Retinal exam & head CT (suspected shaking or head injury)
  - Elevated LFTs: abdominal CT to R/O intra-abdominal trauma
- Suspected sexual abuse:
  - If w/in 72 h, obtain consent from child & parent and use rape kit
  - If >72 h & asymptomatic, refer to specialized clinic for exam
  - Sample all contact areas for gonorrhea, chlamydia, & do wet prep
  - Lesions present: HSV culture
  - Urine pregnancy test

➤ Suspected penetration: blood for RPR, hepatitis B panel, HCG, HIV

DIFFERENTIAL DIAGNOSIS
■ Physical abuse:
  ➤ Infections
  ➤ Bleeding disorders
  ➤ Metabolic/nutritional diseases
  ➤ Allergic diseases
  ➤ Osteogenesis imperfecta
■ Sexual abuse:
  ➤ Nonspecific vaginitis
  ➤ Normal variation

MANAGEMENT
■ Report suspected abuse to state authorities
■ Treat prophylactically for STDs & pregnancy if penetration occurred

SPECIFIC THERAPY
■ Mental health services to prevent post-traumatic stress disorder
■ Pain treatment
■ STD prophylaxis/treatment:
  ➤ Gonorrhea:
    • Ceftriaxone
    • Cefixime
    • Ciprofloxacin (age >18 yr)
  ➤ Chlamydia: azithromycin or doxycycline (age >7 yr)
  ➤ *B. vaginalis* or trichomoniasis: metronidazole
  ➤ PID: IV antibiotics
  ➤ HIV prophylaxis:
    • Combivir
    • High-risk exposures: nelfinavir
■ Pregnancy prevention:
  ➤ Preven kit
  ➤ Ovral tablets
■ Consider hepatitis vaccine, tetanus if indicated
■ Antiemetic (e.g., prochlorperazine or dimenhydrinate) w/ HIV, pregnancy prevention

FOLLOW-UP
■ Mental health weekly

- Follow up any physical injuries
- Reculture any positive STD w/in 2–4 wks of completed treatment
- Consider Pap smear if penetration

COMPLICATIONS AND PROGNOSIS
- Post-traumatic stress disorder
- Encopresis/enuresis
- Chronic pain syndromes
- Eating disorders
- Psychological complications minimized by early treatment

CHRONIC ASTHMA

SUZANNE F. STEINBACH, M.D.

HISTORY AND PHYSICAL

History
- Symptoms (duration, frequency, seasonal/diurnal variation, constant vs. episodic):
  - Wheeze
  - Chronic cough
  - Difficulty breathing
  - Chest tightness
  - Exercise/activity level
  - Sleep disturbance
  - School absence
  - Drug side effect
- Identify triggers:
  - Allergen:
    - Feathers
    - Dust mite
    - Cockroaches, mice
    - Mold
    - Pollen
  - Nonallergen:
    - Exercise
    - Cold
    - URI
    - Rhinitis

- Sinusitis
- Emotion
- Smoke
- Weather
- Airborne chemicals
- Dusts
- Drugs
- GER
■ Family history of asthma/allergy

Physical signs
■ Hyperexpanded chest
■ Retractions
■ Poor air entry, prolonged expiration, wheeze
■ Allergic rhinitis, atopic dermatitis

TESTS
■ Peak expiratory flow (PEF)
■ Spirometry:
  ➤ FEV-1
  ➤ FEF 25/75
■ Allergy tests:
  ➤ Radioallergosorbent test
  ➤ Skin test
■ CXR: exclude other diseases

DIFFERENTIAL DIAGNOSIS
■ Foreign body aspiration
■ Vocal cord dysfunction
■ Vascular ring/sling
■ Laryngotracheomalacia
■ Tracheobronchostenosis
■ Airway compression:
  ➤ TB
  ➤ Lymph nodes
  ➤ Tumor
■ Bronchiolitis
■ Cystic fibrosis
■ Bronchopulmonary dysplasia
■ Heart disease
■ Aspiration:

➤ GER
➤ TEF

MANAGEMENT
■ Rate chronic asthma severity
■ Educate:
  ➤ Skills:
    • Inhaler
    • Peak flow meter
    • Spacer
  ➤ Therapy:
    • Goals
    • Monitor PEF
    • Daily medications & plan
    • Step-up for mild symptoms
    • Avoid triggers

SPECIFIC THERAPY
Daily controller & side effects:
■ Anti-inflammatory:
  ➤ Cromolyn: none
  ➤ Nedocromil: bad taste
  ➤ Leukotriene receptor antagonist (LTRA): head/abdominal pain
  ➤ Inhaled corticosteroids (ICS):
    • Thrush
    • Dysphonia
    • Cataracts & growth suppression (high dose)
  ➤ Oral steroids:
    • Growth suppression
    • Osteoporosis
    • Cataracts
    • Obesity
    • Adrenal suppression
    • Hyperglycemia
    • Bruising
    • Hypertension
    • Disseminated varicella
■ Long-acting bronchodilators:
  ➤ Salmeterol
  ➤ Theophylline, sustained release

Emergency meds & side effects:
- Beta-2 agonist:
  - Hyperactivity
  - Tachycardia
  - Anxiety
  - Tremor
  - Head/abdominal pain
  - Arrhythmias

Mild intermittent
- Symptoms:
  - Daytime <3/wk
  - Nocturnal <3/mo
- Asymptomatic/normal PEF between brief exacerbations
- FEV-1 or PEF >80% predicted
- No daily anti-inflammatory

Mild persistent
- Symptoms:
  - Daytime 2–6/wk
  - Nocturnal 3–4/mo
- Exacerbations may affect activity
- FEV-1 or PEF > 80% predicted
- 1 daily anti-inflammatory:
  - Age 0–5: cromolyn, low-dose ICS; age >2: + LTRA
  - Age >5: low-dose ICS, LTRA, or cromolyn/nedocromil

Moderate persistent
- Symptoms:
  - Daily; beta-agonist
  - Nocturnal >1/wk
- Exacerbations: >1/wk, last days, & affect activity
- FEV-1 or PEF 60–80% predicted
- >=1 daily controller medications:
  - Medium-dose ICS
  - Low-dose ICS + long-acting bronchodilator
  - Low-dose ICS + LTRA

Severe persistent
- Symptoms:
  - Continual; beta-agonist
  - Nocturnal: frequent

- Limited activity
- Frequent exacerbations
- FEV-1 or PEF <60% predicted
- Use multiple controller:
  - High-dose ICS
  - Long-acting bronchodilator
  - LTRA
  - Oral steroid qd or qod

FOLLOW-UP
- Unstable: q2–4 wks
- Initial: q1–3 mo
- Stable: q 6–12 mo
- Good control:
  - No symptoms or beta agonists
  - Normal PEF/spirometry
  - Reduce ICS 50%
  - F/U 1 mo
- Acceptable control:
  - Symptoms:
    - Daytime <3/wk
    - Nocturnal <2/wk
  - Normal activity, ± mild attacks, no school absences
  - Beta-agonist use <3/wk
  - PEF/FEV-1 >90%
  - Consider stepping up regimen
- Poor control:
  - Worse than acceptable
  - Step up regimen
  - F/U 1 mo

COMPLICATIONS AND PROGNOSIS
- Poor quality of life
- Rare: respiratory failure
- 500 deaths/y in U.S.

Prognosis
- One-fourth resolve
- One-fourth remit in adolescence, recur in adulthood
- One-fourth only exercise-induced as adults
- One-fourth lifelong asthma

CHRONIC RENAL FAILURE

MELANIE S. KIM, M.D.

HISTORY AND PHYSICAL

History

- Growth failure
- Symptoms:
  - Fatigue
  - Polyuria or oliguria
  - Bone deformities, rickets, abnormal teeth eruption
  - Anemia
  - Pruritus
  - Vomiting, nausea
  - Paresthesia
  - Rare: seizures, coma

Physical signs

- Short stature
- Pallor
- Edema
- Hypertension
- Systolic flow murmur due to anemia
- Volume overload:
  - Increased pulmonary interstitial fluid
  - CHF
- Rickets
- Dental abnormalities
- Peripheral neuropathy
- Anorexia

TESTS

- Serum creatinine, BUN, electrolytes, calcium, phosphorus
- CBC
- PTH level
- Renal ultrasound

DIFFERENTIAL DIAGNOSIS

- Chronic glomerulonephritis:
  - Primary:

- Focal segmental glomerulosclerosis
- Membranoproliferative glomerulonephritis
➤ Secondary:
  - Lupus nephritis
  - Goodpasture
  - Henoch-Schönlein purpura
■ Congenital/hereditary disease:
  ➤ Hereditary nephritis
  ➤ Renal dysplasia
  ➤ Polycystic kidney disease
■ Obstructive uropathy
■ Interstitial nephritis
■ Hemolytic uremic syndrome
■ Chronic pyelonephritis
■ Diabetes mellitus

MANAGEMENT

What to do first
■ Assess cardiorespiratory status, fluid/electrolyte balance, & degree of uremia
■ Acute intervention:
  ➤ Severe fluid overload w/ pulmonary edema or CHF
  ➤ Hyperkalemia w/ risk for arrhythmias
  ➤ Severe uremia
  ➤ Seizure from hypocalcemia

General measures
■ Diet:
  ➤ Low phosphorus, sodium, potassium
  ➤ 100% RDA caloric requirement: may need NG supplementation
  ➤ Protein content controversial; current recommendation is to limit to RDA requirement
■ Fluid management; restrict if oliguria
■ Treat hypertension

SPECIFIC THERAPY
■ Calcium/phosphorus:
  ➤ $CaCO_3$ for calcium supplementation & phosphorus binding
  ➤ 1,25-dihydroxycholecalciferol

- Anemia:
  - Erythropoietin
  - May require iron
- ACE inhibitors:
  - To slow renal failure
  - Diabetic nephropathy
- Dialysis: Peritoneal or hemodialysis
  - Management as above, except no ACE inhibitors
  - Folic acid supplementation:
    - Increase protein intake, esp. w/ peritoneal dialysis (loss of protein)
    - Frequent assessment of caloric intake & nitrogen balance (aim for positive nitrogen balance)
- Renal transplant

FOLLOW-UP
- Depends on renal function & treatment used

COMPLICATIONS AND PROGNOSIS
- Arrhythmias (hyperkalemia)
- CHF
- Pulmonary edema
- Encephalopathy (hypertension or uremia)
- Seizures (encephalopathy or hypocalcemia)
- Bleeding disorder
- Growth failure
- Developmental delay
- Infection:
  - Hemodialysis: hepatitis B
  - Peritonitis from peritoneal dialysis
  - Renal transplant; increased risk w/ immunosuppression
- Hypertension, side effect of cyclosporine & prednisone (renal transplant)
- Restrictive pericardial effusions
- Renal osteodystrophy

Prognosis
- Goal: renal transplantation; best quality of life
- 50% cadaveric & 60% living related donor transplant functioning 10 y posttransplant

COARCTATION OF THE AORTA

SHARON E. O'BRIEN, M.D.

HISTORY AND PHYSICAL

History
- Varies depending on pt's age & severity of obstruction
- Infants:
  - Tachypnea
  - Feeding intolerance
  - Diaphoresis
  - Lethargy
  - Oliguria
- Older children:
  - Usually asymptomatic
  - Occasional leg pain

Physical signs
- Varies depending on pt's age & severity of obstruction
- Male predominance (56%)
- Infants:
  - Tachypnea
  - Blood pressure differential between arms & legs
  - O_2 saturation differential between arms & legs in ductal dependent lesion
  - Hyperdynamic precordium
  - Murmur of coarctation (low pitch, systolic ejection murmur heard best over back at left scapular region)
  - Ejection click of bicuspid aortic valve (85%)
  - Murmur of associated lesion:
    - Aortic stenosis
    - Subaortic stenosis
    - Mitral regurgitation
    - Weak or absent distal pulses
    - Gallop rhythm
    - Congestive heart failure
    - Shock
- Older children:
  - Hypertension
  - Blood pressure differential between arms & legs
  - Hyperdynamic precordium

➤ Systolic ejection click of bicuspid aortic valve
➤ Murmur of coarctation
➤ Murmur of associated lesions:
  • Aortic stenosis
  • Mitral regurgitation
  • Collaterals
➤ Weak or delayed distal pulses

TESTS
■ Pre- and postductal measurements of blood pressure & O_2 saturation
■ ECG:
  ➤ May be normal
  ➤ RVH in infant
  ➤ LVH in older child
■ CXR:
  ➤ May be normal
  ➤ Cardiomegaly
  ➤ Pulmonary edema in infants
  ➤ Prominent aortic knob in older children
  ➤ "3-sign"
  ➤ Rib notching late (after 5–10 y)
■ Echocardiography:
  ➤ Anatomy of coarctation
  ➤ Severity of obstruction
  ➤ Associated cardiac defects
  ➤ Ventricular function

DIFFERENTIAL DIAGNOSIS
■ L ventricular outflow tract obstruction
■ Other causes of hypertension (see "Hypertension" entry)
■ Other causes of cardiac murmurs (see "Heart murmurs" entry)

MANAGEMENT
■ Medical management of hypertension & CHF as necessary
■ Prostaglandin therapy in neonates w/ ductal dependent lesion

SPECIFIC THERAPY
■ Relief of obstruction:
  ➤ Balloon angioplasty of coarctation
  ➤ Repair of coarctation via thoracotomy:
    • End-to-end anastomosis
    • Subclavian flap

■ Subacute endocarditis prophylaxis (see "Subacute endocarditis prophylaxis" entry)

FOLLOW-UP
■ Yearly:
  ➤ Pre- and postductal blood pressure measurements: assess residual gradient
  ➤ Echocardiography: assess area of coarctation repair, assoc. cardiac defects
  ➤ MRI: assess for aneurysm

COMPLICATIONS AND PROGNOSIS
■ Postoperative hypertension
■ Recurrence of coarctation
■ Aneurysm formation
■ Complications of assoc. defects

Prognosis
■ Varies depending on age at treatment & presence of associated cardiac or noncardiac defects
■ Isolated coarctation status post repair: 10-y survival rate: 91%

COLIC

JULIE LUMENG, M.D.
MARILYN AUGUSTYN M.D.

HISTORY AND PHYSICAL
■ Classically described as unexplained paroxysmal bouts of fussing & crying that last >3 hr/d for >3 d/wk for >3 wk in duration between ages 3 wk and 3 mo
■ Peaks at 6 wk
■ Observed in approximately 15% of healthy infants
■ Occurs equally in infants fed breast milk & formula
■ Requires careful history & physical exam to rule out organic etiology

History
■ Usually occurs in diurnal pattern, late evening or afternoon

Physical
■ Abdomen often distended & tense, legs drawn up, hands clenched, & baby often seems to be in pain

TESTS
- Consider stool guaiac & urinalysis

DIFFERENTIAL DIAGNOSIS
- Broad; includes any disturbance that may cause pain:
  - Intussusception
  - Incarcerated hernia
  - Corneal abrasion
  - Hair tourniquet
  - Fracture
  - Child abuse
  - Lactose intolerance
  - Cow's milk protein sensitivity
- Gastroesophageal reflux (more likely if crying worse 1–2 hr after feeding & worsens as infant approaches 4 mo of age)

MANAGEMENT
- Initial advice
  - Check if baby is hungry, needs a diaper change, has a temperature, is bored or overstimulated
  - Check to make sure nothing is causing pain (e.g., a pin)
  - Try rocking, going for a walk, swaddling, pacifier, car ride, sitting in car seat atop running dryer, white noise (hair dryer, vacuum cleaner)
  - If nothing effective, allow baby to cry
- May need appointment during "crying time" to enable doctor to assist in interpreting cries & exploring methods of soothing

SPECIFIC THERAPY

Treatment
- No single treatment universally effective
- Close follow-up by phone may help reassure parents & manage the problem earlier & more effectively
- Treatments shown to have a beneficial effect: possibly
  - Calming measures as above
  - If mother is breastfeeding, reduce her intake of lactose-containing foods
  - Educate parents about the normal amounts of crying in a newborn
  - Teach the parents to read the infant's cues regarding stimulation
  - Change to soy or hypoallergenic formula
- Treatments shown to have no significant effect:

- ➤ Simethicone
- ➤ Early introduction of rice cereal or solids
- ➤ Lactase enzymes
- ➤ Fiber-enriched formulas
- ➤ Increased carrying of the infant
- ➤ Reduced stimulation of the infant
- ➤ Car ride simulator device
- ■ Older treatments no longer used because of adverse side effects:
  - ➤ Dicyclomine
  - ➤ Methylscopolamine
  - ➤ Low-iron formula can make colic worse
- ■ Common treatments with unproven efficacy:
  - ➤ More frequent feeds & burping
  - ➤ More rapid response to baby's cries
  - ➤ Warm pack or hot water bottle applied to abdomen
  - ➤ Massage, pacifier, or swaddling
  - ➤ Herbal teas; sometimes effective but there are some potential side effects, including reduced caloric intake leading to poor growth

FOLLOW-UP
- ■ Visits are for parental support
- ■ Visit interval determined on individual basis

COMPLICATIONS AND PROGNOSIS
- ■ Colic peaks at 6 wk, usually resolves by 3 mo
- ■ Infants who have had colic frequently develop sleep disturbances later, possibly due to persistence of the same factors in the child & parent that produced the colic earlier

---

CONGENITAL ADRENAL HYPERPLASIA (CAH)

ANDREW W. NORRIS, M.D., PH.D.
MARK R. PALMERT, M.D., PH.D.

HISTORY AND PHYSICAL
- ■ Block in cortisol synthesis:
  - ➤ Compensatory elevation in ACTH
  - ➤ Affected enzymes:
    - • 21-hydroxylase (21OH): 90%
    - • 11-hydroxylase (11OH): 5–8%
    - • 3-BetaOH-steroid dehydrogenase (3-Beta): <5%

History
- Depends on enzyme affected/severity of block:
- Salt-wasting crisis:
  - 21OH, 3-Beta
  - Lack of mineralocorticoid
  - Age: 1–4 wks
  - Vomiting, poor weight gain, hypotension, hyponatremia, hyperkalemia
- Ambiguous genitalia:
  - Virilized female infant:
    - 21OH, 11OH, 3-Beta
    - Excess adrenal androgens
  - Undervirilized male infant: 3-Beta (insufficient testosterone)
- Late-onset "nonclassic" CAH:
  - 21OH, 11OH, 3-Beta
  - Excess adrenal androgens
  - Presents anytime after infancy
  - Precocious puberty, menstrual abnormalities, infertility
- Hypertension: 11OH (excess mineralocorticoids)
- Abnormal newborn screen:
  - 21OH, 11OH
  - Elevated spot 17-OH-progesterone
- Positive family Hx; consanguinity

Physical signs
- Salt wasting/adrenal crisis: dehydration, shock
- Ambiguous genitalia:
  - Virilized female infant:
    - Range: clitoromegaly, labial fusion to male appearing
    - Uterus/ovaries intact
    - No testes
  - Undervirilized male infant
    - Range: hypospadias to near-female appearing
- Late-onset "nonclassic":
  - Acne, hirsutism, growth acceleration, early pubic hair, adrenarche
  - Clitoromegaly or penile enlargement

TESTS
- Electrolytes
- Elevated ACTH

- Adrenal steroids:
  - ➤ Enzyme block determines pattern
  - ➤ Elevated precursors
  - ➤ ACTH-stimulated steroids (definitive test)
- Plasma renin activity (PRA): elevated in salt-wasting CAH
- Screen for late-onset 21-OH: 8am 17-OH-progesterone
- Prenatal screen
- Bone age: advanced if excess androgens

DIFFERENTIAL DIAGNOSIS
- Late-onset:
  - ➤ Polycystic ovarian syndrome
  - ➤ Virilizing tumor
  - ➤ Premature adrenarche
- Elevated newborn 17-OH-progesterone:
  - ➤ Prematurity
  - ➤ Stress
  - ➤ Low birthweight

MANAGEMENT
- Consult pediatric endocrinologist
- Salt-wasting crisis:
  - ➤ Isotonic fluids
  - ➤ Stress-dose steroids: 50–100 mg/m^2/d hydrocortisone IV q6h
- Ambiguous genitalia: specialty team consultation
- Abnormal newborn screen:
  - ➤ Risk of salt-wasting, death
  - ➤ Monitor weight & electrolytes
- Adrenal crisis:
  - ➤ Preventive Rx, stress-dose steroids:
    - Fever >101F
    - Vomiting, dehydration
    - Surgery
    - Sedation, anesthesia
    - Bone fracture, trauma
    - Oral: 50–100 mg/m^2/d hydrocortisone divided tid, qid
    - Low threshold: IV steroids/fluids

SPECIFIC THERAPY
- Daily glucocorticoids
- Salt wasting:

➤ Mineralocorticoid agonist
➤ Supplemental NaCl during infancy
- Ambiguous genitalia:
  ➤ Surgery (controversial)
  ➤ Outcomes under study
- Prenatal treatment:
  ➤ Oral glucocorticoids to mother:
    • May reduce virilization of female infants if started at 4–6 wks gestation
    • Maternal complications frequent

FOLLOW-UP
- Monitor growth, virilization
- Lifelong monitoring of ACTH, PRA, adrenal androgens

COMPLICATIONS AND PROGNOSIS
- Adrenal crisis
- Precocious puberty
- Nonmalignant, testicular:
  ➤ Adrenal-rest tumors

Prognosis
- Short stature (improves w/ treatment)
- Increased female infertility; relative risk unclear

CONGENITAL SYPHILIS

COLIN MARCHANT, M.D.

HISTORY AND PHYSICAL
- Most infants: no physical signs, but if mother had syphilis before or during pregnancy, usually manifest by positive nontreponemal serologic test (RPR, ART, or VDRL) & treponemal test (FTA-ABS, MHA-TP)

HISTORY
- Document adequate maternal treatment for syphilis:
  ➤ >2.4 million units benzathine penicillin, before or during pregnancy & >1 mo before delivery, <u>and</u>
  ➤ 4-fold subsequent decline in VDRL or RPR
- All other scenarios = inadequate treatment

Physical signs
- Clinical disease:
  - Prematurity
  - Hydrops fetalis
  - Stillbirth
- At birth:
  - Rash
  - Snuffles
  - Lymphadenopathy
  - Hepatosplenomegaly

TESTS
- Neonates w/ seropositive mothers: treponemal & nontreponemal antibody test
- Neonate antibody tests usually reflect passive maternal antibody: nontreponemal test higher than mother's or rising indicates congenital infection
- CBC, LFTs, LP, and long bone films: for infants w/ clinical findings or suspected congenital syphilis (inadequate maternal treatment)
- Hemolytic anemia, thrombocytopenia, liver dysfunction
- CSF: pleocytosis, elevated protein, or positive VDRL (neurosyphilis)

DIFFERENTIAL DIAGNOSIS
- False-positive serology: (+) nontreponemal tests but (–) treponemal test: may be due to pregnancy or inflammatory disease
- False-positive treponemal test but (–) nontreponemal test: may be due to infection with other spirochete (e.g., Lyme disease)

MANAGEMENT
- Identify extent of disease
- Screen for other congenital infections
- Antibiotic therapy

SPECIFIC THERAPY
- Untreated mother or failed treatment; infant has clinical or lab evidence of disease: IV penicillin for 10 d or procaine penicillin IM for 10 d
- If maternal regimen appropriate but response to treatment not documented, treated <1 mo before delivery, or w/ nonpenicillin (e.g., erythromycin): single IM dose of benzathine penicillin
- Adequate maternal treatment, no clinical or lab evidence of congenital syphilis, & infant follow-up can be guarenteed: no antibiotic

FOLLOW-UP
- See infants at age 1, 2, 3, 6, & 12 mo
- Infants w/ proven or possible congenital syphilis: document decline in titers at age 3, 6, & 12 mo w/ nontreponemal test

COMPLICATIONS AND PROGNOSIS
- Late manifestations of untreated syphilis:
  - CNS, eye, bone, & dental abnormalities
  - CN VIII deafness

CONGESTIVE HEART FAILURE (CHF)

SHARON E. O'BRIEN, M.D.

HISTORY AND PHYSICAL

History
- History of :
  - Murmur
  - Congenital heart disease
  - Palpitations
  - Rheumatic fever
  - Prolonged febrile illness
  - Weight loss
- Infants:
  - Tachycardia
  - Tachypnea
  - Diaphoresis with feeds
  - Feeding intolerance
  - Failure to thrive
  - Lethargy
  - Vomiting
  - Poor perfusion
  - Cough
- Children:
  - Easily fatigued
  - Tachypnea
  - Orthopnea
  - Dyspnea
  - Tachycardia
  - Cough

- Pallor
- Normal or hyperdynamic precordium
- Wheezing/rales
- Gallop rhythm
- Murmur
- Hepatomegaly, distended neck veins
- Bounding or weak pulses
- Cool extremities
- Edema: facial or peripheral

TESTS
- Electrolytes, Hb, arterial blood gas
- CXR: assess cardiac silhouette & pulmonary vasculature
- ECG: assess for atrial enlargement or ventricular hypertrophy
- Echocardiogram:
  - ➤ Delineate congenital heart disease
  - ➤ Assess ventricular function

DIFFERENTIAL DIAGNOSIS
- Congenital heart disease: large left-to-right shunts (VSD, PDA, AV canal)
- Aortic stenosis
- Severe valve regurgitation
- Coarctation of aorta
- Cardiomyopathy:
  - ➤ Hypertrophic or dilated
  - ➤ Assoc. w/ metabolic defects
  - ➤ Assoc. w/ anomalous coronary arteries
- Large AV malformations
- Arrhythmia: unrecognized reentrant supraventricular tachycardia in infants; complete heart block
- Rheumatic heart disease:
  - ➤ Severe aortic or mitral regurgitation
  - ➤ Severe aortic or mitral stenosis
- Endocarditis
- Drugs, esp. antineoplastics
- Severe anemia
- Prolonged hypertension
- Pulmonary disease

MANAGEMENT
- Treat underlying cause

SPECIFIC THERAPY
- Depends on etiology:
  - Antiarrhythmic
  - Antihypertensive agent
- Inotropes (digoxin): enhance myocardial contractility
- Diuretics (furosemide): reduce volume load on heart w/ large L-to-R shunts
- ACE inhibitors (captopril): reduces systemic afterload; diminishes L-to-R shunting & increases stroke volume

FOLLOW-UP
- Frequent, esp. in infants w/ adjustment of medications

COMPLICATIONS AND PROGNOSIS
- Failure to thrive
- Death

Prognosis
- Variable; depends on etiology

CONJUNCTIVITIS

JACK MAYPOLE, M.D.

HISTORY AND PHYSICAL
- Watery, burning, swollen eyes
- Bacterial etiology: often find mucopurulent discharge
- Allergic conjunctivitis
  - Itchy, scratchy eyes w/o discharge
  - Family history for allergy; may occur with rhinitis
  - Swollen lids, hyperemia, & conjunctivitis irritation
- Giant papillary conjunctivitis with contact lenses
- Chemical: improves rapidly; refer if concerned
- Neonates
  - Consider evaluation for serious illness (meningitis, sepsis)
  - Other etiologies
    - Chlamydia: mucoid discharge: may have respiratory symptoms
    - Gonococcus also mucopurulent
    - Viral often adenovirus

- HSV: serous discharge, may have hazy cornea; other evidence of HSV infection

TESTS
- Culture of discharge in older infants & children only if treatment fails
- Blood culture if child ill or periorbital cellulitis present
- Neonates
  - Gram stain purulent discharge; infant seriously ill; no history of neonatal prophylaxis
  - No evidence of gonorrhea, then consider culture for bacteria & chlamydia
- Gram stain positive for gonorrhea, then confirm with culture

DIFFERENTIAL DIAGNOSIS
- Bacterial etiology
- Allergic etiology
- Viral etiology
- Cat-scratch disease
- HSV
- Molluscum contagiosum
- Congenital glaucoma
- Corneal abrasion
- Nasolacrimal obstruction
- Trauma

MANAGEMENT
- Ophthalmologic drops: patient must lie down & drops should be placed in medial cul-de-sac
- Viral infections with corneal involvement: cool, artificial tears

SPECIFIC THERAPY
- Child with suspected bacterial etiology:
  - Trimethoprim/polymyxin B or ofloxacin ointment/drops
  - Conjunctivitis with AOM; oral antibiotics as per for AOM
- HSV: if suspect, refer to ophthalmologist to clarify diagnosis & treatment
- Allergic: tailor treatment to patients
  - Cold compress/artificial tears
  - Topical antihistamines (e.g., levocabastine)
  - Mast cell stabilizers (e.g., cromolyn)

- ➤ Antihistamine/mast cell stabilizer (e.g., olopatadine)
- ➤ Topical steroids: most aggressive treatment; avoid for prolonged use (glaucoma, cataracts) & avoid worsening fungal/viral ulcers
- ■ Newborn
  - ➤ No evidence of gonorrhea: erythromycin
  - ➤ Evidence of gonorrhea: ceftriaxone

FOLLOW-UP
- ■ Return for evaluation if no change or worse after 3 d of treatment, develop photophobia, foreign body sensation, loss of vision
- ■ Refer to ophthalmologist if failure to respond to treatment or if vision loss or patients with immune compromise, or history of trauma
  - ➤ Newborn follow-up depends on etiology

COMPLICATIONS AND PROGNOSIS
- ■ Complications rare and prognosis good for common bacterial, viral, allergic conjunctivitis
- ■ HSV: if disease progresses to keratitis can cause scarring/corneal blindness

---

CONSTIPATION

SAMUEL NURKO, M.D., M.P.H.

HISTORY AND PHYSICAL

History
- ■ 5% of school-age children
- ■ Withholding behavior common
- ■ Stool accidents
- ■ May also have urine accidents
- ■ Abdominal pain
- ■ Red flags:
  - ➤ Fever
  - ➤ Abdominal distention
  - ➤ Delayed passage of meconium
  - ➤ Constipation in infancy
  - ➤ Bloody stools
  - ➤ Vomiting
  - ➤ Poor growth

> Urinary incontinence
> New-onset constipation
> Neurologic difficulties
> Family history of Hirschsprung, cystic fibrosis (CF), celiac, hypothyroidism

Physical signs
- Growth & development
- Thyroid
- Abdomen: stool & masses
- Rectal exam:
  > Anal position & tone
  > Fissures
  > Patency
  > Evidence of stool impaction
- Spine: pigmented areas, hair tufts
- Neurologic:
  > Cremasteric reflex
  > Anal wink

TESTS
- Usually clinical diagnosis
- Plain abdominal x-ray
- Intractable cases (before referral):
  > Thyroid function tests
  > Celiac disease screening
  > Sweat test
  > Calcium
- GI referral:
  > Intractable patients or red flags
  > May need:
  > Anorectal manometry and/or rectal biopsy to R/O Hirschsprung
  > Colonic transit, spine MRI, & colonic manometry
- Behavioral /psychological eval.

DIFFERENTIAL DIAGNOSIS
- Beyond newborn period, most cases functional
- Anatomic:
  > Anal stenosis
  > Anorectal malformations

- Endocrine/metabolic:
  - Celiac
  - Hypercalcemia
  - Hypothyroidism
  - CF
  - Allergy
- Hirschsprung
- Spinal cord disease
- Drugs/toxins:
  - Lead
  - Opiates
  - Anticholinergics
  - Botulism

MANAGEMENT
- Infants:
  - Check formula dilution
  - Add prune juice or other osmotic feeds
- Older children:
  - Explain etiology & pathogenesis of stool accidents
  - Behavior therapy:
    - Regular sitting on toilet
    - Calendar & praise
  - Disimpaction: evacuation of stool impaction necessary for successful treatment
    - Osmotic or lubricant laxatives + stimulant laxatives
    - Occasionally enema/suppositories
    - PEG solutions
    - Hospitalization (rarely)

SPECIFIC THERAPY
- Osmotic and lubricant laxatives:
  - Mineral oil 1–3 mL/kg
  - Milk of magnesia 1–3 mL/kg
  - Lactulose 1–3 mL/kg
  - MiraLax (PEG solution) 0.5–1 g/kg
- Stimulants (use for short periods):
  - Senna (age 2–6 y): 2.5–7.5 mL/d; (age 6–12 y): 5–15 mL/d
  - Bisacodyl (age >=3 y): 1 tablet; (age 3–12 y) 1–2 tablets; (age > 12 y) 1–3 tablets/dose

FOLLOW-UP
- Frequent communication w/ pt/family
- Frequent visits, medication adjustments

COMPLICATIONS AND PROGNOSIS

Prognosis
- Prolonged therapy needed; initially 12 wks, but possibly longer
- Long-term prognosis good
- 30–50% may still require intermittent laxatives

CROUP (LARYNGOTRACHEOBRONCHITIS)

ILAN SCHWARTZ, M.D.

HISTORY AND PHYSICAL

History
- Insidious onset of mild upper respiratory illness with low-grade fever, coryza, & cough
- During next 48 h, child develops signs of upper respiratory obstruction (stridor, hoarseness, barking cough)
- Symptoms often worse at night

Physical signs
- Generally nontoxic
- Mild to moderate respiratory distress
- Low-grade fever (38°–39° C)
- Tachycardia & tachypnea (rarely exceeds 40 breaths/min)
- Stridor, often expiratory & unchanged with positioning
- Suprasternal & subcostal retractions
- Absence of drooling

TESTS
- Usually not needed
- AP & lateral neck x-rays:
  - ➤ To R/O foreign body
  - ➤ May demonstrate subglottic narrowing ("steeple" sign)
  - ➤ Does not correlate with degree of airway obstruction

DIFFERENTIAL DIAGNOSIS
- Epiglottitis
- Foreign body aspiration

- Retropharyngeal abscess
- Bacterial tracheitis
- Congenital/acquired subglottic stenosis

MANAGEMENT
- Make pt comfortable and avoid unnecessary procedures
- Pulse oximetry
- Humidified air or mist therapy

SPECIFIC THERAPY
- Corticosteroids: single dose of dexamethasone (Decadron) 0.6 mg/kg IV/IM/PO
- Racemic epinephrine or L-epinephrine:
  - Vasoconstrictive effects decrease mucosal edema
  - 2.25% solution @ 0.05 mL/kg (max, 0.5 mL) in 3 mL normal saline
- Nebulized budesonide (2 mg) as effective as oral dexamethasone

FOLLOW-UP
- Most managed as outpatients
- Admit for dehydration and/or signs of respiratory compromise (e.g., stridor at rest)
- Racemic epinephrine: observe for 3–4 h after treatment to determine respiratory status before discharge

COMPLICATIONS AND PROGNOSIS
- May develop worsening disease and respiratory failure (rare):
  - Change in mental status:
    - Depressed level of consciousness
    - Restlessness
    - Hypotonicity
      - Increased retractions
      - Decreased inspiratory breath sounds
      - Tachycardia out of proportion to fever
      - Cyanosis
- Bacterial tracheitis: high fever & respiratory distress
- Intubation required in <1% of cases

Prognosis
- Recovery usually complete with no long-term complications

CYANOTIC HEART DISEASE

SHARON E. O'BRIEN, M.D.

HISTORY AND PHYSICAL

- Cyanosis: presence of deoxygenated hemoglobin at a concentration of 5 g/dL
- Degree of hypoxemia may not correlate w/ cyanosis depending on hemoglobin type & level
- Cyanotic congenital heart disease (CHD): intracardiac right-to-left shunt is present
- Pulmonary blood flow may be diminished

History

- Family history of CHD
- Maternal history of illness (diabetes) and drugs (lithium)
- Complicated pregnancy
- Meconium staining/aspiration
- Tachypnea
- Cyanosis
- Poor feeding
- Other organ system defects

Physical

- Tachypnea
- Respiratory distress in total anomalous pulmonary venous return (TAPVR)
- Hyperdynamic precordium in pressure or volume overload lesions
- Normal first heart sound
- Usually single second heart sound
- Widely split second heart sound with Ebstein's anomaly
- Murmur may be present
- Brachial/femoral delay w/ associated coarctation or interruption of aortic arch

TESTS

- Pre- and post-ductal O_2 saturation
- Pre- and post-ductal blood pressure measurements
- Hyperoxia test
- ECG: Assess for axis deviation, pre-excitation, atrial enlargement, & ventricular hypertrophy

- CXR: assess pulmonary blood flow & heart size
- Echocardiogram: delineate anatomy

DIFFERENTIAL DIAGNOSIS
- Pulmonary
  - Respiratory distress syndrome
  - Pneumonia
  - Meconium aspiration
  - Pneumothorax
  - Diaphragmatic hernia
  - Effusion
  - Airway obstruction
- Metabolic: shock
- Hematological: methemoglobinemia
- Cardiac lesions most commonly associated w/ cyanosis:
  - Tetralogy of Fallot
  - Transposition of great arteries
  - Tricuspid atresia
  - Truncus arteriosus
  - TAPVR
  - Tricuspid atresia
  - Ebstein's anomaly
  - Pulmonary atresia
  - Univentricular heart

MANAGEMENT
- Variable depending on cause of cyanosis; see specific lesion

SPECIFIC THERAPY
- Medications to control CHF if present (see "CHF" entry)
- Prostaglandins to maintain patency of ductus arteriosus in ductal dependent lesions
- Interventions: cardiac catheterization or surgery to relieve obstruction
- Surgery to correct anatomy & physiology

FOLLOW-UP
- Variable depending on cause of cyanosis (see specific lesion)

COMPLICATIONS AND PROGNOSIS
- Variable depending on cause of cyanosis (see specific lesion)

CYSTIC FIBROSIS

LAWRENCE RHEIN, M.D.

HISTORY AND PHYSICAL

History
- Pulmonary:
  - Recurrent/chronic infections
  - Chronic cough, wheeze
  - Mucopurulent sputum
  - Chest pain
  - Respiratory distress
  - Hemoptysis
- Upper respiratory:
  - Chronic nasal congestion
  - Rhinitis
  - Sinusitis
  - Nasal polyps: mouth breathing, epistaxis
- GI:
  - Meconium ileus or plug
  - Obstructive jaundice
  - Rectal prolapse
  - Steatorrhea
- Dehydration
- Failure to thrive
- Family history
- Exercise intolerance

Physical
- Tachypnea, cyanosis, use of accessory respiratory muscles
- Rhonchi or wheezes
- Nasal polyps
- Digital clubbing
- Hepatosplenomegaly
- Abdominal distention
- Growth retardation
- Rectal prolapse
- Barrel chest
- Infants: edema, bulging fontanel
- Dehydration

TESTS

- Neonatal screen: serum trypsinogen; if positive, further testing necessary
- Genetic screen by serum or cheek brush, prenatal diagnosis
- Sweat test (gold standard)
- CBC, PT/PTT
- Sputum culture and Gram stain
- Electrolytes, Ca, Mg, phos
- Albumin, serum protein analysis
- Vitamins A and E
- Pulmonary function tests (PFTs)
- Chest x-ray

DIFFERENTIAL DIAGNOSIS

MANAGEMENT

- Assess cardiopulmonary status; stabilize as needed
- Comprehensive intensive longitudinal treatment program

SPECIFIC THERAPY

- Pulmonary:
  - Chest physiotherapy
  - Antibiotic therapy based on sputum culture, sensitivities, symptoms: 2–3 wk IV or oral/aerosol therapy for mild/moderate disease
  - Consider bronchodilators
  - Chronic suppressive antibiotic therapy: decrease exacerbations
  - Mucolytic agents: recombinant human DNase
  - Anti-inflammatory
    - NSAIDs
    - Systemic steroids: severe airway disease unresponsive to NSAID therapy
    - Aerosolized steroids: clinical trials
- Hemoptysis:
  - Airway & IV access
  - CBC, PT/PTT, type/cross-match
  - Consider empiric vitamin K, fresh frozen plasma
  - Hold chest physiotherapy
  - IV vasopressin or conjugated estrogens
- Allergic bronchopulmonary aspergillosis:
  - Diagnosis: IgE, skin test
  - Consider steroids, itraconazole
- Malabsorption: enzyme replacement

- Meconium ileus/equivalent: stool softener or N-acetylcysteine enema
- Nutritional support

FOLLOW-UP
- Monitor symptoms, exam
- Follow PFTs
- Follow growth curves

COMPLICATIONS AND PROGNOSIS
- Cor pulmonale, cardiac failure
- Respiratory failure
- Distal intestinal obstruction syndrome: up to 15% w/ recurrent bowel obstruction
- Small-bowel volvulus or intussusception: 1%
- Gastroesophageal reflux
- Peptic ulcer disease
- Cirrhosis:
  - 4–6% multilobular biliary cirrhosis
  - 1–2% portal hypertension
- Gallbladder abnormalities: 60% of adult patients
- Infertility: 98% of males

Prognosis
- Improving with time:
  - 1996 data: median age of survival: 31 y
  - Lung transplantation: 55% survival, 3 y after transplant

DEPRESSION

SUSAN O'BRIEN, M. D.

HISTORY AND PHYSICAL
- Often unrecognized by clinicians

History
- General:
  - Depressive mood
  - Loss of interest in usual activities
  - Poor appetite
  - Sleep disturbance
  - Agitation
  - Poor concentration

➤ Somatic complaints
➤ Fatigue
➤ Poor self-esteem
■ Infant/toddler/preschool:
➤ Passivity
➤ Irritability
➤ Failure to thrive
■ School age/adolescent:
➤ Withdrawal
➤ Overactivity
➤ Impulsivity
➤ School problems
➤ Isolation
➤ Loss or gain in weight
➤ Morbid preoccupations
➤ Suicidal ideation
➤ Risk-taking behavior
➤ School drop-out
➤ Running away
➤ Sexual acting out
➤ Substance use

Physical signs
■ Anthropometric measurements (weight loss)
■ Evidence of self-mutilation
■ Signs of substance use
■ Dentition & nails (evidence of bulimia/anorexia)
■ Thyroid exam

TESTS
■ Based on history & physical
■ CBC, urinalysis, ESR, electrolytes, BUN, Ca
■ T4, TSH
■ Liver enzymes
■ VDRL
■ Lead (age <5 yrs)
■ Drug screen

DIFFERENTIAL DIAGNOSIS
■ Neurologic:
➤ ADHD
➤ Learning disability

- Child neglect/abuse
- CNS injury/lesion
- Epilepsy
- Metabolic/endocrine:
  - Thyroid
  - Parathyroid
  - SLE
  - Wilson
  - Cushing or Addison
  - Eating disorder
  - Premenstrual syndrome
- Infection (eg, mononucleosis)
- Other:
  - Anemia
  - Pregnancy
  - Substance abuse
  - Medication toxicity

MANAGEMENT
- Assess severity:
- Mild: response to acute identifiable situation or loss
- Moderate: longer history of behavior change
- Severe:
  - Suicidal ideation
  - Inability to contract for safety
- Very severe:
  - Gestured suicide
  - Suicide plan

SPECIFIC THERAPY
- Initiate counseling
- Consider school evaluation (IQ, academic performance)
- Psychiatric referral (moderate or severe symptoms)
- Hospitalize:
  - Severe symptoms
  - Suicidal ideation
  - Suicidal gestures
  - Inability to contract for safety
- Parent guidance: support, parent skills training
- Family therapy
- Medication

FOLLOW-UP
- Reassess in 12 wks
- Ensure continued therapy
- Ensure appropriate school plan in place

COMPLICATIONS AND PROGNOSIS
- Average duration of major depressive episode: 32 wks
- Recovery: 92% of children w/in 18 mo
- Recurrence: 72% w/in 5 yrs
- Early onset associated with protracted course & poorer outcome
- Prepubertal onset: is more severe, more resistant to treatment; assoc. w/ 32% risk of future bipolar or manic symptoms
- Suicide:
    - Adolescent males more likely to complete suicide (use more lethal means)
    - Rate of attempts is higher in females

DEVELOPMENTAL DYSPLASIA OF THE HIP

DONNA PACICCA, M.D.

HISTORY AND PHYSICAL

History
- History of associated abnormalities such as myelodysplasia, arthrogryposis, or proximal femoral focal deficiency
- Breech delivery
- Oligohydramnios
- Typical or postnatal DDH has hip that is dislocatable
- Females at high risk
- Family history may be positive in sibling
- Bilateral in 1/3
- Associated conditions
    - Congenital muscular torticollis
    - Metatarsus adductus

Physical
- Examine one hip at a time!
- In infants <= 2 mo perform Barlow test, which will dislocate or subluxate an unstable hip:
    - Stabilize pelvis
    - Flex hip to 90°, adduct to 20°

- Apply posterior force
- Feel for motion
- Subluxation vs. dislocation
- May also use the Ortolani test, which reduces a dislocated hip:
  - Stabilize pelvis
  - Flex hip to 90°, abduct & lift femoral head into acetabulum
  - Apply gentle anterior force with finger on greater trochanter
  - Feel the "clunk" of relocation
- Ortolani & Barlow signs lost after age 2–3 mo
- Hip clicks not pathologic & produced by:
  - Break in surface tension across hip joint
  - Snapping of tendons
  - Patellofemoral motion
  - Knee rotation
- Asymmetric skin folds unreliable in this age group
- Child >2–3 mo has limitation of abduction at the hips
- Older infant, child has uneven knee level with feet together, hips & knees flexed to 90° (Galeazzi sign); may have associated asymmetric thigh folds, limp, or waddling gait & hyperlordosis of lumbar spine

TESTS
- Ultrasound: not recommended for general screening due to high false-positive rate in infants <2 wks of age
- Plain radiographs
  - Useful in older infants & children
  - Evaluate position of ossific nucleus in relation to acetabulum

DIFFERENTIAL DIAGNOSIS
MANAGEMENT

General measures
- Triple diapers ineffective
- Orthopedic consult

SPECIFIC THERAPY

Specific treatment
- Application of Pavlik harness
- US to confirm hips in proper alignment
- Harness remains in place for weeks to months

FOLLOW-UP
- Confirm hips in proper position after application of harness with hip ultrasound

- Weekly orthopedic follow-up
- Harness left on full time until weaning schedule established by orthopedics
- Parents may remove harness during weaning but only under orthopedic direction
- Repeat radiographs after 3 mo of age
- May need long-term orthopedic follow-up
- Some patients may go on to need surgical intervention

COMPLICATIONS AND PROGNOSIS
- Most children will do well if identified early & placed in appropriate harness
- Osteonecrosis
- Repeat dislocation
- Residual dysplasia

DIABETES INSIPIDUS (DI)

MELANIE S. KIM, M.D.

HISTORY AND PHYSICAL

History
- Polyuria
- Excessive thirst & polydipsia
- Nocturia or enuresis
- Pale or clear urine
- Positive family Hx
- Two forms:
    - Central: lack of arginine vasopressin (AVP):
        - Symptoms depend on etiology (often hypothalamic lesion)
        - Headache
        - Poor growth
        - Weight loss
        - Obesity
        - Hyperpyrexia
        - Sleep disturbance
        - Sexual precocity
        - Emotional disturbances
        - Head trauma or surgery

➤ Nephrogenic: lack of renal tubular response to AVP to absorb water & concentrate urine
  - Infants: signs of chronic dehydration
  - Irritability
  - Poor feeding
  - Growth failure
  - Hyperpyrexia
  - Constipation

Physical signs
- Exam often normal
- Central DI: signs of CNS etiology
- Failure to thrive

TESTS
- Serum electrolytes: hypernatremia
- Serum osmolality: hyperosmolar
- Urine specific gravity <=1.005 or osmolality <=200 mmol/L when serum osmolality >285
- AVP levels: measure in hyperosmolar state w/ inappropriate dilute urine
  ➤ Water deprivation test (no fluids for 4–8 h): AVP level
    - Low: central DI
    - High: nephrogenic DI
- Test-administration of DDAVP: to see if urine-concentrating ability & hyperosmolar state are correctable
- MRI for suspected CNS disease

DIFFERENTIAL DIAGNOSIS
- Central DI:
  ➤ Genetic defects (rare)
  ➤ Brain tumors in sellar region:
    - Craniopharyngioma
    - Optic glioma
    - Germinoma
  ➤ Trauma, esp. basal skull fracture
  ➤ Brain surgery
  ➤ Systemic disease:
    - Encephalitis
    - Histiocytosis
    - Sarcoidosis

- Tuberculosis
- Leukemia
- ➤ Newborn:
  - Asphyxia
  - Intraventricular hemorrhage
  - Meningitis
- ■ Nephrogenic DI:
  - ➤ Genetic:
    - X-linked
    - Autosomal recessive
  - ➤ Drug-induced:
    - Lithium
    - Demeclocycline
  - ➤ Metabolic: prolonged hypercalcemia or hypokalemia
  - ➤ Systemic disease:
    - Sickle cell anemia
    - Chronic pyelonephritis
    - Urinary tract obstruction
  - ➤ Other renal disorder:
    - Polycystic kidney disease
    - Renal dysplasia
- ■ Primary polydipsia:
  - ➤ Can concentrate urine during water deprivation test
  - ➤ Psychogenic polydipsia
  - ➤ CNS disease (multiple sclerosis)
  - ➤ Idiopathic

MANAGEMENT

What to do first
- ■ Fluid resuscitation if hypovolemic

General measures
- ■ IV fluids
- ■ Replace deficit over 48 h
- ■ Assess type of DI

SPECIFIC THERAPY
- ■ Central DI: intranasal DDAVP
- ■ Nephrogenic DI:
  - ➤ Decrease renal solute load; limit Na intake (<1 mmol/kg/d), protein (2 g/kg/d)

➤ Drugs to decrease urine output:
  • Thiazides (may produce hypokalemia)
  • Prostaglandin synthesis inhibitors (indomethacin): used w/ thiazides; GI, CNS, or bone marrow side effects
  • Amiloride (used w/ thiazides)

FOLLOW-UP
■ Depends on etiology

COMPLICATIONS AND PROGNOSIS
■ Hypertonic encephalopathy
■ Seizures: too-rapid correction of hypernatremia, resulting in cerebral edema
■ Failure to thrive

Prognosis
■ Nephrogenic DI:
  ➤ Good w/ early diagnosis & follow-up
  ➤ Mental retardation if delay in diagnosis during infancy w/ repeated bouts of hypernatremia & dehydration
  ➤ Isolated reports: Chronic renal failure
■ Central DI: depends on underlying etiology

DIABETES MELLITUS (DM)

DAVID WEINSTEIN, M.D.

HISTORY AND PHYSICAL

History
■ Hyperglycemia:
  ➤ Polyuria/polydipsia
  ➤ Blurred vision
  ➤ Weight loss
  ➤ Nocturia
  ➤ Yeast infections
■ Family Hx
■ Vomiting/abdominal pain suggests diabetic ketoacidosis (DKA)
■ Check medications

Physical signs
■ Assess hydration status
■ Weight, height

- Acanthosis: Type 2 DM (T2DM)
- Tachypnea in DKA
- Nonfocal abdominal pain
- Pubertal status
- Neuro and mental status exam

Tests
- Plasma glucose/electrolytes:
  - Criteria for diagnosis:
    1. Classic symptoms: glucose >200
    2. Fasting glucose: >=126 mg/dL*
    3. 2-hr glucose: >=200 mg/dL*
       *on 2 d if no symptoms
- Urine ketones
- HbA1c
- Pancreatic antibodies if unclear type
- If ketones present or ill:
  - Venous pH
  - Ca/Mg/phos
  - Consider insulin level if obese
- If no ketones:
  - Consider LFTs, BUN/Cr (T2DM)
  - Insulin level if etiology unclear
  - No other labs if consistent w/ T1DM

DIFFERENTIAL DIAGNOSIS
- May be confused w/:
  - GI illness (abdominal pain, emesis)
  - Respiratory illness (increased respiratory rate)
  - Infection (elevated WBC)
- Hyperglycemia DDx:
  - Stress response
  - Suspected hypoglycemia
  - Glycogen storage disease
  - Fanconi-Bickel
  - Medications

MANAGEMENT
- Rehydration (oral or IV)
- Insulin therapy (T1DM)
- Insulin or metformin (T2DM)
- Intensive teaching

SPECIFIC THERAPY

- DKA (see "DKA" entry)
- Rehydrate over 48 h
- Starting insulin dose (T1DM):
  - Prepubertal: 0.4–0.5 U/kg/d
  - Pubertal: 0.75–1 U/kg/d
  - Use higher dose if DKA suspected
  - Insulin divided bid or tid:
    - AM: 2/3 total insulin
    - PM: 1/3 total insulin
  - Divide 2/3 NPH w/ 1/3 Regular (R) or Humalog (H)
  - If tid: PM NPH moved to h.s.
- Sliding scale (high glucose/ketones):
  - Use H or R
  - % of total insulin
  - No ketones:
    - 250–400: +5%
    - 400+: +10%
    - Moderate/high ketones (non-DKA):
      - 250–400: +10%
      - 400+: +15%
- T2DM therapy:
  - Insulin if ketones
  - Metformin if normal LFTs, BUN/Cr
  - Exercise & diet counseling

FOLLOW-UP

- Target blood sugars (mg/dL):
  - Infant: 100–200
  - Child: 80–180
  - Adol: 70–150
- ADA-recommended screening:
  - HbA1c: q3 mo
  - TFTs: yearly
  - Lipids: q5y minimum
  - Dilated eye exam: after puberty
  - Urine microalbumin: yearly after puberty

COMPLICATIONS AND PROGNOSIS

Complications

- Hypoglycemia:

➤ Seizures if severe
➤ Lowered IQ if recurrent in age <5
➤ Avoid in young children
- Cerebral edema (DKA)
- Long-term:
  ➤ Retinopathy
  ➤ Neuropathy
  ➤ Nephropathy
  ➤ Macrovascular disease
- Co-morbidities (T1DM):
  ➤ Thyroid disease (5–20%)
  ➤ Celiac disease (3–5%)
  ➤ Adrenal insufficiency

Prognosis
- Depends on blood glucose control

DIABETIC KETOACIDOSIS

ROBERT VINCI, M.D.

HISTORY AND PHYSICAL

History
- Possible Hx of diabetes mellitus
- Coma, change in mental status
- Polyuria, polyphagia, polydipsia
- Abdominal pain/vomiting
- Often, weight loss or growth failure

Physical signs
- Assume 10% dehydration
- Kussmaul respiration
- Fruity odor on breath
- Neurologic status
- Search for precipitant, esp. infections

TESTS
- Rapid bedside glucose test
- ABGs
- Serum electrolytes and glucose
- Urinalysis
- Serum insulin levels, glycosylated hemoglobin

DIFFERENTIAL DIAGNOSIS
- Nonketotic hyperosmolar coma
- Head injury
- Sepsis
- Drug overdose

MANAGEMENT
- IV fluids
- IV insulin
- Correct hyperosmolarity

SPECIFIC THERAPY
- IV fluids (think hyperosmolar):
  - Serum osm. $= 2 \times Na + BUN/2.6 + glucose/18$
  - Restore circulating volume w/ normal saline or lactated Ringer's solution
  - Do not overhydrate
- Calculate IV fluid rate:
  - Estimate degree of dehydration
  - Calculate maintenance fluid
  - Assess ongoing losses (1–2 mL/kg of urine output; replace excess)
- Replace fluid deficit over 48 h
- After restoring circulating volume:
  - Na conc.: 100–125 mEq/L
  - After 12–18 h: Na conc. 50–75 mEq/L
- Serum Na should increase as hyperglycemia resolves:
  - For every 100-mg/dL decrease in serum glucose, serum Na should rise 1.6 mEq/L
  - If Na does not increase as glucose falls, pt may be receiving too much free water
- Limit fluid intake to <4 L/m^2/24 h
- Correct acidosis w/ IV fluids; bicarbonate not generally indicated
- Serum K:
  - Not reflective of total body K^+
  - Replace with IV K^+ with conc of no more than 40–60 mEq/L (max, 0.5 mEq/kg/h)
- Hyperglycemia: low-dose insulin infusion (0.1 units/kg/h)

FOLLOW-UP
- Admit to ICU
- Transition to subcutaneous insulin:
  - Await clearance of urinary ketones

- ➤ 0.5–1 units/kg/d
- ➤ Less insulin required for:
  - Younger pts
  - No ketosis at presentation
- ➤ Divide: 2/3 in am, 1/3 in pm
- ➤ Divide each dose into 2/3 long-acting and 1/3 short-acting
- ➤ As ketotic state resolves, insulin requirement may decrease
- ▪ Monitor growth

COMPLICATIONS AND PROGNOSIS

- ▪ Complications rare
- ▪ Cerebral edema:
  - ➤ 2–3% of pts
  - ➤ Esp. age <5 yr
- ▪ Avoid tight control in hospital to avoid hypoglycemia as outpatient

Prognosis

- ▪ Generally excellent with ICU care & careful fluid management.
- ▪ Avoid repeat episodes of DKA
- ▪ Growth failure, peripheral vascular disease from long-term DM not well controlled with insulin

---

DIAPER DERMATITIS

BARBARA L. PHILIPP, M.D., I.B.C.L.C.

HISTORY AND PHYSICAL

- ▪ Skin breakdown allows secondary infection with yeast, bacteria
- ▪ Jacquet dermatitis: severe form, erosions

History

- ▪ Prolonged contact & irritation from urine, feces, excessive moisture
- ▪ Friction from diaper

Physical

- ▪ Rash occurs where skin is in greatest contact with diaper, convex surfaces of skin in diaper area
- ▪ Rash erythematous, scaly, papulovesicular or bullous lesions, fissures, erosions

Tests

- ▪ Often treat empirically based on history & physical
- ▪ Microscopic examination of skin scraping plus potassium hydroxide reveals pseudohyphae

- Can also send off culture
- For both take samples from newer satellite lesions

DIFFERENTIAL DIAGNOSIS
- Contact dermatitis
- Candida dermatitis:
  - Often follows contact dermatitis
  - May be history of antibiotic use
  - 1–2-mm shallow pustules that erode, leaving a donut-shaped lesion with scales on periphery (satellite lesions or collarettes)
- Atopic dermatitis: area under diaper may be less affected than rest of body
- Seborrheic dermatitis:
  - Found in creases
  - Spares convex surfaces
  - Rash also found on face, neck, or other body part
  - May get secondarily infected with Candida
- Psoriasis (consider this diagnosis for the diaper rash that won't go away)
  - Sharply demarcated, red plaques occurring on convex surfaces & in creases
  - Characteristic silvery micalike scales may or may not be present under diaper
  - Other areas of body may be involved
- Ask for family history
- Koebner reaction – lesions of psoriasis erupt in areas of epidermal injury
- Acrodermatitis enteropathica:
  - Autosomal recessive disorder of zinc metabolism
  - Presents 1–2 wks after weaning from breast milk or at 4–10 wks of life if formula fed
  - Triad of dermatitis, diarrhea, alopecia
- Histiocytosis X (Letterer-Siwe):
  - Hemorrhagic seborrhea-like eruption in diaper area, axilla, retroauricular, & scalp areas
  - Creases affected
  - Chronic ulcerations
  - Diarrhea
  - Anemia
  - Low-grade fever
  - Hepatosplenomegaly

- Bullous impetigo:
  - Quick-spreading bullous lesions
  - Causative agent: *S. aureus*
- Congenital syphilis:
  - Rash in diaper area at birth or postnatally
  - Copper-colored reddish macules/papules
  - Perianal condyloma lata (papular eruption)
  - Hepatomegaly
  - Bony involvement
  - Jaundice
  - Anemia
  - Snuffles

MANAGEMENT
- Key: minimize wetness
- Timely change of wet & soiled diapers
- Gently clean area with water or mild soap/cleansing agent; rinse thoroughly
- Allow area to dry completely
- Apply protective barrier ointment & creams with diaper changes (petrolatum, zinc oxide)
- If unresponsive, use topical low-potency corticosteroid preparations
- If both used, apply corticosteroid before barrier preparation

SPECIFIC THERAPY
- Good hygiene as noted for irritant contact dermatitis
- Anti-yeast preparation: clotrimazole, miconazole, ketoconazole, econazole, nystatin
- Other therapy depends on specific diagnosis

FOLLOW-UP
- Should resolve in 5–10 d; if not, patient should be seen

COMPLICATIONS AND PROGNOSIS
- Prognosis generally excellent with no complications, unless unusual underlying disease

DISSEMINATED INTRAVASCULAR COAGULATION (DIC)

BEAU MITCHELL, M.D.

HISTORY AND PHYSICAL
- Occurs only as secondary event

- Must identify and treat underlying cause
- Sepsis is most common cause
- Other causes:
    - Head trauma
    - Cancer
    - Post-transplant
- Giant hemangioma (Kasabach-Merritt)

History
- May present as bleeding, clotting, or both

Physical signs
- Mucosal bleeding, oozing from IV site
- Petechiae if low platelets
- Ecchymotic fingers or toes

TESTS
- Platelet count: low and dropping a strong indicator of DIC
- PT and PTT: usually prolonged
- Fibrin degradation products (FDP): usually present
- Fibrinogen: may be low or declining
- Antithrombin III and protein C: may be low
- Coagulation factors: may be low

DIFFERENTIAL DIAGNOSIS
- Severe liver disease, although coagulopathy of liver disease tends to be more stable than DIC
- Hemolytic uremic syndrome: peripheral smear usually shows marked schistocytosis (usually mild or no schistocytosis in DIC)

MANAGEMENT
- Treat underlying disorder
- Initial management will depend on whether patient is currently bleeding or thrombosing

SPECIFIC THERAPY
- Bleeding:
    - Transfuse platelets for thrombocytopenia <20,000 and/or bleeding
    - Fresh frozen plasma to correct coagulation defect
    - Fibrinogen <100: may give cryoprecipitate
- Thrombosis:
    - Supraphysiologic doses of AT-III concentrate administered with heparin

- Up to 150% correction of AT-III
- Low-dose continuous heparin infusion
- Experimental: protein C concentrates and anti-tissue-factor protein

FOLLOW-UP
- Monitor platelets, PT/PTT, fibrinogen, FDP

COMPLICATIONS AND PROGNOSIS

Prognosis
- Depends on underlying condition and severity of coagulation defect
- DIC in sepsis or severe trauma: twice the risk of death

DOWN SYNDROME

JEFF MILUNSKY, M.D.

HISTORY AND PHYSICAL
- 1/660–1/800 live births

History
- May have history of advanced maternal age
- Developmental delay/mental retardation (moderate)

Physical signs
- Neonatal cardinal features:
    - Flat facial profile
    - Upslanting palpebral fissures
    - Excess nuchal (neck) skinfold
    - Clinodactyly/hypoplastic mid-phalanx 5th finger
    - Hypotonia

TESTS
- Chromosome analysis

DIFFERENTIAL DIAGNOSIS
- Other chromosome abnormalities
- Zellweger (similar face and hypotonia)

MANAGEMENT
- Genetics consultation
- Echocardiogram/cardiology

- TFTs (serial)
- Down syndrome growth charts
- Early intervention, speech and language, occupational and physical therapy
- Parental support groups

SPECIFIC THERAPY
- Surgery (significant cardiac disease)
- Levothyroxine (hypothyroidism)
- Screening for participation in Special Olympics

FOLLOW-UP
- Multiple medical problems
- Help coordinate care

COMPLICATIONS AND PROGNOSIS
- ~ 50% cardiac disease
- ~20% thyroid dysfunction: levothyroxine
- ~1–2% atlanto-occipital dislocation (neck films)
- ~ 1% leukemia (ALL): monitor CBC
- ~6% acquired hip dislocation
- Myopia/strabismus/cataracts
- Periodontal disease
- Recurrent otitis media: hearing loss (audiology)
- Constipation: treat aggressively
- Short stature
- Obesity as teenager
- Premature aging
- ~ 45% survive to age 60

DYSFUNCTIONAL UTERINE BLEEDING

PAULINE SHEEHAN

HISTORY AND PHYSICAL
- Clinical syndrome of frequent, irregular periods, often assoc. w/ prolonged & excessive, painless vaginal bleeding w/out demonstrable organic lesion
- 90% occurs in adolescents
- Usually result of anovulatory cycles
- Diagnosis of exclusion

History

- Onset & severity of menstrual bleeding
- Family & personal Hx of bleeding disorders
- Symptoms or Hx of thyroid disease
- Other systemic diseases
- Stress, eating disorders, excessive exercise
- Medication use:
  - Aspirin
  - NSAIDs
  - Depo-Provera
  - OCPs
  - Anticonvulsants
  - Anticoagulants

Physical signs

- Orthostatic vital signs
- Inspection of thyroid gland
- Breast exam (galactorrhea)
- Evidence of androgen excess or liver disease
- Bruising or petechiae
- Abdominal, pelvic, rectal exam

TESTS

- CBC, reticulocyte count
- If indicated:
  - Pregnancy test
  - LFTs
  - TFT
  - Cervical cultures (gonococci/Chlamydia)
  - Pap smear
  - LH, FSH, prolactin
  - Free & total testosterone, DHEA-S
  - PT, PTT, platelets, bleeding time
  - Von Willenbrand's panel (if abnormal bleeding time)

DIFFERENTIAL DIAGNOSIS

- Complications of pregnancy
- Genital tract infections
- Thyroid disease
- Hyperprolactinemia
- Chronic anovulation
- Adrenal disease

- Coagulation abnormalities
- Vaginal, cervical, uterine, ovarian abnormalities
- Severe chronic illness
- Medications
- Foreign body
- Trauma or sexual assault

MANAGEMENT
- Ensure hemodynamic stability
- Control excessive bleeding
- Correct anemia
- Prevent future episodes

SPECIFIC THERAPY
- Depends on severity of bleeding
- Mild:
  - Patient hemodynamically stable
  - Hb: 12 g/dL
  - Menses mildly prolonged
  - Interval between menses shortened
  - Menstrual calendar, iron supplement, re-evaluation in 3–6 mo, NSAIDs
- Moderate:
  - Menses prolonged, heavy
  - Interval between periods shortened
  - Hb: 10–12 g/dL
  - Iron supplement
  - Low-dose estrogen-progestin OCP
  - If not sexually active, medroxyprogesterone acetate
  - Norethindrone acetate
- Severe:
  - Asymptomatic, not actively bleeding, Hb <10 g/dL:
    - Low-dose estrogen-progestin monophasic OCP
    - One pill qid for 4 d, 3 pills tid for 3 d, 2 pills bid until bleeding stops; immediately follow w/ next pack of OCP
    - Can give continuously 1 pill/day for 6–8 wks if Hb very low
    - Antiemetics
    - Iron supplement for 3 mo
  - Symptomatic, actively bleeding, Hb <9 g/dL:
    - Inpatient management: blood transfusion PRN, monophasic OCP qid, antiemetics

- Consider IV conjugated estrogen if unable to tolerate OCPs
- Iron supplement for 3 mo to replenish stores
- D&C if hormonal therapy does not stop or substantially decrease bleeding w/in 24–48 hrs

FOLLOW-UP
- Re-evaluate Hb, pt needs q3 mo

COMPLICATIONS AND PROGNOSIS
- Most respond well to treatment
- 50% have regular cycles 4 yrs after menarche; otherwise consider polycystic ovary syndrome
- Low morbidity w/ proper evaluation, diagnosis, & treatment

DYSMENORRHEA

LINDA GRANT, M.D., M.P.H.

HISTORY AND PHYSICAL
- Crampy, recurrent abdominal pain occurring at menses, often associated w/ nausea, vomiting, and headaches beginning 6–12 mo after menarche
- Majority is functional
- Primary dysmenorrhea prevalence increases over adolescence, decreases with increasing parity
- Distinguish primary (functional, no underlying structural abnormality) from secondary (evidence of a specific cause)

History
- Degree of debilitation (missed school, work, social)
- History of STDs, instrumentation (adhesions)
- Systemic symptoms:
  - Nausea
  - Vomiting
  - Headache
- Intensity of symptoms:
  - Duration
  - Begin prior to menses
  - Entire cycle or first 2 d

Physical signs
- Sexually active: pelvic exam
- Not sexually active:
  - No speculum

- ➤ Ultrasound preferred over bimanual exam
- ■ Rectal exam
- ■ Tender nodular cul-de-sac or thickened sacrouterine ligaments (endometriosis)

TESTS
- ■ Pelvic culture for gonococci, chlamydia
- ■ Suspected PID: dCBC with differential

DIFFERENTIAL DIAGNOSIS
- ■ Primary:
  - ➤ Normal exam
  - ➤ Pain first days of menses
  - ➤ Usually relieved by NSAIDs (anti-prostaglandins)
- ■ Secondary:
  - ➤ Obstruction (imperforate hymen, abnormal structure): pain throughout menses
  - ➤ Endometriosis: no relief w/ ovulatory suppression or NSAIDs
  - ➤ Psychogenic: diagnosis of exclusion

MANAGEMENT
- ■ Pharmacologic:
  - ➤ NSAIDs
  - ➤ OCP
- ■ Exercise (w/ adequate bra support)
- ■ Diet/supplements: little known effectiveness
- ■ Stress reduction
- ■ Laparoscopy if no improvement

SPECIFIC THERAPY
- ■ NSAIDs:
  - ➤ 3–4 cycles
  - ➤ If one not effective try another
  - ➤ Begin at menses onset
  - ➤ Mefenamic acid & meclofenamate: theoretical therapeutic advantage
- ■ OCP:
  - ➤ Causes decreased flow
  - ➤ May decrease pain by decreasing blood flow, contractions
  - ➤ Trial of 3–6 mo
  - ➤ Additional benefit of pregnancy prevention in sexually active adolescent
- ■ Central-acting analgesic: use with care

FOLLOW-UP
■ Every 3–4 mo to adjust management

COMPLICATIONS AND PROGNOSIS
■ NSAID, OCP side effects

EBV DISEASE/INFECTIOUS MONONUCLEOSIS

JO-ANN S. HARRIS, M.D.

HISTORY AND PHYSICAL
■ Asymptomatic in infants and young children

History
■ Prodrome:
  ➤ Malaise
  ➤ Fatigue
  ➤ Fever for 2–5 d
■ Fever
■ Rash: associated with ampicillin

Physical signs
■ Exudative pharyngitis (mimics strep)
■ Lymphadenopathy:
  ➤ Diffuse, nontender
  ➤ Most prominent in cervical chains
■ Splenomegaly:
  ➤ 50% cases
  ➤ Seen on ultrasound, 2nd–4th wk
■ Hepatomegaly (less common)

TESTS
■ CBC with differential: lymphocytosis with atypicals >10%
■ Liver enzymes
■ Monospot/heterophil antibodies: often (-) in children age <6 yrs
■ EBV serology

DIFFERENTIAL DIAGNOSIS
■ Other causes:
  ➤ Adenovirus
  ➤ Cytomegalovirus
  ➤ *Toxoplasma gondii*
  ➤ Human herpes virus 6

- ➤ HIV
- ➤ Rubella

MANAGEMENT
- Supportive care
- Fever control and analgesia
- Rehydration if indicated
- Avoid contact sports until spleen not palpable (4–6 wks)

SPECIFIC THERAPY
- Corticosteroids: only for cases with complications:
  - ➤ Impending airway obstruction
  - ➤ Massive splenomegaly
  - ➤ Myocarditis
  - ➤ Hemolytic anemia
  - ➤ Hemophagocytic syndrome
- If receiving immunosuppressive therapy helpful if dose can be reduced

FOLLOW-UP
- Splenomegaly may persist for several weeks
- Fatigue may persist for months
- Patients with recent history of infectious mononucleosis should not donate blood

COMPLICATIONS AND PROGNOSIS
- Usually self-limited; complete recovery in 4–6 wks
- Adults: more severe and protracted course
- Long-lasting immunity
- Immunodeficient patients: higher risk for complications
- Streptococcal pharyngitis: 5–25%
- Antibiotic-induced rash: resolves when drug removed
- Splenic rupture: 1/1,000 patients, 50% spontaneous
- Airway obstruction
- Rare CNS illnesses:
  - ➤ Guillain-Barre syndrome
  - ➤ Bell palsy
  - ➤ Aseptic meningitis
  - ➤ Meningoencephalitis
  - ➤ Optic neuritis
- Rare hematologic disorders:
  - ➤ Aplastic and hemolytic anemias

- ➤ HUS
- ➤ Thrombocytopenia
- ➤ Agranulocytosis
- ➤ Hemophagocytic syndrome
- Rare:
  - ➤ Orchitis
  - ➤ Myocarditis
  - ➤ Atypical pneumonia
  - ➤ Pancreatitis
  - ➤ Nephritis
- Other disorders:
  - ➤ X-linked and posttransplantation lymphoproliferative disorders
  - ➤ Burkitt lymphoma
  - ➤ Nasopharyngeal carcinoma
  - ➤ Undifferentiated B-cell CNS lymphoma

ELECTRICAL INJURIES

IRENE TIEN, M.D.

HISTORY AND PHYSICAL

History

- Events surrounding electrocution:
  - ➤ Wet vs. dry electrocution
  - ➤ High (>1,000 volts) vs. low voltage
  - ➤ Type of current (AC or DC)
  - ➤ Associated trauma
  - ➤ Duration of contact to electrical source
  - ➤ Need for CPR at scene
  - ➤ ? LOC

Physical signs

- Completely undress patient:
  - ➤ Burns to head/torso: high mortality
  - ➤ Burns to extremities: may produce serious musculoskeletal injury
  - ➤ Hand-to-hand current flow may produce spinal cord injury
- Shocks under water may result in no cutaneous manifestations
- Cutaneous injury may underestimate extent of subcutaneous damage
- Maintain C-spine immobilization if significant mechanical injury

- Evaluate for compartment syndrome
- Oral exam for lip burns from biting on wires
- Detailed neurologic exam

TESTS
- ECG
- Radiographs for trauma
- Labs:
  - Urine myoglobin
  - CBC
  - Electrolytes: beware hyperkalemia
  - BUN/creatinine
  - LFTs
  - CK-MB fractionation
- Consider echocardiography if evidence of myocardial dysfunction

DIFFERENTIAL DIAGNOSIS
- Thermal burns
- Crush injuries
- Mechanical trauma
- Child abuse/neglect

MANAGEMENT
- ABCs, supportive care, aggressive fluid resuscitation (beware cerebral edema)

SPECIFIC THERAPY
- Asymptomatic children with minor household electrical injury: no lab evaluation and may be discharged home
- AC injuries:
  - Hospitalize if LOC, change in mental status, or cardiac arrest at scene
  - Orthopedic evaluation for underlying muscle necrosis and compartment syndrome
  - Aggressive fluid resuscitation: urine output at least 3 mL/kg/h
  - Consider mannitol, sodium bicarbonate, diuretics for rhabdomyolysis
  - Frequent neurologic exam
  - Head CT for mental status changes or peripheral neuropathy
  - Ophthalmologic evaluation
  - Careful evaluation for acute abdomen

- DC injuries (lightning strikes):
  - Admit for cardiac monitoring & evaluation of associated mechanical injuries
  - Treatment similar to AC injuries

FOLLOW-UP
- Dictated by severity of electrical injury & associated injuries

COMPLICATIONS AND PROGNOSIS
- Orthopedic issues primarily related to severity of muscle necrosis
- Cataracts may develop in those electrocuted by >200 Volts, 6% in first year
- Mood lability, anxiety reactions, loss of appetite, sleep disorders, difficulties in concentration
- Transient or permanent peripheral neuropathy
- Potential damage to coronary arteries: later aneurysm development and/or thrombosis

Prognosis
- Survivors generally do well despite need for cardiopulmonary resuscitation

---

ENDOCARDITIS AND PROPHYLAXIS

CELIA GILLIS, R.N.
SHARON E. O'BRIEN, M.D.

HISTORY AND PHYSICAL
- At-risk patients:
  - Neonates
  - Immunocompromised
  - Central lines
  - Congenital heart disease
- Persistent fever
- Anorexia, weight loss
- Fatigue, pallor
- Recent dental work
- Splenomegaly
- New or changing murmur
- Skin:
  - Petechiae
  - Splinter hemorrhages

➤ Osler nodes
➤ Janeway lesions
■ 50% embolize to other site:
➤ Hematuria
➤ Hemiparesis
➤ Seizures
➤ Pulmonary embolus

TESTS
■ Gold standard for diagnosis:
➤ Multiple positive blood cultures
➤ 3–6 blood cultures taken over 24–48 h from different sites
■ CBC: anemia, leukocytosis
■ Elevated ESR
■ Echocardiography: may demonstrate vegetation or valve regurgitation
■ Eye exam for Roth spots
■ Urinalysis

DIFFERENTIAL DIAGNOSIS
■ Collagen vascular diseases
■ Acute rheumatic fever
■ Lymphoma
■ Cardiac myxomas
■ Miliary tuberculosis
■ Drugs

MANAGEMENT
■ 4–6 wks of IV antibiotics

SPECIFIC THERAPY
■ Initial treatment for likely organism: *Streptococcus* and *Staphylococcus*
■ Final antibiotic choice: once organism isolated
■ No obvious source: IV penicillin (PCN) or ampicillin w/ IV gentamicin or IM streptomycin
■ PCN allergy: IV vancomycin
■ Consider surgery:
➤ Resistant organism
➤ Progressive CHF
➤ Significant valve regurgitation
➤ Severe renal dysfunction

- Prophylaxis:
  - At-risk:
    - Prosthetic valve
    - Previous bacterial endocarditis
    - Congenital heart disease, except isolated secundum ASD
    - Acquired valve dysfunction
    - Hypertrophic cardiomyopathy
    - Mitral valve prolapse w/ mitral regurgitation and/or thickened leaflets
  - Good oral hygiene
  - Oral prophylaxis:
    - Amoxicillin
    - Dental, oral, respiratory tract, esophageal procedures
    - Allergy to PCN: clindamycin, cephalexin, or clarithromycin
  - IV prophylaxis:
    - GU or GI procedures
    - Ampicillin & gentamicin
    - Allergy to PCN: vancomycin & gentamicin
  - Procedures *requiring* prophylaxis:
    - Dental cleaning, extractions, surgery
    - Tonsillectomy/adenoidectomy
    - Rigid bronchoscopy
    - Urethral dilation
    - Surgery involving intestinal mucosa.
  - Procedures *not* requiring prophylaxis:
    - Shedding of primary teeth
    - Fluoride treatments
    - Endotracheal intubation
    - Flexible bronchoscopy w/o biopsy
    - Vaginal delivery
    - Circumcision

FOLLOW-UP
- Blood culture:
  - After 3 d of antibiotics
  - Before stopping antibiotics
  - 1 wk after stopping
- Follow-up echocardiogram

COMPLICATIONS AND PROGNOSIS
- Abscess
- Valve destruction

- CHF
- Conduction defects
- Emboli

Prognosis
- ~100% cure rate:
  - ➤ Early therapy
  - ➤ PCN-sensitive *Streptococcus*
- Overall recovery rate: 80%
- Mortality often result of CHF

ENURESIS

SUSAN O'BRIEN, M.D.

HISTORY AND PHYSICAL
- More common in males than females

History
- Fever
- Polyuria, polydipsia
- Constipation
- Dysuria
- Daytime wetting
- Abdominal or back pain
- Impulsivity, hyperactivity
- Stress incontinence

Physical signs
- Vital signs (fever assoc. with UTI)
- Labial fusion
- Rectal exam

TESTS
- Urinalysis and culture
- Absence of glucose in urine R/O clinically significant diabetes mellitus
- Specific gravity >=.015 R/O diabetes insipidus
- Consider VCUG, renal ultrasound, or IVP (suspected urinary tract malformation)

DIFFERENTIAL DIAGNOSIS
- Diurnal enuresis (daytime wetting):
  - ➤ Neurogenic bladder

- ➤ Congenital urethral obstruction
- ➤ Ectopic ureter
- ➤ Congenital diabetes insipidus
- ➤ UTI
- ➤ Constipation
- ➤ Holding urine to last minute
- ➤ Vaginal reflux of urine
- ➤ Labial fusion
- ➤ Postvoid dribble syndrome
- ➤ Daytime frequency syndrome
- ➤ Giggle incontinence
- ➤ Stress incontinence
- ➤ Emotional stress
- ➤ Urge syndrome
- ➤ Acquired neurogenic bladder
- ➤ Traumatic or infectious urethral obstruction
- ➤ Diabetes mellitus
- ➤ Acquired diabetes insipidus
- ■ Nocturnal enuresis (nighttime wetting):
  - ➤ Not awakening to micturition urge
  - ➤ Small bladder capacity
  - ➤ Incomplete bladder filling (constipation)
  - ➤ Incomplete bladder emptying:
    - • UTI
    - • Neurogenic bladder
    - • Dysfunctional voiding
  - ➤ Polyuria
  - ➤ Nocturnal ADH deficit
  - ➤ Urgency of urination

MANAGEMENT
- ■ Identify predisposing medical conditions
- ■ Assess pattern of enuresis: diurnal more serious than nocturnal
- ■ Measure bladder capacity (nocturnal enuresis only)

SPECIFIC THERAPY
- ■ Nocturnal only:
  - ➤ Enuresis alarms
  - ➤ Bladder stretching exercises
  - ➤ Positive reinforcement
  - ➤ Responsibility for morning cleanup

- Urgency incontinence: stream interruption exercises
- Psychogenic (deliberate) daytime wetting: counseling, motivation program
- Infrequent voiders:
  - ➤ VCUG, renal ultrasound
  - ➤ If abnormal:
    - Timed voiding
    - Prophylactic antibiotics
    - Urologist consult
  - ➤ Drug therapy:
    - Desmopressin
    - Imipramine
    - Oxybutynin

FOLLOW-UP
- As needed depending on etiology
- Ensure therapy is in place and effective: follow frequently (1 wk after initial plan; then in 2–4 wk and as needed)
- Ask parent (or child) to keep diary of progress

COMPLICATIONS AND PROGNOSIS
- 15% of bedwetters become dry each year
- Enuresis alarms successful in 70–80%
- Relapse rate high with medication

EPIDIDYMITIS

DAVID H. DORFMAN, M.D.

HISTORY AND PHYSICAL

History
- Scrotal pain, more gradual in onset than testicular torsion
- Common in sexually active adolescents
- 90% of cases unilateral
- Dysuria & urethral discharge often absent
- May occur in prepubertal children

Physical signs
- Fever usually absent
- Pain, tenderness, & swelling localized to epididymis, posterior to testicle

- Cremasteric reflex usually intact
- With progression, scrotal skin becomes erythematous & edematous
- Reactive hydrocele may develop
- Prehn's sign (pain relief with elevation of the scrotum) is unreliable

TESTS
- Urinalysis
- Urine culture in prepubertal pts
- Gonorrhea & chlamydia testing in sexually active pts
- Doppler ultrasound
  - R/O testicular torsion
  - Shows swollen epididymis, with increased blood flow

DIFFERENTIAL DIAGNOSIS
- Testicular torsion: Doppler ultrasound or nuclear medicine scan demonstrates decreased blood flow
- Torsion of appendix testes
- Orchitis
- Trauma
- Henoch-Schonlein purpura
- Incarcerated hernia
- Acute idiopathic scrotal edema:
  - Benign
  - Occurs in prepubertal boys
- Testicular tumor with hemorrhage (rare)
- Adenitis

MANAGEMENT
What to do first
- Assess for testicular torsion

General measures
- Analgesics
- Sitz baths
- Antibiotics

SPECIFIC THERAPY
- Treat adolescents for gonorrhea and chlamydia
- Outpatient antibiotics; if severe, admit for IV antibiotics

FOLLOW-UP
- Treat partners of pts with sexually acquired epididymitis
- Pain and edema generally resolve w/in 1 wk of therapy
- Epididymal induration may take wks to resolve

COMPLICATIONS AND PROGNOSIS
- Excellent with early treatment
- Prepubescent boys may need evaluation of urinary tract

EPIGLOTTITIS

ILAN SCHWARTZ, M.D.

HISTORY AND PHYSICAL

History
- Rapidly progressive bacterial infection of supraglottic structures
- Brief duration, often as short as 6 h
- Sore throat, dysphagia, high fever, minimal cough
- Determine vaccine status against *Haemophilus influenzae* type B, especially if recent immigrant

Physical signs
- Appears toxic and anxious
- High fever ($>= 40°C$)
- Stridor
- Tachycardia and tachypnea
- Signs of respiratory distress with marked retractions
- Drooling
- "Sniffers" position (sitting and leaning forward)
- Cyanosis may be present

TESTS
- Child at high risk for epiglottitis should be managed in secure setting such as operating room to stabilize airway
- Delay diagnostic tests until airway has been secured
- CBC: often elevated WBC count (range 15,000–25,000) with left shift
- Blood culture: may yield bacterial pathogen
- Lateral neck x-ray not required if presentation is classic:
  - Swollen epiglottis (thumb sign)
  - Thickening aryepiglottic folds
  - Obliteration of the vallecula

DIFFERENTIAL DIAGNOSIS
- Croup
- Foreign body aspiration
- Toxic ingestion
- Allergic reaction (angioedema)
- Retropharyngeal abscess

- Bacterial tracheitis
- Congenital abnormality of airway

MANAGEMENT

General measures
- Avoid excess stimulation
- Keep child with a parent
- No painful procedures
- Blow-by oxygen
- Airway management team

SPECIFIC THERAPY
- Endotracheal intubation
- Tracheotomy (needed rarely)
- IV antibiotics: ceftriaxone (100 mg/kg/d)
- Sedation/paralysis after airway secure

FOLLOW-UP
- ICU admission
- Restrain, sedate, and/or paralyze to prevent self-extubation
- Extubate within 24–48 h of antibiotics

COMPLICATIONS AND PROGNOSIS
- Sudden respiratory obstruction
- Extra-epiglottic dissemination of the infection (e.g., meningitis, pneumonia)

Prognosis
- Mortality:
  - When treated with antibiotics alone: as high as 20%
  - When airway is secured: less than 1%

ETHANOL POISONING

SOPHIA DYER, M.D.

HISTORY AND PHYSICAL

History
- Ingestion of ethanol-containing product:
  - Mouthwash
  - Cough & cold remedies
  - Cologne & aftershave
- Altered mental status

Physical signs
- Loss of balance, slurred speech
- Traumatic injuries
- Ethanol odor on breath
- Symptoms depend on ethanol level:
  - Ataxia
  - Emotional lability
  - Mild tachycardia
  - Mydriasis
  - Vomiting
  - Agitation
  - Coma
  - Rarely hypothermia, seizures

TESTS
- Bedside glucose testing, esp. in young children and if seizures are present
- Breath alcohol analyzers for alert, cooperative pts
- Blood alcohol levels
- Electrolytes, BUN, creatinine, glucose, serum osmolality (esp. if other toxic alcohols possible)
- Can estimate ethanol level: 1 mL/kg (100% ethanol) elevates blood level by 100–150 mg/dL
- Head CT to rule out intracranial process as cause of altered mental status

DIFFERENTIAL DIAGNOSIS
- Intracranial lesion or bleed
- Intoxication caused by other substances:
  - Barbiturates or benzodiazepines
  - Methanol, isopropanol, or ethylene glycol
  - Gamma-hydroxybutyric acid or gamma-hydroxybutyrolactone
- Carbon monoxide poisoning
- Hypoglycemia

MANAGEMENT
What to do first
- Assess level of consciousness
- Rapid glucose assessment
- Assess for reversible causes of lethargy

General measures
- Assess for co-ingestions

- Activated charcoal only if indicated for co-ingestion
- Electrolyte replacement (Mg, K) in chronic alcoholics
- Frequent reassessment to confirm mental status improvement as ethanol is metabolized
- Continuous cardiovascular monitoring for pts w/ depressed mental status

SPECIFIC THERAPY
- Naloxone for depressed mental status
- Thiamine IV if hypoglycemia & Wernicke's encephalopathy is considered
- Hemodialysis to remove ethanol; rarely indicated

FOLLOW-UP
- Confirmation of substance ingested
- Frequent reassessment of mental status
- Family counseling re: poison prevention in the home
- Family & individual counseling for the older child presenting w/ alcohol intoxication
  - ➤ Assess older child or adolescent for alcoholism

COMPLICATIONS AND PROGNOSIS
- Hypoglycemia can recur or develop over the time of intoxication
- Alcoholic ketoacidosis: seen in chronic alcoholics recovering from recent binge
- Pancreatitis
- Alcoholic hepatitis
- Gastritis
- Alcohol withdrawal seizures: in chronic alcoholic who decreases or stops ethanol intake

Prognosis
- Acute ethanol intoxication: good, assuming supportive care & early survey to avoid missed traumatic injuries

EVALUATION OF DYSMORPHIC CHILD

JEFF MILUNSKY, M.D.

HISTORY AND PHYSICAL

History
- Birth defects

- Mental retardation
- Multiple miscarriage
- Neonatal/infant death
- Stillbirth
- Consanguinity
- Medical conditions in mother (i.e., seizures)
- Prenatal history:
  - Teratogens
  - Abnormal ultrasound, maternal serum screen, amniocentesis
  - Oligohydramnios or polyhydramnios
  - Abnormal fetal movement (i.e., decreased)
  - Multiple gestation
  - IUGR
- Birth history:
  - Prematurity
  - Fetal position
  - Mode of delivery
  - Umbilical cord length
  - Apgar
  - Anthropometrics
- Neonatal history:
  - Jaundice
  - Seizures
  - Developmental history
  - Metabolic history (i.e., prolonged vomiting/diarrhea/lethargy)
  - Abnormal behaviors (i.e., stereotypy)
- Medical history (i.e., seizures)
- Surgical history (i.e., birth defects)
- Audiology/vision evaluation

Physical signs
- Anthropometrics
- Major congenital anomalies
- Minor congenital anomalies (>3: ~20% chance of major anomaly)
- Asymmetry: bone/soft tissue
- Abnormal facial features:
  - Compare all features to parents
  - Beware normal variants and normal ethnic traits
- Heart murmur
- Organomegaly

- Hernia
- Abnormal skin pigmentation
- Abnormal neurologic exam, especially tone
- Genital abnormality

TESTS
- Chromosome analysis
- Further testing depends on specific dysmorphism

DIFFERENTIAL DIAGNOSIS
- Chromosome abnormality
- Genetic syndrome
- Teratogenic effects
- Rare metabolic disorders

MANAGEMENT
- Genetics
- Surgery for major congenital anomalies
- Consider neurology consult
- Screening for major congenital anomalies if pattern of minor anomalies or recognizable syndrome
- Developmental delay: early intervention services, speech and language assessment, occupational therapy, physical therapy

SPECIFIC THERAPY
- Depends on diagnosis

FOLLOW-UP
- Genetics
- Based on specific diagnosis
- Specific type of anticipatory guidance depending on diagnosis

COMPLICATIONS AND PROGNOSIS
- Depends on diagnosis

EXTERNAL OTITIS (SWIMMER'S EAR)

PETER J. GERGEN, M.D.

HISTORY AND PHYSICAL
- Infection of outer ear canal
- Moisture in external ear canal enhances chance of infection

■ Variety of organisms (e.g., *Pseudomonas aeruginosa, Staphylococcus aureus*)

History
■ Complaints of pain or itching of ear, usually accompanied w/ discharge from ear canal

Physical signs
■ Ear pain on movement of outer ear
■ External ear canal filled with pus & debris
■ External ear canal may be swollen
■ Decrease in hearing acuity secondary to swollen canal

TESTS
■ None needed

DIFFERENTIAL DIAGNOSIS
■ Otitis media w/ rupture of tympanic membrane
■ Foreign body or insect in outer ear canal
■ Watery, dilute discharge: possible CSF leak, esp. after trauma
■ Chronic infection:
  ➤ Allergic skin condition (eczema or seborrhea)
  ➤ Repeated trauma to skin of middle ear (e.g., cotton swabs)
  ➤ Chronic drainage from middle ear disease
  ➤ Tumor (rare)

MANAGEMENT
■ Topical ear drops:
  ➤ Containing antibiotics/steroids
  ➤ Generally considered safe, even in presence of tympanostomy tubes
■ Clean external canal enough to allow room for otic drop penetration & to ascertain foreign body
■ Cotton wick often necessary to ensure ear drops penetrate external canal
■ Pain relief

SPECIFIC THERAPY
■ Ear drops:
  ➤ Neomycin, polymyxin B, & hydrocortisone 4–5×/d
  ➤ Fluoroquinolone +/− hydrocortisone bid
  ➤ Give sufficient number of drops to fill canal

- Mild cases: 50:50 solution of rubbing alcohol & vinegar or vinegar diluted 50:50 w/ water
- Treat for 7–10 d
- May require analgesic: acetaminophen or ibuprofen
- Warm cloth or heating pad applied to ear to reduce pain
- Oral antibiotics: only if otitis media/cellulitis

FOLLOW-UP
- To prevent recurrence, after swimming or bathing fill external ear canal w/ rubbing alcohol, 50:50 mixture of rubbing alcohol & vinegar, or vinegar diluted 50:50 w/ water to dry out canal
- Use of earplugs when swimming or bathing
- Avoid cleaning ear canals w/ small objects or cotton swabs; damage to skin in ear canal can predispose to additional infections

COMPLICATIONS AND PROGNOSIS
Complications
- Rare
- Allergic dermatitis (neomycin-containing ear drops)
- Malignant or necrotizing external otitis (immunocompromised)

Prognosis
- Usually requires 7–10 d of treatment
- Can recur, esp. with certain activities (i.e., swimming)

FAILURE TO THRIVE

LAKSHMI KOLAGOTLA, M.D.

HISTORY AND PHYSICAL
- Failure to grow at expected rates for age & sex
- Results from interaction of environmental & medical factors
- Weight crosses 2 or more major percentiles within 6 mos or remains at or below third or fifth percentile

History
- Focus on underlying etiology:
  - ➤ Medical:
    - Prenatal/birth
    - Postnatal
    - Review of systems
  - ➤ Developmental: complete assessment
  - ➤ Nutritional: early, current feeding

➤ Social:
  • Income
  • Family support
  • Caretaker illness

Physical signs

■ Careful serial measurements of weight, height, & head circumference; use same instruments at each visit
■ Focus on signs consistent w/ diagnoses suggested by history

TESTS

■ CBC, lead, urinalysis
■ Other tests based on history & physical exam (extensive testing unnecessary):
  ➤ Sweat test if suspect CF
  ➤ RAST if suspect food allergy
■ Consider bone age in children age $>=1$ yr with weight <5th percentile & height >10th percentile

DIFFERENTIAL DIAGNOSIS

■ Vast; includes every organ system
■ Psychosocial FTT most common: poverty single greatest risk factor
■ So-called organic FTT less common: based on history & exam
■ Kwashiorkor, marasmus rare in U.S.

MANAGEMENT

■ Assess severity of malnutrition w/ percent standard weight (actual weight/median weight for age):
  ➤ Mild: 76–90%
  ➤ Moderate: 60–75%
  ➤ Severe: <60%
■ Hospitalize:
  ➤ Severe malnutrition
  ➤ Lack of catch-up growth
  ➤ Suspected child abuse
  ➤ To observe feeding interactions

SPECIFIC THERAPY

■ Treat underlying pathology
■ Daily multivitamins w/ zinc & iron
■ Yearly influenza vaccine
■ Developmental referral if delayed
■ Goal: achieve catch-up growth (1.5 times normal growth)

- Primary steps:
  - Restrict juice
  - Increase milk intake
  - Provide 3 meals & 3 snacks daily
- Instruct on effective feeding techniques
- Calorie-dense foods (i.e., corn oil, cheese, peanut butter, whole milk)
- Consider supplements:
  - Pediasure, Sustacal
  - Duocal added to solid & liquid foods to increase caloric density
  - For infants (may add to formula):
    - Polycose powder
    - MCT oil
- If necessary, arrange financial support for WIC, food stamps, welfare
- Consider SSI for children who qualify

FOLLOW-UP
- See q2–4 wks depending on degree of malnourishment
- Monitor weight & development status
- Refer to interdisciplinary team if fails to demonstrate catch-up growth

COMPLICATIONS AND PROGNOSIS
- Higher risk of infection
- Greater likelihood of developmental delay, short stature

FEBRILE INFANTS

ERIC FLEEGLER, M.D.

HISTORY AND PHYSICAL

History
- Fever >38.0°C (100.4°F)
- Pregnancy & birth history:
  - Maternal group B strep status
  - Maternal antibiotic Rx during delivery
  - Maternal & paternal HSV status: primary or recurrent disease during pregnancy
  - Vaginal vs. c-section
  - Other complications
- Neonatal course:
  - Home w/ mother vs. NICU

>– Mechanical ventilation
>– In-dwelling lines
■ Ill contacts in home or environment, esp. day care
■ Immunization status of infant
■ Irritability, lethargy, vomiting, diarrhea, rash
■ Oral intake & urine output

Physical signs
■ Temperature, heart rate, & blood pressure
■ Assessment of perfusion
■ Bulging fontanel
■ Identify focus for fever

TESTS
■ CBC + differential
■ Blood culture
■ Urinalysis & urine culture (suprapubic or catheter)
■ Lumbar puncture, CSF analysis
>– Culture, Gram stain, cell count, protein, glucose
>– Latex agglutination for GBS or *Pneumococcus*
>– HSV or enterovirus PCR
■ Electrolytes, BUN, creatinine, glucose
■ Chest x-ray if WBC >20,000/cu mm or abnormality on physical exam
■ Stool for white cells if diarrhea Hx

DIFFERENTIAL DIAGNOSIS
■ Sepsis, meningitis
■ Pneumonia, pyelonephritis, bacterial enteritis, cellulitis, osteomyelitis
■ Otitis media, URI

MANAGEMENT
What to do first
■ Identify infant w/ clinical sepsis
■ Establish IV access, if poorly perfused or septic appearing
■ Complete sepsis evaluation
■ Antipyretics

SPECIFIC THERAPY
■ Age 0–28 d:
>– Complete sepsis evaluation

- ➤ IV antibiotics
- ➤ Hospitalization
- ■ Age 29–90 d:
  - ➤ Complete sepsis evaluation
  - ➤ Hospitalization & IV antibiotics if pt meets high-risk criteria for sepsis:
    - CSF pleocytosis >10
    - WBC >15,000 or <5,000 mm^3
    - Bands: neutrophil ratio >0.2
    - Bands > 1,500 mm^3
    - Pyuria, WBCs in stool, or abnormal CXR
  - ➤ Negative workup (absence of all high-risk criteria):
    - Discharge to home with parenteral antibiotics
    - Second option: admit for observation w/o antibiotics
  - ➤ Close FU w/ primary doctor essential for outpatient Rx
  - ➤ IV acyclovir for suspected HSV; IV hydration required w/ IV acyclovir

Treatment options
- ■ Age <28 d: ampicillin + (cefotaxime or gentamicin); consider acyclovir if <3 wks
  - ➤ If age >14 d, well-appearing w/ no CSF pleocytosis: consider cephalosporin alone
- ■ Age 29–90 d: ceftriaxone (in older, ill-appearing child, consider ampicillin or vancomycin)

FOLLOW-UP
- ■ Continue IV antibiotics for 48 h for high-risk infants
- ■ Low-risk infants: repeat exam by primary doctor w/in 24 h
- ■ Return to primary doctor or ER if decreased feeding, increased lethargy, increased fever, vomiting, irritability, or other concerns

COMPLICATIONS AND PROGNOSIS
Complications
- ■ Bacteremia: may seed other sites (bone, CSF, urine)
- ■ UTI: renal ultrasound & voiding cystourethrography (VCUG) to identify structural abnormality
- ■ Meningitis:
  - ➤ Subdural empyema
  - ➤ SIADH
  - ➤ Ischemic brain injury

> Hearing loss
> Neurocognitive impairment

Prognosis
- Most with serious bacterial infections treated early recover w/o complications

---

FEBRILE SEIZURES

ROBERT VINCI, M.D.

HISTORY AND PHYSICAL

History
- Simple febrile seizure:
    > Generalized
    > Duration <15 min
    > No recurrences w/in 24 h
    > Age at onset: 6 mo to 6 y
    > No CNS infection or metabolic disturbance
- Complex febrile seizure:
    > Focal
    > Duration >15 min
    > Recurrence w/in 24 h
    > Atypical age at onset
- Key points:
    > Age of patient
    > Duration of seizure, focality
    > History of ingestion/trauma
    > Risk for metabolic disorders

Physical signs
- Vital signs, esp. fever
- Evidence of meningitis:
    > Irritability
    > Full fontanel
    > Meningismus
- Complete neurologic exam
- Identify focus of infection

TESTS
- Routine lab eval not necessary
- CBC, blood culture for evaluation of fever & bacteremia

- Urine culture:
  - ➤ Febrile males <6–12 mo
  - ➤ Febrile females <24 mo
  - ➤ History of renal abnormality or previous UTI
- Lumbar puncture if high suspicion for meningitis:
  - ➤ Age <12–18 mo
  - ➤ Prior antibiotic use (i.e., partially treated meningitis)
  - ➤ Meningeal signs
- EEG not helpful
- Neuroradiology studies: not indicated in simple febrile seizure

DIFFERENTIAL DIAGNOSIS
- Meningitis
- Simple vs. complex febrile seizures
- Afebrile seizure disorder
- Head trauma/child abuse/CNS lesions
- Toxin ingestion
- Metabolic disturbance

MANAGEMENT
General measures
- ABCs
- Oxygen via non-rebreather mask
- Prevent aspiration
- Antipyretics

SPECIFIC THERAPY
- Most pts do not require routine anticonvulsants
- Standard anticonvulsants for febrile status
- Prophylactic anticonvulsants:
  - ➤ Not generally indicated
  - ➤ Decrease recurrence rate to ~12%
  - ➤ Not clear whether they prevent development of afebrile seizures
- Drugs:
  - ➤ Diazepam: intermittent at time of fever
  - ➤ Oral or rectal
- Valproic acid: use continuously
- Phenytoin and carbamazepine: not effective
- Phenobarbital: not indicated

FOLLOW-UP
- Simple febrile seizure: discharge to routine follow-up

- Complex febrile seizures:
  - ➤ Admit for 24 h
  - ➤ May require neuro consult

COMPLICATIONS AND PROGNOSIS
- Risk of recurrence ~33%
- Rate of recurrence varies with age at presentation & history of previous febrile seizure:
  - ➤ Age <12 mo: 50%
  - ➤ Age >12 mo: 33%
  - ➤ Pts w/ second febrile seizure: 50%
- Time frame for recurrence:
  - ➤ 50% w/in 6 mo
  - ➤ 75% w/in 12 mo
  - ➤ 90% w/in 24 mo
- Risk factors for subsequent afebrile seizures:
  - ➤ Complex febrile seizure
  - ➤ Abnormal neurologic exam before febrile seizure
  - ➤ Family history of afebrile seizures
- Risk for developing afebrile seizures:
  - ➤ No risk factors: 1–2%
  - ➤ 1 risk factor: 1–2%
  - ➤ 2 risk factors: 10%
  - ➤ 3 risk factors: >25%
- Consider prophylactic anticonvulsants if 2 or more risk factors

Prognosis
- Simple febrile seizures: most have no further events after age 3–4 yr

FEVER AND BACTEREMIA

ROBERT VINCI, M.D.

HISTORY AND PHYSICAL

History
- Fever: >39.0 °C (102.2 °F)
- In immunocompromised hosts any temp elevation significant
- Sick contacts? Day care?
- Immunization Hx, esp. conjugate pneumococcal vaccine
- Parent's assessment of degree of illness, level of activity, irritability, lethargy

- Oral intake, urine output
- Associated Sx: vomiting, diarrhea, cough, coryza, rash
- Hx of chronic disease:
  - Sickle cell anemia
  - HIV
  - Immunodeficiency

Physical signs
- Does pt look toxic?
- Vital signs:
  - Degree of fever
  - BP
  - Tachycardia or tachypnea in excess of degree of fever
- Identifiable source of infection?
- Rash, esp. petechiae

TESTS
- CBC w/ differential
- Blood culture
- Urinalysis & urine culture:
  - Males <6 mo
  - Uncircumcised males <12 mo
  - Females <24 mo
  - All pts w/ known structural renal disease or Hx of previous UTI
- Lumbar puncture (meningitis)
- Chest x-ray if abnormality on exam or unexplained elevated peripheral WBC count
- Electrolytes if clinically dehydrated

DIFFERENTIAL DIAGNOSIS
- Sepsis, meningitis, epiglottitis
- Pneumonia
- Pyelonephritis/cystitis
- Bacterial enteritis
- Cellulitis
- Osteomyelitis
- Acute otitis media, pharyngitis, sinusitis, URI

MANAGEMENT
What to do first
- Identify infant w/ clinical sepsis, meningitis: cardiovascular support if hypotensive

General measures
- Antipyretics
- Antibiotics (identified bacterial source of infection [e.g., otitis media])
- Close follow-up with primary care clinician essential

SPECIFIC THERAPY
- Inpatient admission & IV antibiotics for serious infections:
  - Presumed sepsis
  - Meningitis
  - Osteomyelitis
  - Pneumonia w/ hypoxia or respiratory distress
  - Epiglottitis
- Outpatient antibiotics to treat focus of infection:
  - Otitis media
  - Community-acquired pneumonia
  - Uncomplicated UTI
- Antibiotics in febrile children w/o a source of infection (controversial) if:
  - Inadequate vaccination Hx
  - WBC >15,000/cu mm
  - Immunodeficiency, esp. sickle cell disease or HIV
  - Other risk factors for bacterial infection

FOLLOW-UP
- If admitted, continue antibiotics to treat focus of infection
- If discharged, contact primary care clinician w/in 24–48 h
- Educate caretakers to return to or contact primary care clinician if child develops decreased feeding, increased lethargy, increased fever, vomiting, irritability

COMPLICATIONS AND PROGNOSIS
- Depends on focus of infection
- Bacteremia: close follow-up to identify secondary complications:
  - Persistent bacteremia
  - Meningitis
  - Arthritis
  - Osteomyelitis

Prognosis
- Fever: most recover w/o complications
- Bacteremia: most spontaneously clear

FOREIGN BODY ASPIRATION (FBA)

ILAN SCHWARTZ, M.D.

HISTORY AND PHYSICAL

History
- High index of suspicion in young children
- Type of object ingested, including size, shape, composition
- Food vs. nonfood
- Coughing, choking, wheezing, gagging
- History of unexplained or recurrent pulmonary symptoms or symptoms that don't respond to usual treatment

Physical signs
- Upper respiratory tract:
  - No phonation or crying
  - Respiratory distress, cough
  - Stridor
  - Cyanosis
  - Apnea
- Lower respiratory tract:
  - Decreased breath sounds on side of foreign body
  - Wheezing, cough
  - May have fever and dyspnea

TESTS
- PA and lateral soft tissue of the neck
- Chest x-ray (inspiratory and expiratory views): hyperinflation of affected lobes during expiration
- Fluoroscopy or lateral decubitus films (for uncooperative child)
- Direct laryngoscopy or rigid bronchoscopy (for definitive diagnosis)

DIFFERENTIAL DIAGNOSIS
- Upper respiratory tract infections
- Bronchiolitis
- Reactive airway disease
- Pneumonitis

MANAGEMENT

What to do first
- Establish airway, breathing, circulation
- Assess for complete airway obstruction; if present, begin BLS:
  - No blind finger sweep

➤ Age <1 yr: back blows or chest thrusts
➤ Age >1 yr: Heimlich
■ Consider intubation

General measures
■ NPO until diagnosis certain
■ Supplemental oxygen

SPECIFIC THERAPY
■ Direct laryngoscopy and rigid bronchoscopy under general anesthesia
■ Nebulizer mist (racemic epinephrine)
■ Consider antibiotics in fever, pneumonia, or vegetable FBA

FOLLOW-UP
■ Repeat radiographs after removal
■ 24-hr observation for airway distress

COMPLICATIONS AND PROGNOSIS
■ Respiratory distress
■ Airway edema
■ Airway stenosis or scarring
■ Postobstructive pneumonia, atelectasis, or bronchiectasis
■ Pneumothorax

Prognosis
■ Generally excellent

FRAGILE X

JEFF MILUNSKY, M.D.

HISTORY AND PHYSICAL
■ 1/4,000–1/6,000 males
■ 1/6,000 females

History
■ Significant learning disability
■ Often speech delay, articulation problems, echolalia
■ Mental retardation (mild to profound)
■ Hypotonia as infants

Physical signs
■ Macrocephaly
■ Craniofacial abnormalities:

- Often large prominent ears
- Long midface
- Prognathism (after age 20)
- High-arched palate
- Overcrowded teeth with malocclusion
- Connective tissue manifestations:
  - Hyperextensible
  - Pectus excavatum
  - Soft velvety skin
  - Hernias
  - Mitral valve prolapse
- Macro-orchidism (>90% after puberty; 15% at 8 y)

TESTS
- DNA analysis for CGG triplet repeat expansion
- Chromosome analysis: recommended if fragile X negative

DIFFERENTIAL DIAGNOSIS
- (Sex) chromosome anomalies

MANAGEMENT
- Genetics
- Neurology consult if indicated
- Behavioral issues (pharmacologic therapy)
- Early intervention, speech and language, occupational and physical therapy
- Parental support groups

SPECIFIC THERAPY
- Anticonvulsants (seizures)
- Specific therapy for behavioral problems (e.g., ADHD)
- Behavioral management (autistic features)

FOLLOW-UP
- Genetics: screening for carriers in family
- Neurology
- Child development or psychiatry

COMPLICATIONS AND PROGNOSIS
- ~10% seizures
- 5–10% autistic spectrum disorder
- 80% mitral valve prolapse (after age 18)
- Scoliosis
- Normal longevity

GI FOREIGN BODY

ILAN SCHWARTZ, M.D.

HISTORY AND PHYSICAL

History
■ Type of object ingested, incl. size, shape, composition
■ Food vs. nonfood
■ Choking episode, vomiting, drooling, dysphagia, difficulty swallowing or handling secretions
■ Chronic abdominal pain
■ Complaint of foreign body sensation (older child)
■ History of esophageal disease, especially stricture

Physical signs
■ Many are asymptomatic; specific physical findings are unusual

TESTS
■ Radiologic exam:
  ➤ Single frontal view that includes neck, chest, & abdomen sufficient if object is radiopaque
  ➤ Esophageal coins oriented in coronal plane
  ➤ Tracheal coins in sagittal orientation
■ Metal detectors (known metallic ingestion)
■ Nonmetallic foreign bodies and/or high-risk situations:
  ➤ AP & lateral neck films: disruption of usual air shadows in upper airway
  ➤ Esophagoscopy

DIFFERENTIAL DIAGNOSIS
■ Pharyngitis
■ Esophagitis
■ Peptic ulcer disease
■ Foreign body aspiration
■ Esophageal stricture

MANAGEMENT

What to do first
■ Assess for respiratory compromise

General measures
■ NPO until diagnosis certain

- Impacted esophageal foreign bodies should be promptly removed, except coin in distal esophagus
- Most foreign bodies in stomach and intestines will pass without intervention

SPECIFIC THERAPY
- Esophageal foreign bodies, incl. coins in proximal esophagus:
  - Rigid esophagoscopy under general anesthesia
  - Flexible endoscopy under conscious sedation
  - Medications (benzodiazepines or glucagons) not indicated
- Coins in distal esophagus: leave alone if acute ingestion and no symptoms
- Gastric and intestinal foreign bodies: no specific treatment unless:
  - Very large object that will not pass through pylorus
  - Very sharp object (e.g., sewing needles): surgical consult for monitoring and potential removal

FOLLOW-UP
- If foreign body removed, discharge home from PACU
- Repeat x-ray in 24 h for distal esophageal coins to ensure passage into GI tract
- Most foreign bodies pass harmlessly through GI tract
- Return for GI-related symptoms

COMPLICATIONS AND PROGNOSIS
- Mucosal abrasion
- Esophageal stricture
- Upper airway compromise
- Retropharyngeal abscess
- Esophageal perforation may lead to mediastinitis

Prognosis
- Most children do well after removal or successful passage of foreign body

GASTROESOPHAGEAL REFLUX

ROBERT VINCI, M.D.

HISTORY AND PHYSICAL

History
- Meticulous feeding history, including volume of feeds
- Frequent spitting up after feeds

- Arching while feeding
- Refusal to eat
- Chronic vomiting
- Unexplained crying/irritability
- Poor weight gain
- History of neurologic disorders
- History of apparent life-threatening event (ALTE) or apnea
- Recurrent pulmonary disease
- Older pts: heartburn or chest pain

Physical signs
- Usually well appearing
- Monitor weight gain carefully

TESTS
- Stool guaiac: may be positive
- CBC to evaluate for anemia
- Serum amylase/lipase
- 24-hour pH probe
- Upper GI endoscopy with biopsy to evaluate for esophageal disease
- Barium swallow to R/O anatomic abnormalities

DIFFERENTIAL DIAGNOSIS
- Infantile colic
- Pyloric stenosis
- Intestinal malrotation
- Milk protein allergy
- Gastritis
- Overfeeding

MANAGEMENT
General measures
- Distinguish between gastroesophageal reflux with and without esophagitis
- Elevate head of bed
- Consider lateral position for sleeping with elimination of "puffy" bedding materials
- Thicken feeds with 1 Tbls dry rice cereal/oz of milk formula
- Decrease volume of individual feeds

SPECIFIC THERAPY
- Promotility drugs
- Decrease gastric acidity (more critical if associated esophagitis):

➤ Antacids
➤ H2 antagonists
➤ Proton pump inhibitors
■ Surgery (fundoplication) for:
    ➤ Lack of response to medical therapy
    ➤ Chronic aspiration
    ➤ Failure to thrive
    ➤ ALTE/apnea

FOLLOW-UP
■ Monitor weight gain in infants
■ Monitor for resolution of symptoms

COMPLICATIONS AND PROGNOSIS
■ Failure to thrive
■ Esophagitis
■ Esophageal strictures

Prognosis
■ Generally excellent in infants with optimal medical management
■ Symptoms peak by age 1–4 mo; 55% abate by age 10 mo; 80% by age 18 mo
■ Approximately 1/3 of older children develop chronic GI and pulmonary diseases

GENERAL APPROACH TO BURNS

HANAN SEDIK, M.D., F.A.A.P.

HISTORY AND PHYSICAL

History
■ Mechanism of injury
■ Estimated heat of burning object
■ Length of contact
■ Concurrent trauma
■ Determine if patient was in closed-space confinement
■ Presence of smoke or other toxins
■ First aid measures, if any, initially applied to burn

Physical signs
■ Identify patient at risk for airway injury:
    ➤ Facial burns
    ➤ Singed nares

➤ Airway soot
➤ Stridor or respiratory distress
■ Estimate total body surface area (TBSA) involved:
  ➤ Age >9 y: apply Rule of Nine:
    • Lower extremity: 9% anterior, 9% posterior
    • Upper extremity: 9%
    • Head & neck: 9%
    • Perineum: 1%
  ➤ Younger children: area of child's palm = 1% of TBSA
■ Burn severity:
  ➤ Minor: <10% TBSA
  ➤ Moderate: 10–20% TBSA
  ➤ Major: >20% TBSA
■ Depth of injury:
  ➤ First-degree: pain & erythema
  ➤ Second-degree:
    • Superficial partial thickness: red & moist skin, w/ blister formation, intact touch, pain
    • Deep partial thickness: mottled appearance, waxy-white areas, w/ dry & anesthetic surface
  ➤ Third-degree: dry leathery appearance
■ Distribution: critical areas include face, hands, feet, & perineum
■ Identify circumferential burns & distal neurovascular function

TESTS
■ CBC
■ Blood bank specimen
■ Urinalysis, myoglobin content
■ Carboxyhemoglobin level
■ Radiographs (associated injuries)
■ NG tube and Foley catheter

DIFFERENTIAL DIAGNOSIS
■ Inflicted burns: child abuse

MANAGEMENT
■ Supportative care and pain control as needed
■ Estimate the severity and depth of burn

SPECIFIC THERAPY
Minor burns:
■ Clean using bland soap & water
■ Debride dead tissue

- Apply bacitracin or 1% silver sulfadiazine
- Apply nonstick gauze, sterile wrap
- Tetanus prophylaxis
  Major burns:
- Supportive care/pain control
- IV fluids:
  - Bolus with 20 mL/kg normal saline or lactated Ringer's
  - Fluid resuscitation formulas:
    - *Parkland*: 4 mL/kg × % TBSA, half in first 8 h & half in next 16 h; add maintenance in child <5 y
    - *Carajajal:* 5,000 mL/m^2 × % TBSA, half in first 8 h & half in next 16 h; add 2,000 mL/m^2/d maintenance
  - Withhold potassium

FOLLOW-UP
- Minor burns:
  - Wash daily w/ bland soap & water; repeat steps of wound care
  - Encourage ROM of affected extremity
  - Frequent wound checks
  - Monitor for signs of infection
  - Protect healing skin from sunburn
- Major burns: admit to ICU or transfer to local burn center

COMPLICATIONS AND PROGNOSIS

Complications
- Fluid loss and hypotension
- Myoglobinuria and renal failure
- Smoke inhalation
- Carbon monoxide poisoning
- Wound infection, sepsis

Prognosis
- Good w/ proper fluid resuscitation, early excision & grafting, antiseptic burn care techniques

GIARDIA

ELIZABETH BARNETT, M.D.

HISTORY AND PHYSICAL
- Can occur in many different settings
- May be asymptomatic

■ Chronic infection: may be associated with weight loss and malabsorption syndromes

History
■ Exposure to well water, poor hygienic conditions: increased risk
■ Watery, foul-smelling diarrhea
■ Flatulence
■ Abdominal cramping and bloody stool not typical

Physical signs
■ None specific

TESTS
■ Identification of cysts or trophozoites of organism in properly stained stool specimens
■ Giardia antigen test of stool: 95% accurate
■ String test: obtain sample from duodenum

DIFFERENTIAL DIAGNOSIS
■ Bacterial or viral gastroenteritis
■ Other parasitic infections
■ Celiac disease
■ Cystic fibrosis
■ Lactose intolerance

MANAGEMENT
■ Obtain appropriate stool culture
■ Attention to malabsorption syndromes (esp. lactose intolerance); may occur during or after infection

SPECIFIC THERAPY
■ Metronidazole
■ Furazolidone
■ Paromomycin
■ **Side effects of medications**
  ➤ Metronidazole:
    • Nausea, vomiting
    • Headache
    • Anorexia
    • Metallic taste
    • Diarrhea
    • Insomnia
    • Weakness

> Furazolidone:
  - Nausea, vomiting,
  - Allergic reactions
  - Hypotension
  - Urticaria
  - Fever
> Paromomycin: GI disturbance
■ Contraindications:
  > Alcohol (metronidazole, furazolidone)
  > G6PD deficiency (furazolidone)
  > MAO inhibitors (furazolidone)

FOLLOW-UP
■ Assess resolution of symptoms after treatment
■ Repeat stool test only if recurring symptoms, other causes (i.e., lactose intolerance) ruled out
■ Possible second course of therapy in recalcitrant cases

COMPLICATIONS AND PROGNOSIS
■ Malabsorption, vitamin deficiencies
■ Steatorrhea
■ Urticaria
■ Arthralgia
■ Lactose intolerance may outlast parasitic infection

Prognosis
■ Generally good

GLOMERULONEPHRITIS

MELANIE S. KIM, M.D.

HISTORY AND PHYSICAL

History
■ Hematuria or tea-colored urine
■ Edema
■ Headache
■ Malaise, lethargy
■ Decreased urine output
■ Rare:
  > Somnolence

➤ Seizures
➤ Coma

Related to specific disease:

■ Acute poststreptococcal glomerulonephritis:
  ➤ Hx of recent strep infection: pharyngitis or impetigo
■ IgA nephropathy:
  ➤ Precipitating URI
  ➤ Loin pain

Physical signs

■ Hypertension
■ Volume overload w/ pulmonary edema or CHF
■ Periorbital, peripheral edema
■ Systemic disease & associated findings

TESTS

■ Urinalysis:
  ➤ Hematuria (dysmorphic RBCs)
  ➤ Proteinuria
  ➤ Cellular casts (RBC casts)
■ Serum creatinine, electrolytes, calcium, phosphorus
■ CBC
■ Other tests depend on clinical findings:
  ➤ Complement: C3
  ➤ ASLO titers or streptozyme
  ➤ Serum albumin
  ➤ Urine protein: 24-h collection or spot urine protein/creatinine
    ratio
■ Chest x-ray:
  ➤ Pulmonary interstitial fluid
  ➤ Effusions
  ➤ Cardiomegaly
  ➤ CHF
■ Renal biopsy

DIFFERENTIAL DIAGNOSIS

■ Acute poststreptococcal glomerulonephritis
■ IgA nephropathy
■ Membranoproliferative glomerulonephritis
■ Systemic diseases w/ glomerulonephritis:
  ➤ Henoch-Schönlein purpura
  ➤ Lupus nephritis

➤ Nephritis of chronic bacteremia
➤ Goodpasture syndrome
➤ Wegener granulomatosis

MANAGEMENT
■ Assess cardiorespiratory status & intervene promptly:
  ➤ Hypertensive encephalopathy
  ➤ Cardiac & respiratory failure due to CHF, pulmonary edema, or pericardial effusion
■ Assess electrolyte status; intervene promptly for hyperkalemia

SPECIFIC THERAPY
■ Treat underlying cause if possible
■ Most case: no effective cure; management based on supportive care:
  ➤ Assess volume status
  ➤ Careful fluid & electrolyte management
  ➤ Treat hypertension
  ➤ Treat acidosis
  ➤ Treat hypocalcemia & hyperphosphatemia if present
  ➤ Dialysis:
    • Uremia
    • Refractory hyperkalemia
    • Acidosis
    • Severe volume overload w/ pulmonary edema or CHF
■ Rapidly progressive glomerulonephritis:
  ➤ Rapid decline in renal function, uremia in wks to mo, & often end-stage renal disease (ESRD)
  ➤ Anecdotal use: aggressive immunosuppression, incl. plasmapheresis

FOLLOW-UP
■ Depends on underlying etiology & severity of disease

COMPLICATIONS AND PROGNOSIS
■ CHF
■ Pulmonary edema
■ Hypertensive encephalopathy
■ ESRD
■ Hyperkalemia w/ arrhythmias
■ Hypocalcemia triggering seizures

Prognosis
- Depends on diagnosis:
  - Acute poststreptococcal glomerulonephritis: good, few w/ residual mild sequelae:
    - Microscopic hematuria
    - Proteinuria
    - Hypertension
  - IgA nephropathy:
    - Varies
    - If severe nephritis or nephrotic syndrome, increased risk for ESRD
  - Membranoproliferative glomerulonephritis: 1/3 ESRD
  - Nephritis of chronic bacteremia: resolves w/ treatment

GONOCOCCAL INFECTION

KATHRYN J. QUINN, M.D.

HISTORY AND PHYSICAL
- Newborn:
  - Conjunctivitis, scalp abscess
  - Disseminated disease:
    - Bacteremia
    - Arthritis
    - Meningitis
    - Endocarditis
- Prepubertal children:
  - Vaginitis, anorectal or tonsillopharyngeal infection
  - PID & gonococcal urethritis rare in prepubertal children
  - Strongly consider sexual abuse; must confirm diagnosis with culture
  - Ensure organism isolated before treatment
- Sexually active adolescents:
  - Males:
    - Usually symptomatic
    - Incubation: 2–5 d
    - Urethra primary site
    - Presents w/ mucopurulent penile discharge & dysuria
    - Can progress to epididymitis, presenting w/ unilateral testicular pain & swelling

- ➤ Females:
  - • Frequently asymptomatic
  - • Urethritis
  - • Endocervicitis w/ pruritus and/or purulent discharge
  - • Salpingitis
  - • PID
- ■ Disseminated gonococcal infection: presents as two syndromes:
  - ➤ Tenosynovitis, dermatitis, polyarthralgias without purulent arthritis
  - ➤ Purulent arthritis without skin lesions

TESTS
- ■ Gram stain of endocervical or urethral smear: gram-negative intracellular or extracellular diplococci
- ■ Culture:
  - ➤ Thayer-Martin agar (gold standard)
  - ➤ Collect urethral, rectal, endocervical, and/or pharyngeal specimen on cotton swab
  - ➤ Inoculate immediately on medium & transport rapidly to laboratory
  - ➤ Culture only acceptable method of diagnosis for sexual abuse evaluation
- ■ PCR or ligase chain reaction: on urethral or endocervical swabs or first-void urine; highly sensitive and specific

DIFFERENTIAL DIAGNOSIS
- ■ Depends on age and presenting signs and symptoms
- ■ Generally other viral & bacterial etiologies

MANAGEMENT
- ■ Third-generation cephalosporin or fluoroquinolone over 18 yrs
- ■ Treat empirically for chlamydia; co-infection common

SPECIFIC THERAPY
- ■ Newborns: ceftriaxone or cefotaxime for 7 d (10–14 d if meningitis)
- ■ Uncomplicated cervical, urethral, anorectal, or pharyngeal infection (child/adolescent): cefixime (PO), ceftriaxone (IM), spectinomycin (IM), ciprofloxacin (PO, over 18 yr) as single dose
- ■ Epididymitis:
  - ➤ Treat empirically for chlamydia
  - ➤ Ceftriaxone (IM) as single dose and doxycycline for 10 d

FOLLOW-UP
- No test of cure if uncomplicated & asymptomatic after treatment
- Evaluate sexual partners
- Reportable disease in every state

COMPLICATIONS AND PROGNOSIS
- PID
- Epididymitis
- Disseminated infection

Prognosis
- Generally good

GUILLAIN-BARRÉ SYNDROME

JANET SOUL, M.D., F.R.C.P.C.

HISTORY AND PHYSICAL

History
- Acute to subacute progressive weakness in >1 limb
- Weakness usually symmetric
- Pain in limbs:
  - Cramplike, may be severe
  - Prominent irritability
- Bell's palsy: 30–40%
- Possible antecedent infection:
  - Viral
  - *Campylobacter jejuni*

Physical signs
- Areflexia in affected limbs
- Symmetric weakness of limbs
- No abnormalities of consciousness (may be irritable, withdrawn)
- Sensory abnormalities:
  - Muscle cramps
  - Dysesthesia
- Bell's palsy: unilateral or bilateral
- Bulbar muscles may be involved
- Miller-Fisher variant:
  - Areflexia
  - Ataxia
  - Ophthalmoplegia

- Autonomic dysfunction:
  - Labile blood pressure
  - Arrhythmia
  - GI, and/or bowel/bladder dysfunction
- Respiratory distress

TESTS
- Clinical diagnosis initially (tests may not be diagnostic first few days)
- Pulmonary function tests (PFTs) to R/O respiratory compromise
- CSF exam shows classic albuminocytologic dissociation (may be normal 1st week):
  - Pleocytosis with <50 cells, mostly lymphocytes
  - Elevated protein (80–200 mg/dL)
- Electrophysiology:
  - Early (<5 d) NCV/EMG: absent H reflex & F wave
  - Later study:
    - Slowed conduction velocity
    - Reduced compound muscle action potential
    - Prolonged distal latencies
- Stool:
  - *Campylobacter*, viral cultures
  - Lyme ELISA/titer

DIFFERENTIAL DIAGNOSIS
- Transverse myelitis: upper motor neuron signs present
- Botulism: acute weakness, pupil involvement
- Acute myositis, dermatomyositis:
  - Increased CK
  - Rash
  - Other myopathies or dystrophies
- Lyme disease:
  - Bell's palsy, other cranial nerve palsies
  - Meningitis
  - Radiculoneuritis or mononeuritis multiplex (rare)
- Familial periodic paralysis

MANAGEMENT
General measures
- Monitor & support respiratory function (PFTs q4–12 h)
- Monitor blood pressure, ECG
- ICU admission:
  - Signs of autonomic dysfunction
  - Respiratory compromise

> Bulbar and/or facial weakness
> Rapid onset of weakness
- Supportive care for weakness, pain, bowel & bladder dysfunction
- Physical therapy

SPECIFIC THERAPY
- IVIG 1 g/kg/d for 2 d
- Plasmapheresis (in place of IVIG)
- Steroids not beneficial

FOLLOW-UP
- Discharge when:
  > Clearly improving
  > Ambulating (if ambulatory at baseline)
  > No autonomic or respiratory dysfunction
- Follow up in 1–3 mo, depending on severity, to monitor neurologic recovery

COMPLICATIONS AND PROGNOSIS
- Complications related to severe illness w/ need for ventilatory support
- Death if autonomic dysfunction (arrhythmia, hypotension) not treated aggressively
- Bed sores, contractures from severe prolonged weakness

Prognosis
- Generally excellent in young children, except those with severe weakness, axonal variant
- Rare recurrence or evolution into chronic inflammatory demyelination polyneuropathy

---

HIV INFECTION IN CHILDREN

ALAN MEYERS, M.D., M.P.H.

HISTORY AND PHYSICAL
- ~20% of HIV-infected infants develop rapidly progressive disease:
  > Profound immunosuppression
  > Encephalopathy
  > Opportunistic infections
  > Malnutrition
- Most have more slowly progressive disease; may present with:
  > Adenopathy

> Organomegaly
> Short stature
> Recurrent invasive bacterial disease
> Lymphoid interstitial pneumonitis (LIP)
> Unexplained thrush
- Acute (primary) retroviral syndrome: 50–90% of adol./adults w/in days to weeks after HIV infection; mononucleosis-like syndrome
- *Pneumocystis carinii* pneumonia (PCP):
  > Peak age 4–6 mo
  > Respiratory distress
  > Hypoxia
  > Diffusely abnormal chest x-ray

History
- In U.S., most acquired from HIV-infected mother
- Other routes:
  > Sexual abuse
  > Receipt of infected blood products
  > Sexual transmission
  > Injection drug use

Physical signs
- Infants not distinguishable by physical exam
- Exam of older children depends on presentations noted above

TESTS
- All infants born to HIV-seropositive mothers will be seropositive; maternal antibody disappears by age 18 mo
- Viral test (PCR or viral culture) at minimum:
  > Before age 48 h (not cord blood; possible false-positives)
  > At age 1–2 mo
  > At age 3–6 mo
  > 2 separate (+) tests required for diagnosis
  > 2 (–) tests, one at age >1 mo and one at age >4 mo, establish absence of infection
- After age 18 mo: Dx by HIV serology
- Viral load after age 1 mo: predicts pace of disease progression
- T-helper (CD4+) lymphocyte counts:
  > Higher in normal infants than adults
  > Decline to adult levels by age 6
- IgG: elevated in most infected children; some with rapid progression are hypogammaglobulinemic
- CMV serology/urine culture

■ Syphilis serology
■ ECG, echocardiogram
■ Head CT
■ Ophthalmologic eval.

DIFFERENTIAL DIAGNOSIS
■ Congenital immunodeficiency
■ HIV-2 infection

MANAGEMENT
■ HIV counseling & testing for all pregnant women
■ Maternal-child transmission rates:
  ➣ Average 25% in absence of maternal treatment
  ➣ Prenatal, intrapartum, & postpartum treatment (of infant) w/ AZT alone reduces transmission rate to 8%
  ➣ Highly active antiretroviral therapy (HAART) can reduce rate further
  ➣ Even if mother receives no antiretroviral drugs, treating newborn w/in 48 h of birth can reduce transmission rate
■ Breastfeeding increases transmission rate
■ Immunizations:
  ➣ Adhere to regular childhood schedule, incl. inactivated poliovirus vaccine & pneumococcal conjugate vaccine
  ➣ Add influenza vaccine from age 6 mo
  ➣ Varicella vaccine contraindicated
  ➣ Response to vaccine unreliable; prophylaxis for HIV-infected children exposed to vaccine-preventable disease

SPECIFIC THERAPY
■ Prophylactic antiretroviral therapy from birth to 6 wk or until Dx made
■ Begin HAART:
  ➣ As soon as Dx made in infant
  ➣ For age >1 yr if clinically symptomatic or w/ moderate-severe immunosuppression
  ➣ If >1 yr & asymptomatic: initiate therapy or monitor & begin therapy when viral load high or rising, CD4+ count declining, or clinical symptoms develop
■ Theoretical benefits to initiating HAART in acute (primary) HIV infection
■ Poor adherence leads to viral resistance
■ Suggested initial regimen: 2 reverse transcriptase inhibitors (RTIs) & 1 protease inhibitor (PI) or nonnucleoside reverse transcriptase inhibitor (NNRTI)

- Goal of HAART: suppression of viral load below detectable limits
- Rising viral load or failure to suppress by >1 log from baseline by 8–12 wks:
  - Development of viral resistance or lack of adherence
  - Testing of genotypic resistance may be helpful
  - Consider change of therapy
- Prophylaxis against PCP:
  - All infants born to HIV-infected mothers from age 4–6 wks to age 1 y or until Dx of absence of HIV infection is made
  - First choice: co-trimoxazole
  - Alternatives:
    - Dapsone
    - Atovaquone
    - Inhaled or IV pentamidine
  - Age 1–5 yr: begin at CD4+ count <500 or <15%
  - Age >6 yr: begin at CD4+ count <200 or <15%
- Advanced disease (CD4+ count <50 in child age >6 yr): consider prophylaxis against CMV w/ oral ganciclovir and *Mycobacterium avium* complex (MAC) w/ clarithromycin or azithromycin

FOLLOW-UP
- Determine viral load and T-cell subset levels q 3–4 mo
- Monitor CBC, electrolytes, liver function, renal function q3–4 mo
- Monitor growth & development
- Ophthalmologic exam q6 mo if CMV-positive or advanced immunodeficiency
- Repeat CMV serology or urine culture q12 mo if initially negative
- PPD testing at age 3–9 mo, then q2–3 yr at minimum, preferably annually

COMPLICATIONS AND PROGNOSIS
- Opportunistic infections:
  - Candidiasis
  - PCP
  - Cryptosporidiosis
  - CMV retinitis
  - MAC
  - Histoplasmosis
  - Toxoplasmosis
- Lymphoid interstitial pneumonitis
- Anemia, neutropenia, thrombocytopenia
- Recurrent respiratory infections

- Encephalopathy
- Nephropathy
- Cardiomyopathy
- Hepatitis
- Herpes zoster
- Neoplasms:
  - Burkitt's lymphoma
  - CNS lymphoma
- Parotitis
- Dermatitis
- Infants w/ rapidly progressive disease rarely survive beyond 2 yr w/o HAART
- Median survival:
  - Pre-HAART: 8–9 yr
  - HAART: long-term survival rate still unknown

HEAD TRAUMA

SCOT BATEMAN, M.D.

HISTORY AND PHYSICAL

History
- Mechanism of injury (height of fall, speed, surface)
- Loss of consciousness
- Vomiting
- Change in behavior, lethargy, irritability
- Seizures

Physical signs
- Increased ICP suggested by hypertension or bradycardia, full fontanel, or papilledema
- Hemorrhages on retinal exam
- Localized scalp hematoma or evidence of "step-off" (skull fracture)
- Lacerations or abrasions
- Inability to abduct eye (CN VI)
- Dilated pupil (CN III)
- CSF otorrhea or rhinorrhea, Battle sign, raccoon eyes, hemotympanum (basilar skull fracture)

TESTS
- Skull films:
  - Age <2 yr and fall at least 3 ft

➤ Suspected depressed fracture or unexplained cephalohematoma (unless pt meets criteria for CT)
■ Head CT if:
➤ Glasgow Coma Scale (GCS) < 12
➤ Focal neurologic exam
➤ LOC >15 min
➤ Seizure
➤ Definite depressed fracture
➤ Basilar skull fracture
➤ Persistent vomiting
➤ Age <2 yr w/ skull fracture
■ Skeletal survey for suspected child abuse

DIFFERENTIAL DIAGNOSIS
■ Soft tissue injury
■ Skull fracture
■ Intracranial injury
■ Child abuse

MANAGEMENT
■ Establish airway, breathing, & circulation
■ Stabilize neck
■ Serial neurologic exams and neurosurgical involvement
■ Head of bed at >30°
■ Avoid hyperthermia
■ If sports-related, avoid return to activity until cleared

SPECIFIC THERAPY
■ ICP monitoring for GCS <8
■ Neurosurgical drainage of expanding epidural hematoma
■ Mannitol:
➤ Use acutely for suspected expanding bleed
➤ Not helpful for diffuse injury
■ Elevation for depressed skull fracture >0.5 cm
■ Observation for basilar skull fractures:
➤ No prophylactic antibiotics
➤ 80% of CSF drainage stops w/in 72 h

FOLLOW-UP
■ If initial CT not performed: close observation for 24 h
■ Negative CT: discharge home
■ Positive CT:

- ➤ Neurosurgical consult
- ➤ Repeat CT in 12–24 h
- ■ Skull fracture: may require repeat skull x-ray 3 mo after injury to identify potential leptomeningeal cyst

COMPLICATIONS AND PROGNOSIS
- ■ Post-concussive syndrome:
    - ➤ Memory impairment, headaches, difficulty concentrating
    - ➤ May lead to school difficulty
- ■ Impact seizure (at time of event): no long-term significance
- ■ Early post-traumatic seizure <7 d after head injury: 25% recur
- ■ Late post-traumatic seizure >7 d after head injury: 75% recur

HEADACHES

FRANCIS J. DIMARIO JR. M.D.

HISTORY AND PHYSICAL

History
- ■ Single or multiple types
- ■ Course:
    - ➤ Acute recurrent
    - ➤ Chronic progressive
    - ➤ Chronic nonprogressive
- ■ Pain:
    - ➤ Prodrome
    - ➤ Aura
    - ➤ Quality
    - ➤ Palliatives
    - ➤ Triggers
    - ➤ Radiation
    - ➤ Severity
    - ➤ Location
    - ➤ Timing
- ■ Associated symptoms:
    - ➤ Scotoma
    - ➤ Nausea
    - ➤ Pallor
    - ➤ Photophobia
    - ➤ Sonophobia

- Other neurologic symptoms:
  - ➤ Vertigo
  - ➤ Aphasia
  - ➤ Visual hallucinations
  - ➤ Hemiparesis
- Family Hx

Physical signs
- Symptoms of increased ICP:
  - ➤ Papilledema
  - ➤ CN VI palsy
  - ➤ Meningismus
- Local processes in head & neck
- Signs of systemic disease, trauma
- Neurologic deficits

TESTS
- No routine tests
- Head CT (trauma, increased ICP, or subarachnoid bleed)
- Lumbar puncture (meningitis, papilledema w/o mass, or subarachnoid bleed)
- Brain MRI (mass, brain edema, or vascular lesion)

DIFFERENTIAL DIAGNOSIS
- Migraine +/− aura
- Muscle contraction headache
- Somatoform disorder
- Pseudotumor cerebri:
  - ➤ Normal imaging/CSF
  - ➤ Elevated ICP
- Intracranial mass
- Meningitis
- CNS leukemia
- Headache with systemic disease

MANAGEMENT
- Exclude elevated ICP, meningitis, systemic disease
- Acute symptomatic therapy
- Chronic preventive therapy
- Treat underlying etiology

SPECIFIC THERAPY
Migraine
- First-line drugs:

> NSAIDs
> Antiemetics
- Specific abortive therapy:
  > Selective serotonin receptor agonists:
    - Sumatriptan
    - Zolmitriptan
    - Naratriptan
    - Dihydroergotamine (adolescents)
- Sleep induction:
  > Analgesics + sedative: butalbital, caffeine, & aspirin/acetamino-phen
- Recurrent migraine >3×/mo: consider preventive Rx:
  > Tricyclic antidepressants
  > Anticonvulsants (divalproex sodium, gabapentin)
  > Beta-blockers
  > Calcium channel blockers
  > Cyproheptadine (age <10 y)
- Avoid potential triggers:
  > Fasting
  > Sleep deprivation
  > Caffeine
  > Specific foods
- Nonpharmacologic interventions:
  > Biofeedback
  > Relaxation
  > Visualization

FOLLOW-UP
- Evaluate response to Rx w/in 6–8 wks
- Reexamine for new neurologic signs/symptoms
- Neuroimage if evidence of raised ICP or focal deficits

COMPLICATIONS AND PROGNOSIS
- Complications rare
- 40% of children have headaches by age 7; 1.5% have migraine

---

HEMOLYTIC UREMIC SYNDROME

MELANIE S. KIM, M.D.

HISTORY AND PHYSICAL
- Syndrome a triad:
  > Microangiopathic hemolytic anemia

➤ Thrombocytopenia
➤ Nephropathy

History
■ Prodrome: 5–14 d before acute phase
  ➤ Most cases: bloody diarrhea
  ➤ Upper respiratory infection
■ Pallor
■ Irritability
■ Lethargy
■ Decreased urine output
■ Ingestion of undercooked meat, unpasteurized milk, contaminated apple juice or cider
■ Drug-induced:
  ➤ Cyclosporine
  ➤ Oral contraceptives
  ➤ Mitomycin
■ Pregnancy

Physical signs
■ Pallor
■ Petechiae
■ Hypertension
■ Altered volume state:
  ➤ Dehydration
  ➤ Volume overload
  ➤ Edema
■ Lethargy, seizure, coma, stroke w/ focal deficits

TESTS
■ CBC:
  ➤ Microangiopathic hemolytic anemia: Hgb 5–9 g/dL
  ➤ Helmet & burr cells, RBC fragments
  ➤ Thrombocytopenia: <100,000/cu mm
  ➤ WBC: may rise to 30,000/cu mm
■ Urinalysis: hematuria & proteinuria
■ PTT, PT: usually normal
■ Serum creatinine, BUN, amylase, electrolytes, calcium
■ Stool culture or serologic testing for *E. coli* 0157:H7
■ Imaging if indicated
  ➤ Head CT or MRI: may find hypodensity or hemorrhage, esp. in basal ganglia w/ severe neurologic disease
  ➤ Chest x-ray

DIFFERENTIAL DIAGNOSIS
- Thrombotic thrombocytopenia purpura
- Lupus nephritis
- Bilateral renal vein thrombosis

MANAGEMENT
- Determine cardiopulmonary, hematologic, renal, & neurologic status & need for intervention
- Supportive care as clinically indicated

SPECIFIC THERAPY
- Careful fluid & electrolyte management
- RBC, platelet transfusion as clinically indicated
- Dialysis for uremia, uncontrollable hyperkalemia, metabolic acidosis, or severe fluid overload w/ CHF or pulmonary edema
- Severe CNS disease:
  - Plasmapheresis has been recommended; remains controversial & unproven
  - Anticonvulsants for seizures
- Control of hypertension
- Insulin therapy if severe pancreatic deficiency results in hyperglycemia

FOLLOW-UP
- Depends on severity of acute illness & complications
- After acute phase, assess long-term complications
  - If renal impairment/hypertension: monitor frequently
  - If asymptomatic proteinuria: monitor biyearly
  - If complete recovery: monitor yearly

COMPLICATIONS AND PROGNOSIS
- Toxic megacolon: surgical intervention
- Pancreatitis: glucose intolerance, transient or permanent insulin-dependent diabetes mellitus
- Renal failure
- Major neurologic dysfunction in 1/3 of pts:
  - Seizures: 10–20%
  - Strokelike events or coma: 5%
- Cardiac failure from fluid overload or anemia
- Pulmonary edema
- Rare: myocarditis & cardiogenic shock w/ microthrombi, aneurysms

Prognosis
- 65% complete recovery

- 3–5% mortality rate
- 3–5% end-stage renal disease
- <5% severe neurologic impairment
- Remainder w/ asymptomatic proteinuria and/or mild to moderate renal insufficiency

HEMOPHILIA

BEAU MITCHELL, M.D.

HISTORY AND PHYSICAL
- Hemophilia A, 85%:
  - Factor VIII deficiency
  - 1:5,000 males
- Hemophilia B (Christmas disease):
  - Factor IX deficiency

History
- Hallmarks: hemarthrosis & IM bleeding
- 30% bleed after circumcision
- 1–2% intracranial hemorrhage at birth
- 30%: no family history of hemophilia

Physical signs
- Localize site of bleeding:
  - Joints:
    - May develop "target joint" where they repeatedly bleed
    - Assess ROM compared to baseline
  - Intramuscular bleeds:
    - Difficult to localize
    - High index of suspicion
  - CNS bleeds: can present w/ vague neurologic findings
  - Retroperitoneal bleeds (usually in iliopsoas):
    - May present w/ vague abdominal pain & fixed hip flexion
    - May mimic appendicitis
- Assess, sites, & extent of swelling & pain
- Careful neurologic exam

TESTS
- Initial diagnosis:
  - PT, PTT
  - Platelets
  - Von Willebrand factor (vWF) studies (antigen & activity)

- Prolonged PTT:
  - Factor VIII & IX levels
  - Mixing studies: PTT corrected by normal plasma
- Classification:
  - Severe: bleed spontaneously
    - <1% of factor activity
  - Moderate: 1–5% activity
  - Mild: usually no spontaneous bleeding
    - >5% activity

DIFFERENTIAL DIAGNOSIS
- Von Willebrand disease (vWD): typically mucocutaneous bleeding
- Primary platelet disorder
- SLE w/ autoantibody against clotting factors
- DIC

MANAGEMENT
- Locate site & extent of bleeding
- Possible CNS or retroperitoneal bleed: treat immediately w/ 100% factor correction before continuing with evaluation; do not wait for CT results
- Suspicion of bleed that cannot be found: treat, then CT of head & abdomen, looking for CNS or retroperitoneal bleed
- X-ray of affected joint: not usually necessary, but will demonstrate joint effusion
- Hip joint bleeds:
  - Orthopedic consult
  - May need to be tapped to prevent necrosis
- Retroperitoneal bleeds: often large & life-threatening

SPECIFIC THERAPY
- Recombinant or plasma-derived factor VIII or IX Fresh frozen plasma: only if none of the above available
- Hemarthrosis:
  - Hemophilia A: raise factor VIII by 40% (20 unit/kg)
  - Hemophilia B: raise factor IX by 30% (30 unit/kg)
  - If severe, re-treat next day; consider additional qod. treatment
- IM bleed:
  - Raise factor VIII by 40%, treat qod. until resolved (20 unit/kg)
  - Raise factor IX by 30%, treat q2–3 d until resolved (30 unit/kg)
- Mouth bleed or tooth extraction:
  - Raise factor VIII by 40%

- Raise factor IX by 30%
- Antifibrinolytic therapy: Amacar 50 mg/kg (5 gm max) po q 4–6 h for 1–5 d
- CNS bleed:
  - Maintain 100% correction for 24 h w/ continuous infusion
  - Then maintain 50% correction for 2 wks
  - Then 20–30% correction for another 2 wks
- Retroperitoneal bleed:
  - Correct to 100%
  - Then maintain 50% correction until asymptomatic
  - Then maintain 20–30% correction for 14 d total therapy
- Preoperative measures:
  - Measure factor VIII (or IX) level & test for inhibitors
  - Ensure hospital has appropriate factor available
  - Correct factor level to 100% preop, then maintain at 40–50% for 7 d after surgery, then at 20–30% for 7 more d
- Mild hemophilia:
  - DDAVP:
    - IV (0.3 MICG/kg) or intranasal (Stimate)
    - Raises vWF & factor VIII 3–4-fold

FOLLOW-UP
- Hospitalization:
  - Life-threatening bleeds
  - Most bleeds in infants
  - Large joint bleeds that may require immobilization & pain medication
- Minor bleeds: 1 treatment may be enough
- Larger bleeds: reevaluate following day for further treatment

COMPLICATIONS AND PROGNOSIS
- Chronic arthropathy from destruction of cartilage in target joints:
  - Decreased ROM
  - Deformity
  - Eventual fusion of joint
- Aseptic necrosis of hips after hip bleeds
- Muscle contractions from IM bleeds, esp. calf
- Pseudotumor: large, chronic hematoma that may erode through muscle & bone
- Infections:
  - Screen yearly for HIV, hepatitis A, B, C, non-A, non-B, non-C
  - Immunize against hepatitis A & B

- Development of factor inhibitors:
  - ➤ 15–25% of factor VIII pts & 2–3% of factor IX pts will develop inhibitors

---

HEMOPTYSIS

LAWRENCE RHEIN, M.D.

HISTORY AND PHYSICAL

History
- Coughing: blood or blood-tinged sputum
- Fever
- Respiratory distress
- Chest pain
- Choking episode
- Trauma
- Recent travel
- Calf pain or prolonged inactivity
- Medication use
- Hematuria
- Cystic fibrosis, cardiac or rheumatologic disease

Physical signs
- Fever
- Tachypnea, cyanosis, cough
- Abnormal breath sounds
- Heart murmur
- Weight loss, fatigue
- Digital clubbing
- Bruising or signs of trauma
- Telangiectasia or hemangioma
- Blood in oropharynx
- Deep venous thrombosis

TESTS
- CBC
- ESR
- PT/PTT
- Blood type & cross-match
- Sputum culture & Gram stain
- Urinalysis & serum urea/creatinine
- Consider:
  - ➤ Sweat test

➤ TB testing
➤ ANCA, antiglomerular basement membrane antibodies
➤ Bronchoscopy
■ Imaging: CXR not as helpful as CT

DIFFERENTIAL DIAGNOSIS
■ Pneumonia: bacterial, viral, parasitic, & fungal
■ Lung abscess
■ Pulmonary tuberculosis
■ Cystic fibrosis
■ Foreign body
■ Trauma
■ Arteriovenous malformation
■ Pulmonary embolism
■ Tumor
■ Cardiac disease: left-sided obstruction
■ Vasculitis
➤ Goodpasture
➤ Wegener's granulomatosis
➤ Polyarteritis nodosa
➤ Systemic lupus erythematosus
■ Aspiration from other sources:
➤ Epistaxis
➤ Upper airway trauma
➤ Gastric causes

MANAGEMENT
■ Adequate airway & IV access
■ Provide as needed:
➤ O_2
➤ Fluid resuscitation
➤ Blood transfusion
■ Consider:
➤ Bronchoscopy
➤ Embolization

SPECIFIC THERAPY
■ Embolization
➤ Indications
• Persistent hemoptysis
• >300 cc × 1 episode
• >60 cc × 3 episodes

➤ Complications
  • Transient fever
  • Chest or back pain
  • Dysphagia
  • Bowel necrosis
  • Transverse myelitis

FOLLOW-UP
■ Depends on underlying cause

COMPLICATIONS AND PROGNOSIS
■ Depends on underlying cause
■ Bronchial arterial embolization
  ➤ 90% effective
  ➤ 70% minor recurrence
  ➤ 2% major rebleed

HENOCH-SCHÖNLEIN PURPURA

MELANIE S. KIM, M.D.

HISTORY AND PHYSICAL

History
■ 30–50% preceding upper respiratory infection
■ Malaise
■ Low-grade fever
■ Rash
■ Abdominal pain:
  ➤ Bloody or black stools
  ➤ Vomiting
■ Joint pain, refusal to walk
■ Less common:
  ➤ Scrotal pain
  ➤ Seizure
  ➤ Gross hematuria
■ Clinical findings simultaneous or sequential over days or weeks, recur, & involve multiple organs

Physical signs
■ Purpura over lower extremities & buttocks; may begin as maculopapular rash

- Nonpitting edema:
  - Dorsum of hands & feet
  - More common age <3 y
- Guaiac-positive stools
- Abdominal tenderness
- Swelling of joints:
  - Usually knees & ankles, less frequently fingers & wrists
  - No erythema, effusion, tenderness
- 2–38% boys: scrotal pain, tenderness, swelling
- Hypertension

TESTS
- No confirmatory diagnostic test
- CBC:
  - WBC: usually 10–20,000/cu mm
  - Platelets: normal or elevated
  - Possible anemia from blood loss
- PT, PTT normal
- ESR: possible mildly elevated
- Urinalysis: possible hematuria, proteinuria, pyuria, or casts
- Serum creatinine, BUN
- Renal biopsy if nephrosis, nephritis, or renal insufficiency present

DIFFERENTIAL DIAGNOSIS
- Sepsis:
  - Meningococcemia
  - DIC
- Idiopathic thrombocytopenic purpura
- Juvenile rheumatoid arthritis
- Rheumatic fever
- Systemic lupus erythematosus
- Polyarteritis nodosa
- IgA nephropathy

MANAGEMENT
- Supportive therapy
- Monitor for complications

SPECIFIC THERAPY
- Fluid & electrolyte management
- Treat hypertension
- Nutrition

■ Steroids:
  ➤ Use controversial
  ➤ For abdominal pain & to reduce risk of intussusception; inconclusive benefits (in retrospective reviews)
■ Surgery (intussusception or bowel perforation)
■ No known effective therapy for nephritis/nephrosis; immunosuppressives (anecdotal)

FOLLOW-UP
■ Depends on course of disease, severity, complications
■ Long-term follow-up for renal involvement
■ Recurrences usually within 6 wks but as long as 7 y

COMPLICATIONS AND PROGNOSIS
■ 3–5% severe life-threatening GI disease:
  ➤ Intussusception (usually ileoileal, requiring surgical correction)
  ➤ Massive hemorrhage
■ Less common GI:
  ➤ Pancreatitis
  ➤ Protein-losing enteropathy
■ Renal:
  ➤ 10–15% nephrotic syndrome
  ➤ 5–10% nephritis with hypertension; half progress to chronic renal failure
■ Neurologic:
  ➤ Seizure (hypertension or vasculitis)
  ➤ Rare: focal defects
■ <1% mortality from GI, renal, or neurologic complications

HERNIAS AND HYDROCELES

HAROON PATEL, M.D.

HISTORY AND PHYSICAL
Failure of closure of normal processus vaginalis: allows fluid (hydrocele) or bowel/omentum/ovary (hernia) to accumulate in groin or scrotum

History
Hernia
■ 3–5% of term infants, 10% of preemies (35% if <28 wks gestation)
■ R>L; boys > girls; 15% bilateral

- Risk factors:
  - Prematurity
  - Family Hx
  - Abdominal wall defects
  - Connective tissue disorders (Marfan, Ehlers-Danlos)
  - Increased intra-abdominal pressure:
    - Dialysis
    - VP shunts
    - Obstructive pulmonary disease
- Painless "lump" in groin (rarely in scrotum), usually reducible
- Pain, redness, irreducible if incarcerated ("stuck") or strangulated (compromised blood supply)
- Features of bowel obstruction (distention, vomiting), unexplained irritability

Hydrocele
- Painless swelling in scrotum
- Same risk factors as for hernias
- In ambulatory child, swelling worse at night & better by am (communicating hydrocele)

Physical signs
- Hernias more apparent when child upright or crying
- Lump above groin crease (below in femoral hernias; unusual in children)
- Testicle usually felt posteriorly in hernias
- Hydroceles envelop whole testicle, are soft, nontender, & often transilluminate (caution: neonatal bowel can transilluminate)
- Can often "get above" a hydrocele: cord structures are readily felt above swelling
- "Silk-glove" sign:
  - Thickening of cord when rubbed over pubic tubercle
  - Feels like two pieces of silk rubbed together
  - Useful if groin lump or scrotal swelling not visualized
- Ovary often present in female hernias
- Incarcerated hernias usually obvious; sometimes confusing if assoc. w/ undescended testicle

TESTS
- Clinical Dx; may require repeat exams
- US nonspecific (cannot R/O hernia/hydrocele)

DIFFERENTIAL DIAGNOSIS
- Inguinal lymphadenopathy: usually indurated; often painful & red

- Hydrocele of the cord:
  - Confused w/ hernia
  - US may be useful; surgery needed
- Undescended testicle palpable in groin (empty scrotum)
- Secondary hydroceles (from trauma, tumor, infection): no Hx from birth

MANAGEMENT
Hernias
- Repair on next available operative schedule (few weeks)
- Premature infants: usually before hospital discharge ($\sim$2 kg)
- Incarcerated hernias:
  - Reduce by pulling "lump" toward opposite thigh (to clear external inguinal ring); then simultaneously push & squeeze it posteriorly
  - Surgical consult essential if difficult
  - Most can be reduced, followed by operative correction after 24 h (reduced edema)

Hydroceles
- Most spontaneously resolve by age 1–2
- Repair if persistent after that or if accompanied by hernia

SPECIFIC THERAPY
- Operative repair

FOLLOW-UP
COMPLICATIONS AND PROGNOSIS
Hernias
- Untreated:
  - Incarceration (complication rate increased 20-fold compared to elective repair)
  - Intestinal obstruction (10%)
  - Gonadal infarction: torsion of ovary or thrombosis of testicular vessels
  - Gangrenous bowel (3–7%)
  - Increase in size w/ damage to inguinal floor musculature
- Treated (rate <1.5%):
  - Wound infection
  - Recurrent hernia
  - Injury to vas/vessels
  - Testicular atrophy
  - Undescended/retracted testicle

Hydrocele

- Untreated:
  - Progressive increase in size (abdominoscrotal hydrocele)
  - Confused w/tumor if tense
  - Potential for hernia through processus
- Treated: same as for hernias

HERPES SIMPLEX VIRAL INFECTIONS

KATHRYN J. QUINN, M.D.

HISTORY AND PHYSICAL

Neonatal
- Most infants with HSV disease have no maternal history of herpes
- Initial symptoms from birth to 4 wk of age
- Three patterns of clinical manifestations:
  - Disseminated disease (25%) involving multiple organs, including liver & lungs; may not have skin involvement; consider diagnosis in neonates with sepsis, severe liver dysfunction
  - Localized CNS involvement (35%) fever, irritability, seizures, abnormalities in CSF
  - Skin, eye, & mouth (40%)
- Oral/facial HSV
  - Usually caused by HSV-1
  - Results from contact with infected oral secretions, lesions
  - Primary infection can be asymptomatic, or have gingivostomatitis, perioral vesicles, fever, irritability, & tender submandibular lymphadenopathy.
  - Recurrent infection often preceded by prodrome, triggered by stress, sunlight
- Genital HSV
  - Usually caused by HSV-2
  - Primary infection, results from contact with infected genital secretions, lesions
  - Can be asymptomatic or have systemic symptoms of headache, fever, malaise, abdominal pain, aseptic meningitis, painful inguinal adenopathy
  - Recurrent infections usually less severe
- HSV encephalitis
  - Hallmarks: fever, altered mental status, focal neurologic signs
  - Can result from primary or recurrent infection

TESTS
- Tzanck:
  - ➢ Sensitivity varies by operator
  - ➢ Cannot differentiate HSV-1 or 2 from herpes zoster (varicella)
- Direct fluorescent antibody
- Viral culture can differentiate between HSV-1 & HSV-2, results in 1–3 d
- LP: CSF elevated protein, pleocytosis with RBCs; send for CSF HSV PCR
- EEG: paroxysmal epileptiform discharges
- MRI: temporal lobe involvement

DIFFERENTIAL DIAGNOSIS
- Aphthous ulcers
- Streptococci
- Epstein-Barr virus
- Other viral causes of encephalitis

MANAGEMENT
- Acyclovir
- Neonatal: ophthalmology exam

SPECIFIC THERAPY
- Neonatal:
  - ➢ Acyclovir for all neonates with HSV infection; 14 d for skin, eye, & mouth; 21 d for CNS or disseminated
  - ➢ If eye involvement, topical antiviral drops (3% vidarabine, 1 to 2% trifluridine)
- Genital:
  - ➢ Acyclovir taken for primary episode reduces pain & time to healing
  - ➢ Suppressive acyclovir therapy for frequent recurrences (>6X year)
- Encephalitis: acyclovir for 21 d

FOLLOW-UP
- Follow-up for neurologic sequelae necessary

COMPLICATIONS AND PROGNOSIS
- Neonatal and CNS involvement can have severe sequelae
- Oral and genital infections self-limited; recurrences common, but may diminish in severity and frequency

HIRSCHSPRUNG'S DISEASE

SAMUEL NURKO, M.D., M.P.H.

HISTORY AND PHYSICAL

History

■ Symptoms vary with age of pt and extent of disease:
  ➤ Newborn period:
    • Bilious emesis
    • Abdominal distention
    • Failure to pass meconium or abnormal stool frequency
    • Complete intestinal obstruction & perforation of cecum or appendix
  ➤ Infant:
    • Mild constipation that may be followed by acute obstruction, frequent episodes of fecal impaction, or development of acute life-threatening enterocolitis
    • Failure to thrive
  ➤ Infancy to adulthood: mild to severe constipation
■ Enterocolitis the main cause of death; can present at any age

Physical signs

■ Abdominal distention
■ Failure to thrive
■ Tight rectal exam, with an empty ampulla; may have explosive stools when finger is removed

TESTS

■ Rectal biopsy (confirms absence of ganglion cells)
■ Anorectal manometry:
  ➤ Sensitive & specific after age 3 mo
  ➤ Normal finding rules out Hirschsprung's
  ➤ Abnormal: requires confirmation by biopsy
■ Barium enema (single contrast with unprepared colon): transition zone in older children; may be normal in newborns & infants

DIFFERENTIAL DIAGNOSIS

■ Functional constipation.
■ Anatomic obstruction
■ Intestinal neuropathies (i.e., hypoganglionosis, neuronal intestinal dysplasia)

MANAGEMENT

General measures
- NPO
- IV fluids and antibiotics (enterocolitis)
- Correct electrolyte abnormalities

SPECIFIC THERAPY
- Rectal decompression with rectal irrigation and rectal tubes
- Surgical management:
  - Removal of aganglionic segment with pull-through of ganglionic bowel to anus
  - 3 main types:
    - Swenson (rectosigmoidectomy)
    - Duhamel (retrorectal transanal)
    - Soave (endorectal)

FOLLOW-UP
- Post-operative care per surgery

COMPLICATIONS AND PROGNOSIS
- Long-term survival excellent
- Sudden death from enterocolitis may occur years after successful surgical reconstruction
- Higher than anticipated incidence of complications:
  - Persistent obstruction
  - Fecal incontinence
  - Enterocolitis
  - Laxatives frequently necessary
- Despite successful surgery, pts presenting w/ abdominal distention, fever, & diarrhea should be considered at risk of enterocolitis & treated aggressively with support, rectal decompression, broad-spectrum antibiotics

---

HUMAN BITES

FRANZ E. BABL, M.D., M.P.H.

HISTORY AND PHYSICAL

History
- Circumstances of injury (play, fight, self-inflicted)
- Consider physical & sexual abuse

➤ Measure bite marks between the center of the canines to determine if bite caused by adult or child
  - Distance >3 cm: permanent teeth
  - Distance <3 cm: primary teeth
- Hepatitis status of pt & perpetrator
- HIV status of perpetrator
- Tetanus status of pt

Physical signs
- Signs of local infection
- Location of bite; hand injuries at high risk for infection
- Associated injuries to muscles, nerves, tendons, & vessels
- Closed-fist injury assoc. w/ fighting (closed fist vs. teeth of opponent)

TESTS
- Radiographs
  ➤ Deep injuries
  ➤ Possible fracture or joint involvement
- Closed-fist injuries: x-ray for fractures, embedded teeth, & air in the joint
- Wound culture: if infected or presenting >8 h after injury

DIFFERENTIAL DIAGNOSIS
- Animal bite
- Preschool children:
  ➤ Ringworm
  ➤ Granuloma annulare
  ➤ Other superficial oval skin eruptions

MANAGEMENT
What to do first
- Clean wound, sponge away visible dirt
- Irrigate with copious sterile saline by high-pressure syringe
- Debridement:
  ➤ Remove devitalized tissue
  ➤ Surgical debridement for extensive wounds
- Elevate injured areas to minimize swelling
- Human bite wounds should rarely have primary closure:
  ➤ May consider delayed primary closure

SPECIFIC THERAPY
- Tetanus immunization
- Antimicrobial therapy:

➤ Limited data available re: initiation of antimicrobial therapy for noninfected wounds
➤ Consider antibiotics for most human bite injuries, except abrasions
➤ Oral
  • Amoxicillin-clavulanate
  • Alternative for penicillin-allergic pts: co-trimoxazole + clindamycin
➤ IV
  • Ampicillin-sulbactam
  • For penicillin-allergic patients: extended-spectrum cephalosporin or co-trimoxazole + clindamycin
■ Consider inpatient care for:
➤ Infected wounds
➤ Closed-fist injuries
➤ Extensive wounds
➤ Wound involving joint, tendon, cartilage, or bone
➤ Potential poor pt compliance

FOLLOW-UP
■ Return if redness, discharge, swelling, fever, or chills
■ Follow-up wound inspection w/in 24 h
■ Social service evaluation for abuse suspicion

COMPLICATIONS AND PROGNOSIS
■ Bacterial infection:
➤ Secondary bacterial infection
■ Transmission of other infections:
➤ Hepatitis B virus
➤ HIV

Prognosis
■ Infection after human bite: 25–50%
■ Closed-fist injuries especially high-risk

HYPERCOAGULABLE STATE

BEAU MITCHELL, M.D.

HISTORY AND PHYSICAL
■ 70% of children w/ spontaneous or secondary thrombosis will have genetic thrombophilia

- 20% of these will be homozygous or heterozygous for thrombophilia mutations

History
- Risk factors:
  - ➤ Family Hx of thrombosis
  - ➤ Prior thrombosis during surgery, trauma, or immobilization

Physical signs
- Depends on presentation

TESTS
- Resistance to activated protein C (APC resistance)
- Factor V Leiden mutation
- Prothrombin mutation
- Serum homocysteine level
- PTT:
  - ➤ Elevated by lupus anticoagulant
  - ➤ If elevated, send mixing studies.
- Factor VIII
- Protein C (antigen & activity)
- Protein S (antigen & activity)
- Antithrombin III (AT-III)
- Fibrinogen

DIFFERENTIAL DIAGNOSIS
- APC resistance (V Leiden)
- Prothrombin mutation
- Increased homocysteine level
- Increased factor VIII
- Lupus anticoagulant
- Protein C deficiency
- Protein S deficiency
- AT-III deficiency

MANAGEMENT
- Address underlying cause (e.g., liver disease, sepsis)
- Take adequate blood samples for APC resistance, AT-III levels before starting heparin
- Make sure baseline PT/PTT normal
- Begin heparin therapy for 5–10 d; keep PTT 1.5–2× baseline (all pts)
- Begin warfarin therapy; overlap w/ heparin for 2–3 days; maintain INR of 2–3; do not give loading dose in thrombophilia
- Alternative: low-molecular-weight (LMW) heparin

SPECIFIC THERAPY
- Depends on diagnosis
- Factor V Leiden, prothrombin mutation, or elevated homocysteine levels:
  - 6 mo initial therapy
  - Prophylaxis for high-risk situations
  - Avoid OCPs
  - Prophylaxis during pregnancy (controversial)
- Protein C or protein S deficiency:
  - 1–1.5 yr initial therapy
  - Prophylaxis for high-risk situations
  - OCPs contraindicated
  - Prophylaxis during pregnancy (recommended but controversial)
- Continue therapy indefinitely for:
  - Homozygous factor V Leiden
  - Compound heterozygous states
  - AT-III deficiency
  - Lupus anticoagulant
  - Cerebral thrombosis
- Risks of heparin therapy:
  - Bleeding; may be decreased w/ LMW heparin
  - Decreased bone density; osteoporosis
  - Heparin-induced thrombocytopenia:
    - 15–25% of adults on long-term therapy
    - Much lower risk w/ LMW heparin
- Risks of warfarin therapy:
  - Bleeding
  - Warfarin-induced skin necrosis from depletion of protein C; rationale for heparin therapy before starting warfarin

FOLLOW-UP
- Monitor thrombosis for response to therapy; adjust accordingly
- Monitor for bleeding
- Test immediate family members for pt's defect (controversial); counsel on risk factors for thrombosis

COMPLICATIONS AND PROGNOSIS
- Homozygous & compound heterozygous thrombophilia mutations: recurrent thromboses; and should be on treatment indefinitely
- Heterozygous for factor V Leiden mutation: moderately increased risk of thrombosis under normal circumstances

HYPERTENSION (HTN)

SHARON E. O'BRIEN, M.D.

HISTORY AND PHYSICAL

History

- Etiology varies w/ age
- Assess for other cardiovascular risk factors & for presence of underlying disease
- Family history
- May be asymptomatic
- Neonate:
  - Indwelling lines
  - Bronchopulmonary dysplasia
  - Growth pattern
  - Renal/urologic disorders
  - May present with:
    - CHF
    - Respiratory distress
    - Failure to thrive
    - Irritability
    - Seizures
    - Feeding intolerance
- Older child:
  - Headache
  - Vomiting
  - Seizures
  - Diplopia
  - Encephalopathy
  - Excessive sweating
- Medications:
  - Cyclosporine
  - OCPs
  - Steroids
  - Sympathomimetics

Physical signs

- Screening: start at age 3
- Appropriate cuff size: bladder width 40% of arm circumference
- BP in right arm on 3 separate occasions; HTN defined as systolic or diastolic BP >95% for age/sex/height

- Signs of hyperthyroidism, mineralocorticoid excess
- Papilledema, retinal hemorrhages or exudates
- Hyperdynamic precordium, displaced LV apex
- Cardiac murmurs, renal bruits
- Diminished femoral pulses

TESTS
- Workup tailored to age/probable cause
- Basic studies:
  - CBC, electrolytes
  - BUN/Cr, Ca, uric acid, urinalysis, urine culture
  - Lipid profile
  - Renal ultrasound
  - Echocardiography
- Selected pts:
  - Abdominal CT/MRI
  - Renal DMSA scan
  - Hormonal studies

DIFFERENTIAL DIAGNOSIS
- Neonate:
  - Renal artery thrombosis or stenosis
  - Renal vein thrombosis
  - Congenital renal abnormalities
  - Coarctation of aorta
- Age >1:
  - Coarctation
  - Renovascular or renal parenchymal disease
- Age 1–6:
  - Renal parenchymal or renovascular disease
  - Coarctation
  - Endocrine causes
  - Essential hypertension
- Age 6–12:
  - Renal parenchymal or renovascular
  - Essential hypertension
  - Coarctation
  - Endocrine causes
  - Iatrogenic
- Age 12–18:
  - Essential hypertension

- Iatrogenic
- Renal parenchymal or renovascular
- Endocrine causes
- Coarctation

MANAGEMENT
- Avoid end-organ injury
- Treat underlying cause

SPECIFIC THERAPY
- Differs w/ cause
- Nonpharmacologic:
  - Weight reduction
  - Low-salt diet
  - Exercise
  - Avoid smoking & OCPs
- Pharmacologic:
  - ACE inhibitors
  - Calcium antagonists
  - Beta-blockers (contraindicated in asthma, diabetes)
  - Diuretics
  - Alpha-blockers
  - Central alpha agonists
  - Vasodilators
- Hypertensive emergencies:
  - Nifedipine
  - Sodium nitroprusside
  - Labetalol
  - Hydralazine

FOLLOW-UP
- As necessary

COMPLICATIONS AND PROGNOSIS
- End-organ injury: eyes, kidneys, heart, brain

Prognosis
- Depends on etiology & level of control
- Essential HTN: excellent if controlled

HYPERTHYROIDISM, ACQUIRED (GRAVES' DISEASE)

ERINN T. RHODES, M.D.
MARK R. PALMERT, M.D., PH.D.

HISTORY AND PHYSICAL
Autoimmune disorder w/:
- Diffuse goiter
- Hyperthyroidism
- Ophthalmopathy
- Dermopathy (rare)

History
- Insidious onset possible
- Nervousness, emotional lability, behavioral changes, deteriorating schoolwork
- Fatigue, weakness, dyspnea
- Increased appetite; weight loss; weight gain possible
- Increased stool frequency
- Heat intolerance
- Disturbed sleep
- Palpitations

Physical signs
- Diffuse goiter:
  - Nontender
  - Smooth, firm
  - Bilateral
- Stare, lid lag, exophthalmos
- Tachycardia, wide pulse pressure, hyperactive precordium
- Linear growth acceleration
- Fine tremor, brisk DTRs
- Skin warm/moist, occasionally flushed

TESTS
- TSH: suppressed/undetectable
- T4 (or free T4): elevated
- TBGI (T3 uptake): elevated
- Optional:
  - T3: elevated
  - Anti-thyroid peroxidase antibody: usually present

> ➤ Radioactive iodine uptake: differentiate Graves' & thyroiditis
> ➤ Radionuclide imaging: nodules; fine needle aspiration if needed

DIFFERENTIAL DIAGNOSIS
- Thyroid adenoma
- Subclinical hyperthyroidism
- Thyroiditis; consider if symptoms <2 mo
- Toxic multinodular goiter
- Exogenous thyroid hormone ingestion
- TSH-secreting pituitary adenoma
- McCune-Albright
- Nonautoimmune hereditary hyperthyroidism: TSH receptor gene mutation

MANAGEMENT
- Emergent therapy for thyroid storm (hyperthermia, high output cardiac failure, disturbed mental status):
  - ➤ SSKI
  - ➤ Propylthiouracil
  - ➤ Steroids
- During pregnancy:
  - ➤ Avoid maternal hypothyroidism
  - ➤ Monitor infant for neonatal Graves'

SPECIFIC THERAPY
- Antithyroid drugs:
  - ➤ Propylthiouracil
  - ➤ Methimazole
- Short-term propranolol for symptom control
- Radioiodine:
  - ➤ When drugs not tolerated or definitive therapy desired
  - ➤ 60–95% cure
  - ➤ Complications:
    - Hypothyroidism
    - Rare: thyroid storm, hyperparathyroidism, worse ophthalmopathy, concern for malignancy/genetic damage
- Subtotal thyroidectomy:
  - ➤ Consider if markedly enlarged thyroid or severe ophthalmopathy
  - ➤ Complications:
    - Hypothyroidism
    - Hypoparathyroidism
    - Vocal cord paralysis
  - ➤ 80% cure, 10–15% recurrence

FOLLOW-UP
- Monitor/counsel: drug side effects
- Monitor TFTs q4–6 wks initially
- CBC (pharyngitis, fever, systemic signs of neutropenia)

COMPLICATIONS AND PROGNOSIS
- Persistent/recurrent thyrotoxicosis or thyroid storm
- Hypothyroidism
- Increased thyroid cancer risk
- Minor drug side effects (change drug used):
  - Skin rash
  - Hair loss, nausea, headache, abnormal taste
  - Arthralgia
  - Mild increase in LFTs
  - Transient granulocytopenia:
    - Continue drugs
    - Monitor for decreasing absolute neutrophil count (ANC), systemic signs
- Serious drug side effects (discontinue drugs, use definitive therapy):
  - Lupuslike syndrome:
    - Rash
    - Arthritis
    - Glomerulonephritis
  - Hepatitis
  - Agranulocytosis/neutropenia:
    - ANC <500
    - Pharyngitis, fever, other systemic signs
    - Consider broad-spectrum antibiotics

Prognosis
- Drug therapy: variable rates of remission ~33%
- Drug dose/frequency:
  - May decrease when euthyroid
  - May attempt discontinuation after 6–12 mo

HYPOGAMMAGLOBULINEMIA SYNDROMES

ANDREW KOH, M.D.

HISTORY AND PHYSICAL
- Recurrent sinopulmonary or skin infection

- May have asymmetric arthritis
- Diarrhea & malabsorption (often secondary to infection)
- FTT secondary to recurrent infections

TESTS
- Immunoglobulin levels: <10% normal
- Absence of serum isohemagglutinins
- Absence of antibody response to immunization
- Serum albumin: R/O secondary causes

DIFFERENTIAL DIAGNOSIS
- Secondary hypogammaglobulinemias: nephrotic syndrome, HIV infection, protein-losing enteropathy
- Combined deficiencies of both antibody & cell-mediated immunity
- Severe combined immunodeficiency
- Ataxia-telangiectasia
- Wiskott-Aldrich

MANAGEMENT
What to do first:
- Obtain tests & immunology consult to confirm diagnosis

General measures
- IgG replacement
- Aggressive treatment of infections
- Prevent chronic lung disease (bronchitis, bronchiectasis)

SPECIFIC THERAPY
- IgG usually given IV: specially prepared deaggregated IgG 200–600 mg/kg q4 wk
- Young children: IM injection if IV Rx difficult
- Adults: subcutaneous IgG can be used
- Side effects: headache, back & limb pain, anxiety, chest tightness, fever, tachycardia, chills, rarely shock
  - Premedicate: acetaminophen, antihistamine, or steroids
  - Anaphylaxis can occur in patients with CVI or IgA deficiency (patients with anti-IgA antibody); IgG Rx without IgA can be given
- Treat acute infection: antibiotics

FOLLOW-UP
- Monitor IgG levels

COMPLICATIONS AND PROGNOSIS

Complications

- May develop B-cell hyperplasia in the gut, manifests as diarrhea & malabsorption; mimics Crohn
  - ➤ Exclude infectious cause of diarrhea: *Giardia lamblia*, *Cryptosporidium*
- Gastric atrophy with achlorhydia can develop in adults, followed by pernicious anemia
- Optic atrophy or ataxia, occasionally evolves into fatal encephalitis
- Dermatomyositis-like syndrome: prominent peripheral cyanosis & myopathy, little heliotrope coloration
- Malignancies: lymphoreticular proliferations, may be EBV associated

Prognosis

- Variable: depends on
  - ➤ Adherence to IgG replacement
  - ➤ Number of infections
  - ➤ Development of complications

HYPOGLYCEMIA IN CHILDREN

DAVID A. WEINSTEIN, M.D.

HISTORY AND PHYSICAL

History

- Normal glucose: 70–120 mg/dL
- Glucose <50 rare even with fasting
- Duration of fast critical (hrs), length of longest fast
- Often history of tachypnea
- Feeding Hx critical
- Lethargy
- Medicines or exposures

Physical signs

- Autonomic symptoms common
- Check for midline defects
- Assess skin pigmentation
- Liver size critical (glycogen storage disease [GSD])

- Microphallus (growth hormone [GH] deficiency)
- Cardiac gallop (fatty acid oxidation disorder [FAOD])

TESTS
- Indications for labs:
  - Glucose <60 if not fasting
  - Glucose <50 if prolonged fast
  - Seizure
- Blood:
  - Draw samples before sugar given
  - Confirm w/ plasma glucose
  - Electrolytes, BUN/Cr
  - Cortisol recommended
  - Insulin if low ketones
  - Consider LFTs, urate, lipids
  - Lactate if <1 y or recurrent
  - GH: low specificity
  - Save 3–5 mL serum
- Urine
  - Check 1st urine for ketones, organic acids
  - Store 3–5 mL of 1st urine

DIFFERENTIAL DIAGNOSIS
- Low ketones:
  - Hyperinsulinism
  - FAOD
- Moderate-large ketones:
  - GSD
  - FAOD
  - Adrenal insufficiency
  - GH deficiency
  - Panhypopituitarism

MANAGEMENT
- Get critical sample first
- Glucose bolus (IV/PO)
- IVF w/ 10% dextrose

SPECIFIC THERAPY
- Bolus: 0.3 mg/kg glucose
- Hyperinsulinism/diabetes:
  - Glucagon 0.02 mg/kg IM

- ➤ May cause vomiting
- ➤ No effect if GSD or FAOD
- ■ Run IVF 10% dextrose at 1.25 × maintenance

FOLLOW-UP
- ■ Check sugar in 1 h
- ■ Avoid all fasting
- ■ Specialist referral:
  - ➤ Recurrent hypoglycemia
  - ➤ Plasma glucose <40 mg/dL
  - ➤ Seizure/lethargy
  - ➤ Hypoglycemia not w/ fasting

COMPLICATIONS AND PROGNOSIS
- ■ FAOD must be excluded; may cause sudden death
- ■ Glucose <45: probable pathology
- ■ Recurrent hypoglycemia:
  - ➤ Seizures
  - ➤ Developmental delay
  - ➤ Lethargy
  - ➤ Possible death
- ■ Prognosis excellent if diagnosed

HYPOTHERMIA

ROBERT VINCI, M.D.

HISTORY AND PHYSICAL

History
- ■ Core body temperature <95°F
- ■ Prolonged exposure to cold, wind
- ■ History of hypothyroidism
- ■ Drug use: barbiturates, alcohol, phenothiazines

Physical signs
- ■ Measure core body temperature with hypothermia probe
- ■ Heart rate, blood pressure
- ■ Examine exposed areas for frostbite

TESTS
- ■ Pulse oximetry

- ECG:
  - Arrhythmia
  - Delayed repolarization manifested by J-wave
- ABG, serum electrolytes, glucose
- Renal function tests
- CBC, platelets, clotting studies
- Serum amylase
- Ethanol level & drug screen
- Chest x-ray (aspiration pneumonia)

DIFFERENTIAL DIAGNOSIS
- Sepsis
- Hypothyroidism
- Drug overdose

MANAGEMENT
What to do first
- Confirm hypothermia by measuring core body temperature
- Remove from cold environment
- Remove wet clothes

General measures
- Warm pt
- Supplemental heated oxygen
- Do not break intact blisters
- IV fluids
- Nasogastric tube if gastric distention
- CPR if no pulse or non-perfusing rhythm (i.e., ventricular fibrillation)

SPECIFIC THERAPY
- Rewarming technique:
  - Mild hypothermia: passive external rewarming by covering with insulating material
  - Moderate hypothermia:
    - Active external rewarming with Bear Hugger wrap, warming blankets, heating lamps
    - Not to be used alone if hypothermia occurred over 24 h
  - Severe hypothermia:
    - Active internal rewarming with warm oxygen, IV fluids, possible lavage of peritoneal & chest cavity
    - May also use cardiac bypass
- Frostbite:
  - Meticulous wound care

➤ Elevate injured area
➤ Immerse involved extremities in warm-water bath (104°F)
➤ Avoid re-injury to frostbite areas

FOLLOW-UP
■ Reassess as rewarming is begun
■ Examine frostbite areas for infection

COMPLICATIONS AND PROGNOSIS
■ Excellent for most children with mild hypothermia
■ Frostbite areas chronically sensitive to cold
■ Bony infarcts in digits; require long-term follow-up

HYPOTHYROIDISM

KEVIN STRAUSS, M.D.

HISTORY AND PHYSICAL
■ Most appear normal at birth: 10% diagnosed based on clinical findings
■ Neonate/infant:
  ➤ Prolonged jaundice
  ➤ Poor feeding
  ➤ Hypotonia
  ➤ Hoarse cry
  ➤ Constipation
  ➤ Lethargy
  ➤ Large anterior fontanel, delayed bone maturation
  ➤ Umbilical hernia, abdominal distention
  ➤ Large tongue
■ Children:
  ➤ Tiredness, weakness
  ➤ Cold intolerance
  ➤ Hair loss
  ➤ Constipation
  ➤ Weight gain despite poor appetite
  ➤ Dyspnea
  ➤ Hearing problem
  ➤ Memory disturbances
  ➤ Voice change
  ➤ Menorrhagia, oligomenorrhea, amenorrhea
  ➤ Dry cool skin, cool peripheral extremities

➤ Puffy hands, feet, face (myxedema)
➤ Peripheral edema
➤ Alopecia
➤ Bradycardia
➤ Delayed tendon relaxation, carpal tunnel syndrome
➤ Serous cavity effusion

TESTS
- Newborn screen:
  ➤ Thyroid stimulating hormone (TSH) or T4
  ➤ May not pick up milder cases
- Thyroid panel:
  ➤ Significant age variability
  ➤ TSH (mIFU/mL):
    • 1–4 wks: 0.6–10
    • Infant/child: 0.6–6.3
    • Adult: 0.2–7.6
  ➤ Free T4 (ng/dL):
    • 1–10 d: 0.6–2.0
    • >10 d: 0.7–1.7
  ➤ Reverse T3 (ng/dL):
    • Neonate: 90–250
    • >1 wk: 10–50
  ➤ T3 resin uptake (T3 RU): 25–35%
  ➤ Thyroxine index (T3 RU × total T4): 1.25–4.2
  ➤ Thyroid-binding globulin (mg/dL):
    • Neonate: 0.4–4.5
    • Infant: 1.6–3.6
    • Child: 1.3–2.8
- Antithyroid antibodies (selected autoimmune syndromes)
- Iodine deficiency: 24-hr urine iodine excretion

DIFFERENTIAL DIAGNOSIS
- Hypothalamic disease
- Hypopituitarism
- Ectopic thyroid gland
- Hypoplasia, aplasia, dysgenesis
- Inborn error of thyroid hormone synthesis
- Maternal radioactive iodine treatment
- Autoimmune:
  ➤ Hashimoto or atrophic thyroiditis

- ➤ Polyglandular syndromes
- ■ Iodine deficiency
- ■ Disorders that mimic hypothyroidism:
  - ➤ Growth hormone abnormalities
  - ➤ Chromosomal abnormalities
  - ➤ Genetic syndromes

MANAGEMENT
- ■ Hormone replacement immediately after diagnosis
- ■ Infants: neurologic emergency
- ■ Myxedema coma: levothyroxine 100–500 mcg IV, repeated 24 h PRN
- ■ Determine underlying cause, particularly if multisystem or serious CNS cause

SPECIFIC THERAPY
- ■ Iodine RDA 90–120 mcg/d
- ■ Levothyroxine:
  - ➤ Oral daily dose (mcg/kg/d):
    - • Neonate/infant: 8–15
    - • Infant/child: 5–8
    - • >12 y: 2–3
  - ➤ IV/IM: 50–70% of oral dose
- ■ Immunotherapy: selected cases

FOLLOW-UP
- ■ Assess growth:
  - ➤ Head
  - ➤ Linear growth
- ■ Ongoing development assessment
- ■ Assess adequacy of thyroxine therapy:
  - ➤ T4
  - ➤ TSH

COMPLICATIONS AND PROGNOSIS
- ■ Iatrogenic hyperthyroidism from overtreatment
- ■ Delay in therapy:
  - ➤ Neuron loss & developmental delay
  - ➤ Short stature

Prognosis
- ■ Early recognition & adequate therapy: normal growth & development

HYPOTONIA

JANET SOUL, M.D., F.R.C.P.C.

HISTORY AND PHYSICAL

History
- Acute or chronic
- Axial/appendicular weakness
- Developmental delay: gross motor ± fine motor, cognitive
- Seizures, visual or auditory deficits (central etiology, metabolic/genetic)
- Family history:
  - Hypotonia
  - Developmental delay
  - Seizures
  - Miscarriages

Physical signs
- Central (80%) vs. peripheral (20%) etiology:
  - Peripheral:
    - Areflexia
    - Muscle atrophy
    - Marked weakness
  - Central:
    - Cognitive or marked fine motor delay
    - Dysmorphic features
    - Normal or brisk reflexes (DTRs may also be depressed)
    - Distal appendicular hypotonia
    - Persistent primitive reflexes
- Contractures w/ congenital hypotonia (arthrogryposis)
- Acute-onset hypotonia:
  - Vital signs
  - Mental status/consciousness
  - Brain stem reflexes and DTRs
  - Power, sensation

TESTS
- Suspected peripheral pathology:
  - Serum CK, aldolase
  - NCV/EMG
  - Metabolic studies:
    - Lactate

- • Pyruvate
- • Carnitine
- • Amino & organic acids
- ➤ Specific genetic tests
- ➤ Muscle biopsy if needed
- ■ Suspected central pathology:
  - ➤ MRI brain and/or spine
  - ➤ Electrolytes, LFTs, TFTs
  - ➤ Karyotype & specific genetic tests (e.g., FISH 15q11–13 for Prader-Willi)
  - ➤ TORCH titers (neonate)
  - ➤ Metabolic eval:
    - • Amino & organic acids
    - • Lactate, pyruvate
    - • Very long chain fatty acids
  - ➤ EEG (Hx suggests seizures, disturbed consciousness)
- ■ Ophthalmologic exam, hearing test in either central or peripheral
- ■ Acute: tests per Hx/physical exam (neurologic localization):
  - ➤ ABG, electrolytes, BUN/Cr
  - ➤ CBC
  - ➤ LFTs, TSH
  - ➤ Toxicology screen
  - ➤ CK
  - ➤ CSF
  - ➤ Head CT or brain MRI ± spine

DIFFERENTIAL DIAGNOSIS

- ■ Peripheral:
  - ➤ Spinal muscular atrophy
  - ➤ Neuropathy (usually congenital)
  - ➤ Myasthenia gravis (congenital or acquired)
  - ➤ Congenital myopathy or muscular dystrophy
  - ➤ Metabolic myopathy (rare)
- ■ Central:
  - ➤ Genetic abnormalities (trisomy 21, Prader-Willi)
  - ➤ Cerebral dysgenesis
  - ➤ Fetal/perinatal acquired disorders (congenital infection, rarely hypoxicischemic injury)
  - ➤ Metabolic disorders (peroxisomal, mitochondrial)
  - ➤ Benign congenital hypotonia
- ■ Acute:
  - ➤ Head trauma

> Intracranial hemorrhage
> Meningoencephalitis
> Hypoxic-ischemic encephalopathy
> Ingestion, toxic exposure
> Metabolic encephalopathy
> Spinal cord injury or disease (e.g., transverse myelitis)
> Botulism
> Tick paralysis
> Guillain-Barré

MANAGEMENT

General measures

■ Physical therapy ± occupational or other therapies for gross motor/developmental delays
■ Counseling regarding prognosis for specific disorder, recurrence risk if genetic etiology, testing of siblings

SPECIFIC THERAPY

■ Tailored to diagnosis; most causes of chronic hypotonia have no specific therapy & treatment usually supportive

FOLLOW-UP

■ q3–6 mo depending on severity of hypotonia, weakness, or developmental problem
■ Long-term neuro follow-up: to establish Dx in difficult cases (emergence of new symptoms/signs) or resolution of benign congenital hypotonia

COMPLICATIONS AND PROGNOSIS

Prognosis

■ Related largely to underlying etiology
■ Without specific etiology, related to severity of weakness & developmental delay, other features (e.g., seizures, cognitive or sensory deficits)

IBUPROFEN POISONING

SOPHIA DYER, M.D.

HISTORY AND PHYSICAL

History

■ Amount ingested; time of ingestion

- Over-the-counter analgesics/cold remedies
- Other potential ingestions
- Toxic dose >400 mg/kg in acute ingestion
- Toxic dose manifested by apnea, seizures, & change in mental status; headaches & delirium sometimes seen
- Accidental vs. intentional

Physical signs
- Bradycardia, hypotension, meningismus
- Allergic reaction manifested by wheezing, flushing, rhinorrhea, & angioedema

TESTS
- Serum & urine toxic screen
- Aspirin & acetaminophen level
- Ibuprofen level may be obtained at some reference labs, generally not necessary
- Pregnancy test for patients of childbearing age
- Liver function tests & renal function tests
- CBC for thrombocytopenia as late manifestation of ingestion

DIFFERENTIAL DIAGNOSIS
- Salicylate intoxication
- Bacterial or viral meningitis
- Late-presenting acetaminophen ingestion with elevation of liver function tests

MANAGEMENT
What to do first:
- Assess level of consciousness
- Consider endotracheal intubation if obtundation not reversible

SPECIFIC THERAPY
- GI decontamination
    - Use ipecac if patient at home & within 60 min of ingestion
    - Activated charcoal for ingestions of 200 mg/kg or any intentional ingestion with possibility for co-ingestants or inaccurate history
- Benzodiazepines for seizures
- IV fluids for metabolic acidosis

FOLLOW-UP
- Assess renal function and/or liver function in significant ibuprofen ingestions

- Mental health evaluation for assessment of suicidal ideation/depression

COMPLICATIONS AND PROGNOSIS
- Most pediatric ingestions of ibuprofen have minimal toxicity and recover without sequelae
- Delayed development of thrombocytopenia, acute renal failure, hepatotoxicity

---

IDIOPATHIC THROMBOCYTOPENIC PURPURA

SHARON SPACE, M.D., AND HALLIE KASPER, P.N.P.

HISTORY AND PHYSICAL
- Most common in toddlers and adolescents

History
- Bleeding (nosebleeds, gum bleeding), easy bruising, petechiae
- Usually preceded by viral illness 2–3 wks prior in young children

Physical signs
- Petechiae & bruising in unexpected locations (trunk, abdomen)
- Palatal/mucosal petechiae
- Lymphadenopathy & hepatosplenomegaly (uncommon)

TESTS
- CBC with platelet count: isolated thrombocytopenia
- Large platelets on blood smear
- Antiplatelet antibodies not necessary for diagnosis
- ANA in adolescents

DIFFERENTIAL DIAGNOSIS
- Leukemia
- Aplastic anemia

MANAGEMENT
- Control acute bleeding (pressure for nosebleed)
- Do not transfuse platelets
- Education, reassurance

SPECIFIC THERAPY
- Based on symptoms, not platelet count
- Most treated as outpatients

- Hospitalize for:
  - Significant mucosal bleeding
  - Uncontrolled bleeding
  - Severe anemia from blood loss
- Isolated thrombocytopenia & bleeding in skin only (bruising, petechia):
  - Monitor closely
  - No pharmacologic intervention
  - Avoid trauma, limit activity (no contact sports)
  - Consider bike helmet for active toddlers
- Bleeding in mucosal surfaces (nosebleeds, oral mucosal bleeding, menorrhagia):
  - Potential for significant blood loss
  - Treatment indicated
- Corticosteroids:
  - Prednisone 1–2 mg/kg/d for up to 3 wks
  - Bone marrow aspirate before starting prednisone to verify diagnosis and R/O leukemia
    - Bone marrow normal except increased number of megakaryocytes
  - Response in 7–14 d
- IVIG:
  - 0.5–1 g/kg/dose IV × 2 d
  - Adverse effects: fever, headache, vomiting, myalgia
  - Rapid response
- Anti-D:
  - 50 mcg/kg IV
  - If Hb <10: 25–40 mcg/kg
  - In Rh+ patients only
  - Adverse effects: headache, fever, vomiting, myalgia
  - Risk of positive Coombs & hemolysis, causing severe anemia
  - Response time similar to IVIG
- Splenectomy:
  - Pts w/ severe thrombocytopenia (platelet count $<30 \times 10^9$/L) for <12 mo
  - If medical management not effective
  - >75%: complete remission
- Emergent setting: transfuse w/ platelets after IVIG

FOLLOW-UP

- Monitor platelet count 1–2× weekly until recovery

COMPLICATIONS AND PROGNOSIS

Complications
- Acute ITP:
  - More common in toddlers
  - Self-limited illness
  - >75% complete recovery in 6 mo; most w/in 1 mo
  - Complications unlikely
- Chronic ITP:
  - Duration >6 mo; spontaneous recovery after 6 mo uncommon
  - More common in adolescents
  - R/O underlying disease: SLE, autoimmune disease
  - Prednisone, IVIG, or RhO immune globulin PRN for exacerbations
  - Splenectomy may ultimately be required
- Intracranial bleed:
  - <1% of children w/ ITP
  - IVIG; then platelet transfusion

IMPETIGO

GEOFF CAPRARO, M.D.

HISTORY AND PHYSICAL

History
- Usually age <5 y
- Crowding, poor hygiene
- Warm weather
- Minor trauma, insect bite, or varicella
- Honey-crusted, expanding plaque or bulla
- Contiguous/apposing skin spread
- Mild pruritus
- Occasional contact with same

Physical signs
- Well, usually afebrile
- Honey-crusted, oozing, well-circumscribed, mildly ulcerative lesions
- Bullous lesions possible and likely *S. aureus*
- Scant erythema at margin, base
- No significant inflammation
- Minimal regional adenopathy

TESTS
- Usually clinical diagnosis
- Culture for *S. aureus* or *S. pyogenes*
- HSV test:
  - Atypical history and physical
  - Periorbital lesions
  - Immunocompromised
  - Possible eczema herpeticum

DIFFERENTIAL DIAGNOSIS
- Burn
- Abrasion: "tattooing" with gravel, linear arrays
- HSV:
  - Fever if primary
  - Labial margin
  - Tingle/itch
  - Hx of clustered vesicles
- Eczema herpeticum:
  - Atopic
  - Usually ill
  - Eczema distribution
- VZV/shingles:
  - Hx of VZV
  - Itch/tingle/burn/pain
  - Dermatomal distribution
- Cellulitis:
  - More inflammation
  - Intact skin
- Neonatal:
  - Early staphylococcal scalded skin syndrome
  - Group B strep
  - Bullous mastocytosis

MANAGEMENT

What to do first
- Educate contagious
- Careful hand washing

General measures
- Keep nails short, clean
- Cover PRN, esp. in pm, to limit autoinoculation
- Treat itch PRN

SPECIFIC THERAPY

Indications for treatment
- Confirmed clinical diagnosis

Treatment options
- =1 small patch away from eyes: mupirocin ointment tid 7–10 d or until clear
- Many/large areas, rapid progression, ill, or hands/GU/eye/mouth:
  - ➤ Cephalexin 50–100 mg/k/d divided bid/qid ×10 d
  - ➤ Cloxacillin 50–100 mg/k/d divided qid
- B-lactam-allergic:
  - ➤ Erythromycin ES 50 mg/k/d divided tid
  - ➤ Clindamycin 20–30 mg/k/d divided tid

FOLLOW-UP
- Usually resolves with Rx in 2–4 d
- Parent/MD inspection for improvement/no spread

COMPLICATIONS AND PROGNOSIS
- Fever, cellulitis, lymphangitis: possible hospitalization for IV antibiotics
- Ill, febrile, possible hospitalization
- Myositis/fasciitis: hospitalization for parenteral antibiotics
- Recurrent *S. aureus* infections (rare): may require eradication
- Possible post-strep glomerulonephritis (<1%) even if adequately treated

Prognosis
- Excellent with treatment

INBORN ERRORS OF METABOLISM

MARK KORSON, M.D.

HISTORY AND PHYSICAL
- Altered mental status
- Tachypnea (hyperammonemia, metabolic acidosis)
- Hepatomegaly
- Altered muscle tone
- Ataxia or movement disorder
- Abnormal odor in urine, sweat, earwax (aminoacidopathies, organic acidemias)

- Apnea, seizures, coma, death
- Precipitants:
  - Infection
  - Excess protein intake (organic acidemias, urea cycle defects)
  - Prolonged fasting or poor oral intake (organic acidemias, urea cycle defects, fatty acid oxidation defects [FAOD])
  - Fructose ingestion (fructose intolerance)
  - Constipation (organic acidemias)
- Family Hx: Siblings or maternal relatives
  - Encephalopathy
  - Reye's
  - Childhood deaths
  - Stroke
  - Developmental delay

TESTS
- Perform before or during therapy:
  - CBC: neutropenia and/or thrombocytopenia (organic acidemias)
  - Electrolytes, pH, & bicarbonate:
    - Primary metabolic acidosis w/ increased anion gap (organic acidemias, FAOD, defects in glycogen metabolism, gluconeogenesis, mitochondrial diseases)
    - Primary respiratory alkalosis: hyperammonemia (urea cycle defects)
  - Glucose: low (gluconeogenesis, glycogenolysis defects, fructose intolerance, or FAOD [w/o ketosis])
  - Ammonia:
    - Elevated (urea cycle defects, organic acidemias, FAOD, carnitine disorders)
    - Measure in encephalopathy w/o etiology
  - AST, ALT: elevated (metabolic liver disease, possibly in FAOD, carnitine disorders, glycogen storage disease [GSD], mitochondrial diseases)
  - Bilirubin: indirect hyperbilirubinemia initially in metabolic liver disease; then increase in conjugated bilirubin
  - PT, PTT: metabolic liver disease in infants w/ unsuspected coagulopathy
  - CK: may be elevated (FAOD, carnitine disorders, GSD, mitochondrial disease)
  - Lactic acid: may be elevated (organic acidemias, GSD, defects of gluconeogenesis, mitochondrial disease)

➤ Blood amino acids (quantitative): aminoacidopathies, some organic acidemias
➤ Urinalysis:
  • Ketones (some organic acidemias)
  • Hypoketotic hypoglycemia (FAOD, carnitine transport disorders)
➤ Urine organic acid analysis: organic acidemias, FAOD, carnitine disorders, mitochondrial diseases
■ Initial presentation: save & freeze 2 mL plasma, 10–20 mL urine for further testing
■ If inborn errors of metabolism high concern: perform above tests at presentation
■ If suspicion not high but metabolic disease still possible: obtain specimens & freeze for later use

DIFFERENTIAL DIAGNOSIS
■ Neurologic, neuromuscular, GI, or endocrinologic conditions
■ Acute encephalopathy:
  ➤ Urea cycle disorders
  ➤ Organic acidemias
  ➤ FAOD
  ➤ Disorders of carnitine metabolism/transport
  ➤ GSD
  ➤ Defects in gluconeogenesis
  ➤ Fructose intolerance
  ➤ Mitochondrial disease

MANAGEMENT
■ Maintain airway & breathing, monitor for apnea
■ NPO: avoid intolerable substrate

SPECIFIC THERAPY
■ Fluid therapy: 10% dextrose w/ electrolytes at 1.25–1.5× maintenance:
  ➤ Higher glucose solution for hypoglycemia; reduces catabolic flux through defective pathways
  ➤ Hydration: enhanced renal excretion of toxic metabolic products
■ Consult metabolic specialist
■ Primary metabolic acidosis:
  ➤ Na bicarbonate or K acetate
  ➤ Vitamins and cofactors (may bind toxic compounds, facilitating excretion): thiamine (50–100 mg/d), riboflavin (50–100 mg/

d), biotin (5 mg/d), vitamin B12 (1 mg/d), carnitine (50–100 mg/kg/d)
- Treat precipitating factor (e.g., infection, constipation)
- Dialysis: intractable metabolic acidosis, hyperammonemia (5–6× above normal) or coma (if metabolic diagnosis known or highly likely)

FOLLOW-UP
- Monitor neurologic status and vital signs
- Monitor abnormal initial lab test; if hyperammonemia or acidosis, re-test q4–6 h
- Check urine ketones: if initial test positive or if Dx is organic acidemia

COMPLICATIONS AND PROGNOSIS
- Depends on diagnosis & severity, rapidity of recovery & complications from previous crises or chronic exposure to toxic biochemical disturbances
  - ➤ Milder crisis: complete recovery possible
  - ➤ More severe crisis: cerebral palsy, strokelike episode, death

---

INFAMMATORY BOWEL DISEASE (IBD): CROHN'S DISEASE AND ULCERATIVE COLITIS (UC)

ATHOS BOUSVAROS, M.D.

HISTORY AND PHYSICAL

History
- Abdominal pain
- Change in bowel movements, usually diarrhea
- Rectal bleeding
- Decreased appetite
- Fatigue
- Weight loss/growth failure (Crohn)
- Perianal abscess (Crohn)
- Arthritis/arthralgia

Physical signs
- Poor growth (Crohn)
- Digital clubbing
- Oral ulcers
- Swollen lips/tongue: orofacial granulomatosis

- Iritis/uveitis
- Swollen joints
- Erythema nodosum (rare pyoderma gangrenosum)
- Abdominal mass and/or tenderness
- Stool: occult or visible blood
- Perianal tags or abscesses (Crohn)

TESTS
- CBC:
  - Anemia
  - Low MCV
  - Increased platelets
- Elevated ESR
- Albumin: low
- Liver disease: high AST, ALT, bilirubin, ALP, GGTP
- Stool culture: *Salmonella, Shigella, Yersinia, Campylobacter, E. coli, C. difficile*
- Upper GI/small-bowel series
- Colonoscopy (most useful)
- Upper endoscopy (Crohn gastritis)

DIFFERENTIAL DIAGNOSIS
- UC or Crohn's colitis:
  - Bacterial colitis:
    - *Salmonella*
    - *Shigella*
    - *Yersinia*
    - *Campylobacter*
    - *E. coli*
    - *C. difficile*
  - Amebic colitis
  - Henoch-Schonlein purpura (HSP)
- Crohn's disease of small bowel:
  - *Yersinia*
  - Tuberculous ileitis
  - HSP
  - Lymphoma

MANAGEMENT
SPECIFIC THERAPY
- Depends on type, location, severity:
  - Moderate to severe: steroids

> Mild:
- Aminosalicylates (sulfasalazine, mesalamine)
- Antibiotics
> Refractory disease:
- 6-Mercaptopurine
- Infliximab
- Methotrexate
- Surgery:
  > Abscess
  > Stricture (Crohn)
  > Medical failure (fulminant colitis)
- Antibiotics: metronidazole (perianal abscesses)
- Nutritional therapy for growth failure

FOLLOW-UP
- Remission:
  > q3–6 mo monitor growth, CBC, albumin
  > Yearly monitor AST, ALT, bilirubin, GGTP, ALP
- Chronic therapy or symptomatic:
  > Close follow-up
  > Monitor response to Rx & steroid side effects (weight gain, hypertension)

COMPLICATIONS AND PROGNOSIS

Crohn
- Perianal infection
- Bowel obstruction
- Intra-abdominal abscess
- Growth failure
- Osteopenia, compression fractures, esp. w/ steroids
- Hypersensitivity to medications
- Liver disease (sclerosing cholangitis)
- Increased risk of colon cancer: annual colonoscopy 8–10 y after Dx

Ulcerative colitis
- Refractory/fulminant colitis
- Liver disease (sclerosing cholangitis)
- Increased risk of colon cancer: annual colonoscopy 8–10 y after Dx

Prognosis
- IBD: good prognosis, almost all have normal lifespan

- UC:
  - ➤ 30% pts: surgery w/in 5 y
  - ➤ Surgical cure: removal of colon
  - ➤ Subset develop pouchitis after creation of ileoanal pouch
- Crohn's disease
  - ➤ Depends on disease location, type (mucosal, stricturing, perforating)
  - ➤ Up to 30% will require surgery w/in 5 y

INTUSSUSCEPTION

LISE NIGROVIC, M.D.

HISTORY AND PHYSICAL
- Most cases in children age 6–24 mo
- Older children: consider anatomic abnormality
- Most common cause of GI obstruction age <6 y

History
- Recent viral infection
- Intermittent, colicky abdominal pain; pt may draw legs up during pain episode
- Vomiting earliest sign, especially w/o diarrhea
- Fever, usually low-grade
- Diarrhea less common
- Unexplained lethargy
- Blood per rectum (currant jelly stool)

Physical signs
- Signs of shock
- Tender abdominal mass in RUQ
- Peritoneal signs
- Blood in stool:
  - ➤ 40% gross blood
  - ➤ 40% occult blood

TESTS
- Laboratory studies:
  - ➤ CBC with differential
  - ➤ Electrolytes
  - ➤ Stool guaiac
  - ➤ Stool culture

- KUB and upright abdominal films:
  - ➤ Initially may be normal
  - ➤ With progression:
    - Paucity of gas in RLQ
    - Small-bowel obstruction
    - RLQ soft-tissue mass
- Ultrasound: layered-oval mass with concentric rings and reduced Doppler flow
- Barium or air enema: obstructing lesion (filling defect)

DIFFERENTIAL DIAGNOSIS
- Infectious gastroenteritis
- Constipation
- GERD
- Pancreatitis
- Henoch-Schönlein purpura
- Pyloric stenosis
- Volvulus/malrotation
- Incarcerated hernia
- Neoplasm (lymphoma)

MANAGEMENT
What to do first
- NPO
- Fluid/cardiovascular status
- Careful evaluation for peritonitis

General measures
- IV fluid resuscitation
- Replace electrolyte losses
- Nasogastric suctioning
- Surgical and radiologic consults

SPECIFIC THERAPY
- Barium enema:
  - ➤ Barium exerts backward pressure
  - ➤ Reduces intussusceptum
  - ➤ Risk of barium
- Air enema:
  - ➤ Hydrostatic pressure reduces intussusceptum
  - ➤ Higher success rates w/ experienced radiologist
  - ➤ Lower radiation dose

- ➤ Risk of pneumoperitoneum with microperforations
- ➤ Must have pediatric surgeon available
- ■ Air/barium reduction:
  - ➤ Unsuccessful: 10–30%
  - ➤ Complication rate: 1–3%
- ■ Operative reduction:
  - ➤ When enemas unsuccessful
  - ➤ Bowel resection for necrotic tissue
  - ➤ Appendectomy performed simultaneously

FOLLOW-UP
Complications and prognosis
- ■ With successful reduction, most do well
- ■ Delay in diagnosis:
  - ➤ GI perforation, peritonitis, shock, death
  - ➤ Increasing mortality if delayed >48 h
- ■ Recurrence rates:
  - ➤ 10% after enema reduction
  - ➤ 2–5% after surgical reduction

IRON DEFICIENCY

ALAN MEYERS, M.D., M.P.H.

HISTORY AND PHYSICAL
- ■ Most common nutritional deficiency
- ■ Peak age: 9–24 mo & menstruating females
- ■ Iron deficiency anemia preceded by iron deficiency w/o anemia

History
- ■ High risk (25%):
  - ➤ Low income
  - ➤ Premature
  - ➤ Low birthweight
  - ➤ Poor dietary iron intake
  - ➤ Rapid growth rate
  - ➤ Black or Hispanic
  - ➤ Immigrant from poor country
  - ➤ Low-iron formula intake in 1st year
  - ➤ Vegetarian diet
  - ➤ Early (<12 mo) or high cow milk intake

> Blood loss
> Chronic infection or inflammatory disorder

Physical signs
■ Unreliable; blue sclerae & pale conjunctivae

TESTS
■ Hgb:
  > Age 1–<2 yr: < 11.0 g/dL
  > Age 2–<5 yr: < 11.1 g/dl
  > Age 5–<8 yr: < 11.5 g/dL
  > Age 8–<12 yr: < 11.9 g/dL
  > Males 12–<15 yr: < 12.5 g/dL
  > Males 15–<18 yr: < 13.3 g/dL
  > Females (not pregnant or lactating) 12–<15 yr: < 11.8 g/dL
  > Females 15–<18 yr: <12.0g/dL
■ Adjust up for high altitude, cigarette smoking
■ No single satisfactory test for iron deficiency; each of following tests individually too insensitive to be used as screening test:
  > Ferritin: 15 mcg/L at age >6 mo
  > Transferrin saturation: <16%
  > Erythrocyte protoporphyrin: >80 mcg/dL RBCs, age 1–2 yr
  > Mean corpuscular volume:
    • Age 1–2: <77 fL
    • Age 3–5: <79 fL
    • Age 6–11: <80 fL
    • Age 12–15: <82 fL
    • Age >15: <85 fL
  > Red cell distribution width: >14.0%
■ Increase in Hgb of >1.0 g/dL after 1 mo iron treatment

DIFFERENTIAL DIAGNOSIS
■ Thalassemia minor
■ Lead poisoning
■ Recent infection

MANAGEMENT
■ Primary prevention:
  > Encourage exclusive breastfeeding for infants to age 4–6 mo
  > Iron-fortified formula & no whole milk until age >1 yr
  > Iron-fortified cereal
  > Early introduction of meat (6 mo)

- ➤ Vitamin C-rich foods at age >6 mo
- ➤ Premature infants: 2–4 mg/kg/d of iron drops (max, 15 mg/d) age 1–12 mo
- ➤ Limit milk intake to 24 oz age 1–5 yr
- ■ Secondary prevention:
  - ➤ Screen all high-risk infants at age 9–12 mo, 6 mo later, & annually age 2–5 yr
  - ➤ Therapeutic trial of iron in those with low Hgb or any abnormal test of iron deficiency
  - ➤ Assess risk annually age 2–5 yr
  - ➤ Screen all at risk

SPECIFIC THERAPY
- ■ Age <5 yr: 3 mg/kg/d elemental iron drops, given between meals
- ■ Age 5–<12 yr: 60 mg elemental iron qd
- ■ Age 12–<18 yr: 60–120 mg elemental iron qd

FOLLOW-UP
- ■ Repeat screening in 4 wk
- ■ Hgb should rise 1 g/dL
- ■ Continue treatment for additional 1–2 mo
- ■ Reinforce dietary counseling
- ■ Recheck Hgb at end of therapy & 6 mo later
- ■ If no response: evaluate adherence, consider further tests of iron deficiency
- ■ Poor adherence: try alternative preparations (e.g., iron polysaccharide)
- ■ Severe iron deficiency unresponsive to oral treatment: IV iron dextran

COMPLICATIONS AND PROGNOSIS
- ■ Subtle cognitive deficits
- ■ Diminished work capacity
- ■ Growth delay

IRON POISONING

HANAN SEDIK, M.D., F A.A.P.

HISTORY AND PHYSICAL
- ■ History of ingestion

- Common sources:
  - Children's multiple vitamins with iron
  - Prenatal vitamin preparations
- Toxic dose: >20 mg/kg
- Stage I: GI toxicity (up to 6 h after ingestion):
  - Nausea, vomiting
  - Diarrhea
  - Abdominal pain
  - GI bleeding
- Stage II: apparent improvement: (6–24 h after-ingestion)
- Stage III: systemic injury (12–48 h after ingestion):
  - Hepatic injury
  - Hypoglycemia
  - Metabolic acidosis
  - Bleeding
  - Coma
  - Seizures
  - Shock
- Stage IV: late complications (4–8 wks after ingestion):
  - Pyloric or antral stenosis
  - CNS sequelae

TESTS
- CBC, glucose, renal & hepatic function
- WBC >15,000/cu mm, serum glucose >150 mg/dL may predict elevated serum iron
- Serum iron (2–4 h after ingestion):
  - <350 mcg/dL usually non-toxic
  - >500 mcg/dL potentially toxic
- Abdominal x-ray may show iron tablets
- Deferoxamine challenge test

DIFFERENTIAL DIAGNOSIS
- Other ingestions:
  - Heavy metals
  - Alcohols
  - Salicylates
  - NSAIDs
  - Theophylline
- Hepatotoxins
- Shock

MANAGEMENT
- Supportive care: IV fluids
- Gastric emptying
- Decontamination: whole bowel irrigation
- Chelation (IV deferoxamine): excessive iron chelated; produces pink or "vin rose" colored urine

SPECIFIC THERAPY
- Whole bowel irrigation:
  - Polyethylene glycol solution: 0.5 L/h via NG tube until rectal effluent clear
  - Follow-up radiograph to demonstrate therapy effect
  - Contraindication: GI hemorrhage or obstruction
- IV deferoxamine:
  - Continuous infusion at 15 mg/kg/h
  - Continue chelation until:
    - Serum iron level returns to normal
    - Metabolic acidosis resolves
    - Urine color returns to normal
    - Clinical improvement

FOLLOW-UP
- Admit to ICU setting
- Aggressive replacement of fluid losses
- Monitor for hypotension during chelation
- Monitor renal and hepatic function

COMPLICATIONS AND PROGNOSIS

Complications
- Hypotension
- Metabolic acidosis
- Hypoglycemia or hyperglycemia
- GI hemorrhage
- Renal failure resulting from shock
- Hepatic failure with associated coagulopathy

Prognosis
- Serum iron levels:
  - <350 mcg/dL: predict asymptomatic course
  - 350–500 mcg/dL: often stage I symptoms, but serious complications rare

> \> 500 mcg/dL: significant risk for stage III manifestations; follow-up for development of pyloric/antral scarring & subsequent GI obstruction

JAUNDICE, POST-INFANTILE

MAUREEN M. JONAS, M.D.

HISTORY AND PHYSICAL

History
Unconjugated hyperbilirubinemia
- Anemia or other hematologic condition
- Medications
- Stress or illness (exacerbates)
- Family Hx

Conjugated hyperbilirubinemia
- Direct bilirubin >2.0
- Exposures:
  > Toxins
  > Drugs
  > Ill contacts
  > Travel
- Abdominal pain/surgery
- Acholic stool, pruritus
- Underlying disease:
  > Predisposition (gallstones):
    - Sickle cell
    - Thalassemia
    - Hemolytic anemia
    - Cystic fibrosis
    - TPN

Physical signs
Unconjugated
- Icterus
- Pallor
- Splenomegaly
- Conjugated
- Xanthomas, excoriations (pruritus)
- RUQ tenderness, Murphy's sign (cholecystitis)

- Fever (cholangitis)
- Chronic liver disease:
  - Clubbing
  - Splenomegaly

TESTS
Unconjugated
- CBC, reticulocyte count, haptoglobin, LDH
- G6PD, Coombs, hemoglobin electrophoresis
- Bilirubin (total/direct)
- Urine for urobilinogen

Conjugated
- CBC, AST, ALT, alkaline phosphate (ALP), GGTP, bilirubin (total/direct)
- Amylase
- If elevated ALT $\gg$ elevated ALP: hepatitis workup
- If elevated ALP $\gg$ elevated ALT: biliary tract disease workup:
  - Fasting abdominal ultrasound or CT
  - Cholangiogram
  - HIDA scan

DIFFERENTIAL DIAGNOSIS
Unconjugated
- Hemolytic anemia
- Ineffective erythropoiesis:
  - Thalassemia
  - Sickle cell disease
- Gilbert's syndrome (benign, familial, mild):
  - No hemolysis or splenomegaly
  - Unconjugated bilirubin: <6.0, increased with fasting, stress
  - Autosomal dominant

Conjugated
- Hepatocellular disease:
  - Viral
  - Autoimmune
  - Drug-induced
- Biliary tract disease:
  - Cholangitis: fever, RUQ pain
  - Choledocholithiasis: stones obstructed duct
  - Malignancy (obstructive)
- Drug-induced cholestasis

- Cholestasis of pregnancy
- Familial (Dubin-Johnson, Rotor)

MANAGEMENT
- Treat underlying cause
- Stop all nonessential drugs

SPECIFIC THERAPY
- Hepatitis (see "Hepatitis" entry)
- Cholangitis:
  - Antibiotics, imaging
  - Cholecystectomy when infection controlled
  - Stone in duct or dilated ducts: endoscopic retrograde cholangiopancreatography
  - Stones in gallbladder or gallstone pancreatitis: cholecystectomy

FOLLOW-UP
- Depends on underlying cause

COMPLICATIONS AND PROGNOSIS
- Depends on underlying cause

JUVENILE RHEUMATOID ARTHRITIS (JRA)

AMY L. WOODWARD, M.D.

HISTORY AND PHYSICAL

History
- Age <16
- Joint swelling/effusion or 2 of following:
  - Decreased ROM
  - Tenderness/pain on motion
  - Increased warmth >=1 joint(s)
- Duration: 6 wks
- Exclude other arthritis
- Subtype (disease pattern first 6 mo):
  - Pauciarticular (50%): <5 joints
  - Polyarticular (40%): >=5 joints
  - Systemic (10%): arthritis w/ systemic Sx:
    - Fever: 102–105.8°F, 1–2 spikes/d
    - Rash: salmon-pink, maculopapular, assoc. w/ fever spikes
    - Lymphadenopathy
    - Hepatosplenomegaly

TESTS

May be normal

- CBC:
  - Mild to moderate anemia
  - Thrombocytosis
  - Leukocytosis (esp. systemic JRA)
- ESR, C-reactive protein
- Antinuclear antibody (ANA)
- Rheumatoid factor (RF): prognostic X-rays:
  - Joint effusions
  - Joint space narrowing
  - Bony erosions
  - Periarticular osteopenia

DIFFERENTIAL DIAGNOSIS

Monoarticular

- Acute:
  - Septic arthritis
  - Reactive arthritis
  - Trauma
  - Hemophilia
  - Malignancy
- Chronic:
  - Other chronic arthritis
  - Sarcoidosis
  - Pigmented villonodular synovitis

Polyarticular

- Other chronic arthritis
- Systemic autoimmune disease
- Reactive arthritis
- Serum sickness
- Rheumatic fever (migratory arthritis)
- Septic arthritis (unusual to be polyarticular)

Arthritis assoc. w/ FUO

- Infection
- Malignancy
- Systemic autoimmune diseases
- Periodic fever syndromes

MANAGEMENT

General measures

- Alleviate symptoms

- Control inflammation
- Maximize functional status

SPECIFIC THERAPY

Guided by age, severity, & JRA subtype

- NSAIDs
- Corticosteroids: oral, IV, intraarticular
- Sulfasalazine
- Hydroxychloroquine
- Antiproliferatives:
  - Methotrexate
  - Leflunomide Tumor necrosis factor inhibitors:
  - Etanercept
  - Infliximab

FOLLOW-UP

- Based on severity & treatment response
- Ophthalmologic referral to R/O uveitis

COMPLICATIONS AND PROGNOSIS

- Musculoskeletal:
  - Growth disturbance:
    - Leg length discrepancy
    - Micrognathia
  - Erosive damage (esp. if RF+)
  - Ankylosis
  - Synovial cysts
- Extra-articular:
  - Uveitis (esp. pauciarticular, ANA+)
  - Macrophage activation syndrome: potentially fatal (systemic)
  - Pericarditis, myocarditis (systemic)
  - Pleural effusions (systemic)
  - Airway obstruction secondary to cricoarytenoid arthritis: rare
  - Amyloidosis

Prognosis

- Pauciarticular:
  - Musculoskeletal: good
  - 10–20% ocular damage if uveitis untreated
- Polyarticular:
  - RF+: >50% severe arthritis
  - RF-: 20–40% severe arthritis

■ Systemic:
  ➤ Most systemic features dissipate
  ➤ 30% severe persistent arthritis

KAWASAKI DISEASE (KD)

AMY L. WOODWARD M.D.

HISTORY AND PHYSICAL
■ Acute febrile vasculitis
■ Usually age <5
■ 2:1 male:female
■ Leading cause of acquired heart disease in U.S.
■ Diagnostic criteria:
  ➤ Fever 5 d unresponsive to antibiotics AND
  ➤ 4 of 5 findings:
    • Conjunctivitis (bilateral, nonexudative, limbal sparing)
    • Mucous membrane changes (cracked erythematous lips, strawberry tongue, injected pharynx)
    • Changes of hands/feet (dorsal edema, diffuse erythema of palms/soles in acute phase, periungual desquamation in subacute phase)
    • Polymorphous rash (initially perineal, then primarily truncal; nonvesicular)
    • ervical lymphadenopathy 1.5 cm diameter
■ Pts who do not meet criteria for KD still may develop coronary aneurysms
■ Young (age <6–12 mo) most likely to have "atypical KD"; this age group also at highest risk for coronary involvement
■ Pts with other conditions (esp. strep-, staph-toxin-mediated illnesses) may fulfill criteria for KD

TESTS
■ Elevated ESR, CRP, platelets
■ Leukocytosis with left shift
■ Anemia (normochromic, normocytic)
■ LFTs: transaminitis, hyperbilirubinemia
■ Urethritis with sterile pyuria
■ Ophthalmologic: slit-lamp for anterior uveitis
■ Echocardiogram: coronary artery dilation

DIFFERENTIAL DIAGNOSIS
■ Viral illnesses (including echovirus, adenovirus, measles)

- Toxic shock syndrome
- Scarlet fever
- Stevens-Johnson
- Systemic juvenile rheumatoid arthritis

MANAGEMENT
- Acute: anti-inflammatory
- Convalescent: antithrombotic

SPECIFIC THERAPY
- IV gamma-globulin (IVIG): 2 g/kg IV over 8–12 h
- Aspirin:
  - High dose (80–100 mg/kg/d) during acute phase
  - Low dose (3–5 mg/kg/d) until laboratory studies normalize
  - Ibuprofen or other NSAID if ASA contraindicated
- Management scheme:
  - IVIG × 1 dose + high-dose ASA during acute febrile period
  - May require further treatment if fever persists; Solu-Medrol may be considered if still febrile after IVIG repeated
  - Low-dose ASA after patient afebrile for 48 h

Side effects of treatment
- IVIG:
  - Acute allergic and/or anaphylactic reactions
  - Headache
  - Fever
  - Possible blood-borne pathogens
- ASA:
  - Ototoxic
  - Hepatotoxic

FOLLOW-UP
- Urgent if fever recurs
- Emergent for emesis, chest pain, other symptoms of cardiac ischemia
- Repeat cardiac echo 1 wk & 3 wk after discharge:
  - Normal: discontinue low-dose ASA when lab studies normal; follow-up q1–2 yr
  - Abnormal: individualized follow-up

COMPLICATIONS AND PROGNOSIS
- Coronary artery ectasias/aneurysms:
  - 15–25% of untreated pts
  - Highest in boys age <6 mo

➤ Risk decreased 3–5-fold if treated in first 10 d of illness
- MI:
  ➤ Secondary to thrombotic/stenotic coronary disease
  ➤ Major cause of mortality, most w/in 6 mo
- Vascular obstruction (peripheral ischemia, gangrene) Arthritis (roughly 33%)
- Hydropic gallbladder
- Sensorineural hearing loss (rare)
- Recurrent KD (1–2% w/in 12 mo)

KIDNEY STONES

MICHELLE A. BAUM, M.D.

HISTORY AND PHYSICAL

History
- Dysuria
- Colicky pain
- Nausea, vomiting
- Gross hematuria
- Fever
- Passage of gravel, stone
- Drugs:
  ➤ Furosemide
  ➤ Vitamins C or D
  ➤ Ca
  ➤ Theophylline
  ➤ Antacids
  ➤ Pancrease
- Diet:
  ➤ Fluid, milk, protein intake
  ➤ Vegetarian
  ➤ Caffeine
- Recent surgery, immobilization, or fracture
- Family Hx
- UTI
- Urinary tract abnormalities
- Other:
  ➤ Gout
  ➤ Sarcoidosis
  ➤ IBD
  ➤ CF

- Renal tubular acidosis
- Hyperparathyroidism
- Williams syndrome

Physical signs
- Costovertebral angle, abdominal, or suprapubic tenderness
- Fever

TESTS
- Urinalysis: pH, specific gravity
- Urine culture
- Stone analysis (gold standard)
- Random urine specimen:
  - Ca, Cr, citrate, oxalate, uric acid, possibly amino acids
  - If abnormal: 24-h urine collection for Ca, oxalate, urate, citrate, Cr, volume
- Serum electrolytes, CO_2, BUN, Cr, Ca, Phos, Mg, uric acid, ALP (alk phos)
- Consider 1,25-vitamin D, 25-vitamin D, PTH
- Renal/bladder ultrasound
- Spiral CT
- IVP

DIFFERENTIAL DIAGNOSIS
- Hypercalciuria w/ normocalcemia:
  - Idiopathic
  - Absorptive
  - Drugs:
    - Furosemide
    - Acetazolamide
    - Theophylline
  - Renal tubular acidosis
- Hypercalciuria w/ hypercalcemia:
  - Primary hyperparathyroidism
  - Vitamin D intoxication
  - Immobilization
  - Idiopathic
  - Tumors
  - Sarcoidosis
  - Williams syndrome
- Hypocitraturia:
  - Idiopathic
  - Glycogen storage disease

- Hyperoxaluria:
  - Primary: enzyme deficiency
  - Enteric:
    - Increased oxalate absorption (CF, IBD, short gut)
    - High intake of vitamin C, oxalate-rich food
- Increased production of uric acid:
  - Malignancies
  - Metabolic disorders
  - Lymphoproliferative disorders
- Cystinuria:
  - Autosomal recessive defect
  - Inability to reabsorb dibasic amino acids in proximal tubule
- Sturvite: UTI w/ urease-producing bacteria

MANAGEMENT
General measures
- Hydration:
  - Acute: IV fluids
  - Chronic: oral
- Pain control

SPECIFIC THERAPY
- Hypercalciuria:
  - Identify cause
  - Low-Na diet
  - Thiazide
  - K citrate, Mg, phos
- Hypocitraturia: K citrate
- Hyperoxaluria:
  - Pyridoxine
  - Diet
  - K citrate, Mg
  - Thiazide
- Uric acid:
  - K citrate
  - Acetazolamide
  - Allopurinol
- Cystine:
  - Vigorous hydration
  - K citrate
  - Chelators:
    - Penicillamine

- • Tiopronin
- • Captopril
- ■ Sturvite: sterilize urine
- ■ Surgical:
  - ➤ Lithotripsy:
    - • <3 cm: renal pelvis, proximal ureter
    - • Not for stones in distal ureter
  - ➤ Cystoscopy w/ removal, manipulation, ultrasonic lithotripsy: distal ureter or bladder
  - ➤ Percutaneous nephrolithotomy: >3 cm, if multiple, large, staghorns, or anatomic anomalies
  - ➤ Open approach less common

FOLLOW-UP
- ■ Emphasize hydration
- ■ Urine volume, pH, specific gravity
- ■ Random urine solute values (Ca/Cr ratio)
- ■ Renal US: resolution or formation of new stones

COMPLICATIONS AND PROGNOSIS

Complications
- ■ Obstruction: surgical intervention
- ■ Nephrocalcinosis: poor renal growth & insufficiency
- ■ Infection
- ■ Bleeding
- ■ Renal parenchymal injury

Prognosis
- ■ <4 mm pass spontaneously:
  - ➤ >90% lower ureter
  - ➤ >80% upper ureter
- ■ 4–7 mm: 50% pass spontaneously
- ■ >8 mm rarely pass spontaneously
- ■ Recurrence common, particularly in first few years

KNEE INJURY

ELIZABETH CALMAR, M.D.

HISTORY AND PHYSICAL

History
- ■ Mechanism of injury

- Ability to bear weight
- Timing of knee swelling in relationship to injury:
  - Acute effusion (ACL)
  - Slow effusion (meniscal tear or chondral injury)
- Did pt feel a "pop"?
- "Locked knee" or mechanical catch (possible meniscal tear)
- Lateral blow (possible MCL tear)
- Lateral patellar dislocation
- Motor vehicle accident: dashboard injury (possible PCL tear)
- Dislocation w/ major trauma (possible popliteal artery damage)
- Chronic overuse (stress fracture of distal femoral epiphysis)

Physical signs
- Obvious deformity or fracture
- Passive ROM (compare contralateral)
- Active ROM (compare contralateral)
- Point tenderness
- Effusion
- Patella apprehension test:
  - Knee extended, lateral translation of patella; patient flexes quadriceps
  - Dislocator
- Anterior drawer:
  - Anterior translation w/ knee at 45°
  - Tests ACL
- Posterior drawer:
  - Posterior translation w/ knee at 45°
  - Tests PCL
- Lachman:
  - Patient supine, knee at 10° flex, check anterior translation
  - Best test for ACL
- Valgus: tests medial instability
- Varus: tests lateral instability
- McMurray: mechanical/dynamic test for meniscal tear
- Pulses

TESTS
- X-rays:
  - AP & lateral view for all pts
  - Notch view w/ knee at 45° (best for loose bodies)
  - Sunrise view (patellar subluxation)
- Effusion: sterile aspiration

DIFFERENTIAL DIAGNOSIS

- Strain
- ACL or PCL tear
- MCL tear
- Multi-ligament tear
- Meniscal tear
- Patellar tendon tear vs. tendinitis
- Quadriceps tear
- Subluxation of patella
- Fracture (Salter)
- Septic arthritis:
    - Usually fever
    - Tender knee
    - No history of injury
- Tumor: rare

MANAGEMENT

What to do first

- Assess for neurovascular compromise

General measures

- Reduction of patellar dislocation by extension of knee & medial translation of patella
- Knee immobilizer
- Crutches
- Non-weight bearing
- Tap effusion:
    - Cell count
    - Protein, glucose
    - Crystals
    - Gram stain & culture

SPECIFIC THERAPY

- Sprain:
    - Immobilize
    - Anti-inflammatory drugs
    - Ice, compression, elevation
    - Ortho follow-up w/in 1 wk
- Ligament tear or fracture:
    - Immobilize
    - Ortho consult
- Septic joint: IV antibiotics

FOLLOW-UP
- Acute sprains: initial non-weight bearing followed by physical therapy to restore full mobility
- Quadriceps strengthening exercises
- Fracture/dislocation: depends on extent of initial injury

COMPLICATIONS AND PROGNOSIS
- Depend on extent of initial injury

Prognosis
- Knee sprains usually do well w/ optimal initial care

LANGUAGE DELAY

SUSAN O'BRIEN, M.D.

HISTORY AND PHYSICAL
- Delayed words: fewer than 1–2 words at 1 yr, 50–200 words or not putting words together by 24 mo
- Lack of intelligible speech (<50% at 2 yr, 75% at 3 yr, and 100% at 4 yr)

History
- Aggression
- Overactivity
- History of recurrent otitis media
- Family history of hearing loss
- Other evidence of developmental delay (gross & fine motor, cognition)

Physical
- Evaluate speech (stuttering, dysarticulation)
- Evaluate palate & oral structures
- Assess sucking, swallowing, adenoid or tonsillar hypertrophy
- Neurologic examination (low or high motor tone, reflexes)
- Evidence of autism (poor eye contact, repetitive & stereotypic behaviors)

TESTS
- Audiology evaluation
- Consider CBC, lead (<5 yr of age)

DIFFERENTIAL DIAGNOSIS
- Hearing loss

- Global developmental delay
- Sensorineural hearing loss secondary to congenital infection
- Genetic syndrome (e.g., Cokayne, Down, Goldenhar, Hunter-Hurler, Klippel-Feil, Mobius, Pierre Robin, Treacher Collins, Waardenburg)
- Gentamicin toxicity
- Hyperbilirubinemia
- Autistic spectrum disorder
- Developmental language disorder
- Dysarthria (control disorder of muscles needed for articulation)
- Dyspraxia (inability to use the muscles needed for articulation)
- Stuttering
- Lack of stimulating environment
- Depression

MANAGEMENT
- Assess pattern of language delay (receptive vs. expressive; global developmental delay, autism)
- Assess severity of language delay
- Assess home language stimulation

SPECIFIC THERAPY
- Audiology testing
- Language screen (ELM, Denver)
- Identify & treat middle ear effusion, hearing loss, congenital syndromes
- School evaluation (IQ testing, language evaluation, academic evaluation, occupational & physical therapy evaluation)
- Consider genetics, otolaryngology referral
- Consider counseling, parent skills training
- Consider early intervention (0–3 yr of age), Head Start (3–5 yr of age), other special education program
- Consider speech & language therapy

FOLLOW-UP
- 1–2 wk after developmental testing to discuss diagnosis & prognosis
- 2 mo after initial evaluation to review results of school testing & to ensure speech therapy & counseling in place
- Reassess in 4 to 6 mo

COMPLICATIONS AND PROGNOSIS
- Poor cognitive development
- Behavioral problems

LEAD POISONING

SOPHIA DYER, M.D.

HISTORY AND PHYSICAL

History
- Exposure to decaying paint
- Pica and soil contamination
- Family Hx of lead exposure
- Lead found in:
  - ➤ Lead-glazed pottery & cookware
  - ➤ Degrading painted surfaces, esp. windows
  - ➤ Contaminated pipes
  - ➤ Folk remedies
  - ➤ Industrial exposure
  - ➤ Illicit drug use (methamphetamine)
  - ➤ Hobbies (stained glass, furniture refinishing, target shooting)

Physical signs
- Complete neurologic & developmental exam, may show no appreciable deficits
- Chronic abdominal pain
- Developmental delay or loss of developmental milestones
- Increased ICP (lead encephalopathy)

TESTS
- Serum lead level
- Free erythrocyte protoporphyrin
- CBC: screen for anemia and coexisting iron deficiency
- BUN, creatinine, urinalysis
- KUB: radiopaque foreign material consistent w/ pica
- Plain films of wrist or knee: "lead lines," representing growth arrest & zones of increased calcification after lead exposure
- CT for cerebral edema

DIFFERENTIAL DIAGNOSIS
- Viral encephalopathy
- Learning disability
- Mercury toxicity

MANAGEMENT

General measures
- Remove child from lead exposure

- Family education
- Chelation therapy

SPECIFIC THERAPY
- Consult medical toxicologist or Poison Control Center for guidance prior to chelation
- Lead encephalopathy or serum lead level >70 mcg/dL:
  - First give BAL (75 mg^2/d) 6 times/day
  - After second dose of BAL, CaNa$_2$EDTA IV (1,500 mg/m^2/d) via continuous infusion for 5 d
  - D/C BAL after 3 d
  - Further chelation determined by follow-up lead level
- Outpatient chelation performed only when child is in lead-safe environment
- Serum lead levels 45–69 mcg/dL:
  - CaNa$_2$EDTA IV or succimer 30 mg/kg/d (divided tid for 3 d), then 20 mg/kg (bid for 14 d)
  - Serum lead levels 20–44 mcg/dL:
  - Aggressive environmental controls (CDC, AAP recommendation)
  - Oral chelation with succimer or D-penicillamine

Side effects and complications
- BAL: allergic reaction, hypotension, pain at injection site
- CaNa$_2$EDTA: nephrotoxicity, mild elevations of transaminases
- Succimer: mild elevation of AST
- D-penicillamine: nephrotoxicity, possible allergic reaction if allergic to penicillin

Contraindications to treatment: Relative
- Recent lead ingestion (radiopaque foreign body on plain films): may benefit from whole-bowel irrigation before chelation
- Peanut sensitivity: BAL is solubilized in peanut oil; potential reaction in sensitive pts

FOLLOW-UP
- Repeat lead level 24–48 h after IV chelation to assess response
- Monitor urinalysis, renal function
- Discharge to lead-safe housing only
- Outpatient monitoring of lead level to determine re-exposure

COMPLICATIONS AND PROGNOSIS
- Neurologic complications depend on height of lead level, duration of exposure, & response to treatment

LEGG-CALVE-PERTHES DISEASE

DONNA PACICCA, M.D.

HISTORY AND PHYSICAL

History
- Age 4–8 yr
- 10% bilateral
- Intermittent pain in the groin, thigh, or knee
- Family history may be positive
- Perthes-like picture (osteonecrosis):
  - History of sickle cell disease
  - Trauma to the hip
  - Previous infection of the hip
- May have history of toxic synovitis, but direct correlation uncertain

Physical signs
- Limps with ambulation: Trendelenburg gait (abductor lurch)
- Gait may have antalgic component w/ decreased time in stance on affected leg
- Single leg stance on affected side; trunk will shift over leg to compensate for weak abductors
- External rotation of affected side

TESTS
- X-ray:
  - AP film: subchondral fracture
  - Frog lateral film: collapse of "lateral pillar," which correlates with prognosis
- MRI:
  - May be useful in absence of x-ray findings, with strong clinical suspicion of aseptic necrosis
  - Can demonstrate amount of femoral head involvement
- Ultrasound: may show hip effusion but cannot delineate femoral head involvement

DIFFERENTIAL DIAGNOSIS
- Septic hip:
  - Fever, malaise
  - Increase in WBC, ESR, C-reactive protein
  - Joint aspirate with high WBC

- Toxic synovitis:
  - ➤ Painful ROM
  - ➤ No fever
  - ➤ No increase in septic lab parameters
- Skeletal dysplasia: multiple epiphyseal dysplasia
- Sickle cell disease
- Juvenile rheumatoid arthritis

MANAGEMENT
General measures
- Stop activity
- Crutch walking
- Traction for severe pain, limited motion
- Orthopedic referral

SPECIFIC THERAPY
- Focused on ROM and restoration of full mobility to hip
- Physical therapy
- Surgical management an option

FOLLOW-UP
- Continued orthopedic evaluation
- Return to full activity on individual basis
- Depends on extent of disease and symptoms

COMPLICATIONS AND PROGNOSIS
- Osteoarthritis in 70–90% (with 35-yr follow-up)
- Leg length discrepancy

Prognosis
- Related to age at presentation and degree of femoral head involvement: more favorable age <6 yr

LICE

GEOFF CAPRARO, M.D.

HISTORY AND PHYSICAL
History
- Visualized lice/nits (hatched eggs)
- Contact w/ diagnosed pt
- Three forms:
  - ➤ Head (capitis):

- Children, females, urban, crowding
- Mild/no pruritus
  - Body (corporis):
    - Lives in clothing seams
    - Pts indigent, malnourished (rare in children)
    - Papules, pruritus
  - Pubic (pubis)
    - Pubic area, axillae, eyebrows, beard
    - Sexual contact/abuse

Physical signs
- Well appearing
- Nits 2–4 mm, fixed $\frac{1}{4}''$ from base of hair
- Visualized moving lice, yellow nits
- Wood's lamp
- Erythema, papules, excoriation, adenopathy
- Corporis:
  - Hemorrhagic punctum on papule/wheal
  - Inspect clothing
- Pubis: long-legged, crablike

TESTS
- Usually clinical diagnosis
- May identify nits
- Definitive Dx: identify living, 6-legged louse with low-power microscopy

DIFFERENTIAL DIAGNOSIS
- Persistent nits:
  - No movement
  - White nits
  - No pruritus
- Dandruff:
  - No movement
  - No nits
  - Fine scale on scalp
  - Blue on Wood's lamp
- Seborrheic dermatitis (as for dandruff; scale thicker)
- Dried hair-care products, hair casts:
  - Careful history
  - No movement
  - Hair attachments slide off
- Scabies

MANAGEMENT

What to do first
- Confirm Dx
- Educate contagious/fomites

General measures
- Fine-toothed comb removal of nits, wet hair
- Inspection of close contacts
- Alert teachers/day care
- Hot-water wash hats, clothes, linens or place in plastic bag 7–14 d
- Pediculicides for brushes/combs

SPECIFIC THERAPY

Indications for treatment
- Confirmed new infestation
- Recrudescence of prior infestation (not just retained nits)

Treatment options
- 1% synthetic permethrin cream rinse (NIX) ×10 min, possible second application in 1–2 wks
- Natural pyrethrin (RID, A200) shampoo: 2 applications
- Malathion 0.5% lotion: overnight, age >6 y only
- Lindane shampoo/lotion:
  - Requires prescription
  - Risk of neurologic side effects

Side effects and complications
- Sensitization (RID > NIX)
- Occasional skin or eye irritation
- Rare neurotoxicity (pyrethrins)
- Resistant lice:
  - Rx 5% permethrin (Elimite)
  - Consider Bactrim

Contraindications to treatment: Absolute
- Medicine allergy

Relative
- Prior treatment ineffective

FOLLOW-UP

During treatment
- Parental vigilance usually suffices
- MD for recrudescence

COMPLICATIONS AND PROGNOSIS

Frequency/management
- Infrequent excoriation/secondary infection
- Failure rate NIX ×2: 1/20
- Resistant lice may be local/epidemiologic phenomenon
- Body louse historic (in U.S.) vector of systemic disease: relapsing fever, typhus
- If pubis:
  - ➤ Evaluate for other STDs
  - ➤ Consider abuse in prepubertal child

Prognosis
- Excellent if not body louse, impoverished, or immunocompromised

LOWER GI BLEEDING

MARISA BRETT, M.D.

HISTORY AND PHYSICAL

History
- Ingestion of substances producing red or tarry stools:
  - ➤ Iron
  - ➤ Bismuth
  - ➤ Foods, esp. cranberries & spinach
- Bright-red blood per rectum vs. melena
- Vomiting, intermittent crampy abdominal pain, and/or currant jelly stool (intussusception)
- Diarrhea: bloody vs. mucous
- Presence or absence of abdominal pain
- Recent antibiotic use
- Bleeding disorder
- Travel history
- Weight loss/fever (inflammatory bowel disease [IBD])
- Constipation
- Family history of polyps

Physical signs
- Hemodynamic status
- Evidence of acute abdominal process:

- ➤ Distention
- ➤ Tenderness
- ■ Rectal:
  - ➤ Polyps
  - ➤ Fissure
  - ➤ Tags
  - ➤ Hemorrhoids
- ■ Skin exam:
  - ➤ Eczema (milk allergy)
  - ➤ Erythema nodosum (IBD)
  - ➤ Telangiectasias (GI arteriovenous malformation [AVM])
  - ➤ Purpura (Henoch-Schonlein purpura [HSP])

TESTS
- ■ Hemoccult
- ■ Stool leukocytes & eosinophils
- ■ CBC, PT/PTT (bleeding disorder)
- ■ ESR (IBD)
- ■ Stool cultures:
  - ➤ *Salmonella, shigella, Campylobacter, Yersinia, E. coli* 0157:H7
  - ➤ *C. difficile* if recent antibiotic use
  - ➤ *E. histolytica* if travel history
- ■ KUB/upright films to R/O obstruction or abdominal mass
- ■ Urinalysis, BUN/creatinine (suspected hemolytic uremia syndrome [HUS])
- ■ Air contrast enema (intussusception)
- ■ Consider colonoscopy
- ■ Angiography (AVM)

DIFFERENTIAL DIAGNOSIS
- ■ Allergic colitis (infants)
- ■ Infectious colitis
- ■ Pseudomembranous colitis
- ■ Intestinal polyps
- ■ Hemorrhoids
- ■ Anal fissure
- ■ Meckel's diverticulum (painless rectal bleeding)
- ■ AVM
- ■ Intussusception
- ■ IBD
- ■ HUS

- HSP
- Lymphonodular hyperplasia
- Upper GI bleed with rapid transit
- Coagulopathy
- Trauma/child abuse

MANAGEMENT
What to do first
- Assess hydration status
- Treat shock
- Consider blood transfusion

General measures
- Type & crossmatch blood
- Correct coagulopathy
- NPO until diagnosis certain

SPECIFIC THERAPY
- Intussusception: barium/air enema
- Life-threatening lower GI bleeding: angiography/embolization
- Surgical intervention for recalcitrant severe bleeds, polypectomy, unreducible intussusception
- Allergic colitis: hydrolyzed formula
- Infectious gastroenteritis: antibiotic treatment in select cases
- IBD: anti-inflammatory/immunomodulatory agents, IV antibiotics
- Anal fissure:
  - Treat constipation
  - Topical protection
- Persistent bleeding in stable pts: colonoscopy

FOLLOW-UP
- Hemodynamic status
- Hospitalize for any significant bleed; rate of re-bleed unknown
- Treat associated systemic disorder

COMPLICATIONS AND PROGNOSIS
- Complications related to underlying disorders

Prognosis
- Generally excellent
- Mortality rare in children
- Effective therapy avail for most etiologies, incl. anatomic lesions

LYME DISEASE

EILEEN A. KENECK, M.D.

HISTORY AND PHYSICAL
- Tick needs ~36 h to transmit infection

History
- May have history of tick bite (*Ixodes scapularis* & *Ixodes pacificus*)
- Travel to endemic area:
  - Northeast
  - Upper Midwest
  - Northern California

Physical signs
- Rash (erythema migrans):
  - Earliest manifestation: usually occurs 4–20 d after bite
  - Begins at site of bite
  - Red macule or papule, grows to median of 15 cm in adults
  - Annular, sometimes w/ central clearing
- Fever, headache, myalgias, arthralgias, mild neck stiffness common
- In early disseminated disease:
  - May see multiple erythema migrans
    - Occurs 3–5 wks after bite
    - Lesions usually smaller than primary ones
  - May see arthritis (approximately 50%), cranial nerve palsies (esp. CN VII), meningitis, conjunctivitis, arthralgias, headache, fatigue
  - Carditis (usually heart block) rare
- Late disease:
  - Recurrent arthritis: pauciarticular, large joints (especially knees), occasionally migratory
  - Encephalopathy

TESTS
- If erythema migrans: diagnosis on clinical grounds
- Culture of biopsy from perimeter of lesion: often positive for *Borrelia burgdorferi* (spirochete); difficult to do
- Early treatment interferes w/ testing
- EIA most common test; sometimes IFA
- Confirm w/ Western immunoblot.
- High false-positive rate: pts w/ nonspecific symptoms

DIFFERENTIAL DIAGNOSIS
- Positive titers:
  - Other spirochetes (*Treponema*)
  - Viral infections (varicella)
  - Autoimmune disorders (SLE)
- Cellulitis
- Erythema multiforme
- Erythema marginatum
- Rheumatic fever
- JRA, reactive arthritis
- Multiple sclerosis
- Meningitis from other causes

MANAGEMENT
- Early localized disease: oral antibiotics
- Early disseminated & late disease:
  - IV antibiotics if LP positive, carditis present, or recurrent or persistent disease
  - Oral antibiotics for others

SPECIFIC THERAPY
- Early local disease:
  - Amoxicillin or doxycycline for 14–21 d (age >7 yrs, not pregnant)
  - PCN-allergic: cefuroxime axetil or erythromycin for 14–21 d
- Early disseminated & late disease:
  - Multiple erythema migrans: same as for early, but 21 d
  - Isolated facial nerve palsy: same as for early, but 21–28 d
  - Arthritis: same as for early, but 28 d
- Persistent or recurrent arthritis: ceftriaxone or penicillin for 14–21 d
- Carditis, meningitis, encephalitis: same as persistent arthritis
- Prophylaxis: antibiotic prophylaxis NOT recommended after tick bite, even in endemic areas
- Vaccine:
  - Approved for age 15–70 yrs, at high risk (live, work, play in high- or moderate-risk areas; activities may expose to vector ticks)
  - Not recommended for those age <15 yrs, in low-risk areas, or in higher-risk areas but w/ low-risk activities
- Prevention of initial tick bite prevents disease:
  - detaching infected tick w/in 24–36 h should prevent disease

FOLLOW-UP
- Vast majority treated in early stage recover w/ no sequelae
- No proven pattern of adverse outcomes in pregnancy

COMPLICATIONS AND PROGNOSIS
- Untreated: persistent recurrent arthritis
- Up to 10%: severe, erosive arthritis
- Neurologic symptoms occasionally chronic

LYMPHOMA

JENNIFER MACK, M.D.

HISTORY AND PHYSICAL
- Painless discrete lymphadenopathy; elastic, rubbery
- Systemic symptoms:
  - Fever
  - Anorexia
  - Fatigue
  - Weakness
  - Nausea
  - Night sweats
  - Weight loss
  - Pruritus
- Bone pain
- Neurologic symptoms: cord compression or intracranial disease
- Airway compression or chest pain w/ mediastinal disease
- Persistent nonproductive cough
- Abdominal pain/swelling
- Superior vena caval syndrome
- Splenomegaly

TESTS
- CBC, ESR, LFTs, renal function studies, ALP, LDH, uric acid
- CXR
- Lymph node or mass biopsy
- CT: neck, chest, abdomen, pelvis
- Suspected bone involvement:
  - MRI of bone
  - CT or MRI of spine
- Bone scan
- Gallium scan
- Lymphangiogram
- Hodgkin disease: staging laparotomy w/ multiple lymph node biopsies, splenectomy, liver biopsy

- Bone marrow biopsy
- Non-Hodgkin lymphoma: CSF exam

DIFFERENTIAL DIAGNOSIS
- Hodgkin lymphoma
- Non-Hodgkin lymphoma
- Atypical mycobacterial infection
- Toxoplasmosis
- Infectious mononucleosis
- Other reactive/inflammatory lymphadenopathy
- Metastatic adenopathy of other primary tumors

MANAGEMENT
- Oncologist referral
- Radiotherapy
- Chemotherapy

SPECIFIC THERAPY

Hodgkin lymphoma
- Depends on staging & whether systemic signs present
- B disease (systemic signs):
  - T >100 °F for 3 consecutive days
  - Drenching night sweats
  - Weight loss >10% in 6 mo
- Radiotherapy alone:
  - Stage I: 1 lymph node region or 1 extralymphatic site/organ
  - Stage IIA: 2 lymph node regions or localized involvement of extra-lymphatic organ/site on same side of diaphragm
- Radiotherapy vs. combined modality: IIB
- Combined modality
  - Stage IIIA:
    - Lymph node regions on both sides of diaphragm
    - May involve spleen or localized involvement of extralymphatic organ/site
- Chemotherapy; consider radiotherapy:
  - IIIB
  - Stage IV: diffuse or disseminated involvement of 1 extralym-phatic organ

Non-Hodgkin lymphoma
- Monitor acute, life-threatening complication:
  - SVC syndrome

- ➤ Airway compression
- ➤ Tumor lysis syndrome
- ■ Chemotherapy w/ intrathecal therapy for head & neck tumor:
  - ➤ Stage I: 1 site, excluding mediastinum or abdomen
  - ➤ Stage II: 1 tumor w/ regional nodal involvement or 2 areas on same side of diaphragm, or primary GI site with complete gross resection
- ■ Chemotherapy w/ intrathecal therapy:
  - ➤ Stage III: 2 sites on both sides of diaphragm, primary intrathoracic tumors, unresectable intra-abdominal disease, primary paraspinal or epidural disease
  - ➤ Stage IV: any of above w/ CNS or bone marrow involvement

FOLLOW-UP
- ■ Minimum 10-y period:
  - ➤ Year 1: monthly exam, CBC, ESR, CXR
  - ➤ Following years: decrease frequency
  - ➤ TFTs q6 mo if receive radiation
  - ➤ PFTs, cardiac evaluation yearly
  - ➤ CT, MRI, gallium scan of tumor

COMPLICATIONS AND PROGNOSIS
- ■ Radiation:
  - ➤ Acute:
    - • Skin erythema
    - • Hyperpigmentation
    - • Mild GI symptoms
  - ➤ Late:
    - • Height loss
    - • Avascular necrosis of bone
    - • Pulmonary & cardiac injury
    - • Thyroid dysfunction
    - • Infertility (consider before oophoropexy/sperm storage)
    - • Premature menopause
- ■ Staging laparotomy:
  - ➤ Adhesions
  - ➤ Splenectomy: infection
- ■ Chemotherapy:
  - ➤ Acute:
    - • Nausea/vomiting
    - • Alopecia

- Neurotoxicity
- Myelosuppression
- Infection

➤ Late:
- Pulmonary & cardiac toxicity
- Infertility
- Second malignancies

Prognosis
- Hodgkin lymphoma: 70–90% disease-free survival at 5 y
- Non-Hodgkin lymphoma: 80% cure rate w/ chemotherapy

MALABSORPTION

SAMUEL NURKO, M.D., M.P.H.

HISTORY AND PHYSICAL

History
- Chronic diarrhea (>14 d)
- Abdominal distention
- Failure to thrive
- Weight loss
- Correlate diarrhea w/ ingestion of nutrients
- Associated symptoms:
    ➤ Excessive hunger (cystic fibrosis)
    ➤ Thirst (dehydration)
    ➤ Bloating, abdominal pain, discomfort (fermentation)
    ➤ Weakness, weight loss (celiac, Crohn)

Physical signs
- Weight & height plotted against standard curves
- Malnutrition & vitamin deficiency
- Abdominal distention

TESTS
- Screening for nutrient deficiencies or inflammation:
    ➤ CBC, ESR
    ➤ Albumin & total protein
    ➤ PT/PTT
    ➤ Calcium, phosphate, alkaline phosphatase
    ➤ Vitamin levels, if clinically indicated

- Stool exam for pH (<5.5: sugar malabsorption)
- Reducing substances:
  - Usually positive >0.5%
  - Nonreducing sugars (e.g., sucrose) need to be hydrolyzed
- Stool:
  - Ova & parasites
  - Guaiac
- Sweat test
- IgA, antiendomyseal antibody, antitransglutaminase antibody (R/O celiac)
- IgE, RAST milk/soy and other foods
- D-xylose
- 72-h fat collection:
  - Adequate fat intake necessary
  - Coefficient of absorption varies w/ age
- Lactose breath test
- Small-bowel biopsy
- Radiologic contrast

DIFFERENTIAL DIAGNOSIS
- Chronic nonspecific diarrhea:
  - Normal growth
  - No organic pathology
- Most common causes of malabsorption:
  - Mucosal problems:
    - Lactose intolerance
    - Infections, inflammation
    - Bacterial overgrowth
    - Enteropathies (celiac), allergy
    - Congenital enzyme deficiencies
    - Immunodeficiency
    - Secretory diarrhea
    - Congenital diarrheas
  - Intraluminal problems:
    - Pancreatic insufficiency
    - Bile salt abnormalities
  - Other:
    - Anatomic (short gut)
    - Metabolic
- Malabsorption can be limited to one (e.g., lactose) or multiple nutrients

MANAGEMENT

General measures
- Maintain fluid, electrolytes, nutritional status
- Diet modifications to avoid osmotic diarrhea
- Elemental or semi-elemental diets; supplement w/ MCT oil and vitamins, esp. ADKE in fat malabsorption

SPECIFIC THERAPY
- Gluten-free diet (celiac)
- Pancreatic enzymes (cystic fibrosis)
- Elimination of allergen (allergic enteropathy)
- Possibly TPN

FOLLOW-UP
- Careful monitoring of nutritional status

COMPLICATIONS AND PROGNOSIS
- Those associated w/ underlying disease
- Intestinal failure and growth retardation
- TPN-induced liver disease; may require liver and intestinal transplant

Prognosis
- Good in most cases; may require specialized diets for extended time

---

MALARIA

ELIZABETH BARNETT, M.D.

HISTORY AND PHYSICAL

History
- Travel or residence in area where malaria occurs

Physical signs
- Most common:
  - Fever
  - Chills
  - Malaise
  - Headache
- Other:
  - Cough
  - Anorexia

- ➤ Muscle aches
- ➤ Vomiting
- ➤ Abdominal pain
- Change in mental status or signs of increased ICP (possible cerebral malaria)
- Splenomegaly +/– hepatomegaly (more likely w/ chronic malaria)
- Ill appearance
- Pallor

TESTS
- Giemsa stain: reveals typical forms of *Plasmodium* sp.
- CBC:
  - ➤ Anemia and/or thrombocytopenia
  - ➤ Not assoc. w/ eosinophilia or leukocytosis
- Rapid testing methods under development
- Serologic studies: NOT useful or indicated in Dx of acute malaria

DIFFERENTIAL DIAGNOSIS
- Bacterial or viral sepsis syndromes
- Typhoid fever

MANAGEMENT
- Ensure hemodynamic stability, incl. blood transfusion if severely anemic or exchange transfusion if extremely high-level parasitemia and extremely ill
- Consult with malaria expert

SPECIFIC THERAPY
- Acquired in chloroquine-susceptible area: chloroquine
- Chloroquine resistance suspected or confirmed:
  - ➤ If <9 yrs: quinine + clindamycin or pyrimethamine-sulfadiazine
  - ➤ If 9 yrs: quinine + doxycycline or tetracycline or clindamycin or pyrimethamine-sulfadiazine
  - ➤ Alternatives: mefloquine or halofantrine or atovaquone + proguanil or doxycycline
  - ➤ Parenteral required: quinidine gluconate or quinine dihydrochloride; alternative artemether
- Prevention of relapse (*P. vivax, ovale*): primaquine phosphate

Side effects of treatment
- Mefloquine:
  - ➤ Nausea, vomiting
  - ➤ Diarrhea

> Dizziness, disturbed sense of balance
> Toxic psychosis
> Seizures
> Do not give w/ quinine, quinidine, or halofantrine
- Halofantrine:
  > Lengthening of PR & QTc intervals
  > Fatal cardiac arrhythmias
  > Do not use w/ drugs that affect QT interval (quinine, quinidine, mefloquine)
  > Cardiac monitoring recommended

Contraindications to treatment
- Pregnancy (mefloquine, halofantrine)
- Cardiac conduction defects (halofantrine)
- Malaria due to non-falciparum sp. (atovaquone, proguanil)
- G6PD deficiency (primaquine)
- Do not delay treatment in pt w/ compatible clinical picture & travel Hx while awaiting confirmation of blood smear results, esp. in areas w/ infrequent experience reading such smears

FOLLOW-UP
- Monitor hemodynamic status
- Monitor blood smears frequently during acute phase to ensure that parasitemia is decreasing
- Monitor hematocrit; transfuse for severe anemia accompanied by hemodynamic instability

COMPLICATIONS AND PROGNOSIS
- Anemia
- Hypoglycemia, notably in pregnant women treated w/ quinine
- Cerebral malaria
- Blackwater fever
- Tropical splenomegaly syndrome
- Relapse
- Pulmonary edema, shock
- Nephrotic syndrome
- Resistance to antimalarial drugs

Prognosis
- Best w/ early Dx & treatment, worse w/ severe malaria, shock

MALROTATION AND VOLVULUS

HAROON PATEL, M.D.

HISTORY AND PHYSICAL

- Normal in utero rotation and fixation anchor bowel securely to posterior abdominal wall
- Malrotation (either partial or complete nonrotation): predisposes bowel to twist/volvulize because of inadequate fixation
- Midgut volvulus is a surgical emergency: complete bowel ischemia can develop in ~4 h

History

- Symptomatic most commonly in infants: 30% <1 wk, 66% <1 mo
- Vomiting (bilious): in 95%
- Bloody emesis or stools (28%) are late signs: ischemic necrosis
- Grunting, lethargy, dehydration, shock as condition progresses
- Older pts (chronic intermittent volvulus):
  - Intermittent vomiting
  - Colicky pain (20%)
  - Malabsorption
  - Failure to thrive
  - Chylous ascites

Physical signs

- Bilious aspirates/emesis
- Distention infrequent (and late)
- Tenderness; difficult to elicit in neonates
- Relatively scaphoid abdomen in ill-appearing child
- Hypotension and poor perfusion as ischemia develops

TESTS

- Upper GI series (mandatory and emergent):
  - Malrotation:
    - Contrast fills the duodenum & jejunum, which are to the right of the midline
    - Ligament of Treitz abnormally located
  - Midgut volvulus:
    - Duodenal obstruction
    - Beak of contrast at site of obstruction

> Plain film:
>   • Relative paucity of distal gas
>   • Edema of distal bowel if ischemic

DIFFERENTIAL DIAGNOSIS
■ Other neonatal duodenal obstructions:
> Atresia, stenosis
> Annular pancreas
> Duplication cysts or polyps of duodenum
■ Neonatal sepsis (bilious emesis)
■ Necrotizing enterocolitis
■ Other distal obstructions (usually more distention):
> Atresias
> Meconium syndromes
> Hirschsprung's

MANAGEMENT
■ Malrotation without volvulus:
> Fluid resuscitation
> NPO
> Nasogastric tube
> Surgical correction (open or laparoscopic), preferably during same hospitalization
> Appendectomy universal because of abnormal location in LUQ
■ Midgut volvulus:
> Emergent surgical correction
> Resuscitation in OR
> Goal: gut salvage; may require repeat procedures to assess viability

SPECIFIC THERAPY
FOLLOW-UP
COMPLICATIONS AND PROGNOSIS
■ Few complications if treated
■ Recurrent volvulus rare but possible despite surgery (~3–5%)
■ Chronic malnutrition, pain, vomiting with risk of volvulus if malrotation not diagnosed
■ Delay in treatment of volvulus: often incompatible with life
■ If patient survives complete midgut necrosis:
> TPN cholestasis
> Short gut syndrome
> Liver failure

MENINGOCOCCAL DISEASES

JEROME O. KLEIN, M.D.

HISTORY AND PHYSICAL

History
- Exposure to ill contacts
- Signs/symptoms may be fulminant (hours) or insidious (days)
- Initial presentation may be nonspecific: signs of URI or GI upset

Physical signs
- Rash:
  - ➤ Erythematous round flat macules w/ discrete borders occur early; distinct borders, unlike allergic or viral rashes
  - ➤ Initial rash often overlooked as nonspecific or viral
  - ➤ Hemorrhagic rashes (from a few petechiae to purpura to ecchymoses) hallmark of meningococcal disease
  - ➤ In febrile child hemorrhagic rashes should be considered presumptive of sepsis unless proven otherwise
- Meningeal signs: may follow hours after onset of nonspecific or specific signs of sepsis
- Joint signs: direct invasion or immune reaction to organism
- Uncommon:
  - ➤ Pneumonia
  - ➤ Pericarditis
  - ➤ Peritonitis

TESTS
- WBC: normal or low; pt in transition from high to low counts
- Blood culture
- CSF: criteria for lumbar puncture same for any child w/ overt (e.g., nuchal rigidity) or subtle signs (e.g., altered affect)
- Nasopharyngeal cultures: no value; carriage occurs in 1–2% of healthy infants

DIFFERENTIAL DIAGNOSIS
- Nonspecific signs of URI or GI infection (viral infection)
- Hemorrhagic rash (enteroviral rash or noninfectious event [i.e., Henoch-Schonlein purpura])

MANAGEMENT
- Antibiotics

- Maintain hydration, electrolytes, & vital functions if septic shock
- Careful management of fluids if meningitis; avoid overhydration
- Respiratory isolation for 24 h after onset of therapy
- Appropriate prophylaxis of contacts:
  - Rifampin
  - Ceftriaxone
  - Ciprofloxacin
- Meningococcal polysaccharide vaccine: contacts in large-group setting (college dorm, day care) in children >2 y
- Careful attention to skin lesions if necrotic areas appear
- Properdin, complement, & IgG2: to determine genetic susceptibility
- Chemoprophylaxis for close contacts (incl. household, child care, day care center or anyone directly exposed to secretions):
  - Rifampin
  - Ceftriaxone
  - Ciprofloxacin (age >18 y)

SPECIFIC THERAPY
- Penicillin G or appropriate cephalosporin (ceftriaxone, cefotaxime)
- Resistance to penicillins & cephalosporins still rare
- Chloramphenicol if known history of allergy to beta-lactam antibiotics
- Meningococcemia known or suspected:
  - Admit to ICU
  - Burst of inflammatory mediators may follow use of antimicrobial agent
  - Pt may deteriorate for 4–12 h before recovery
- Duration of parenteral antimicrobial therapy for meningococcal meningitis: 7 d
- Steroids: have not been documented to be of value

FOLLOW-UP
- Removed from ICU when vital signs stabilize
- Careful exam of affected areas for skin breakdown, possible need for grafts
- Hearing eval. (meningitis)
- Sepsis alone: no specific follow-up
- Immunization with 4 type (A, C, Y, W-135) polysaccharide: college students, esp. freshmen who live in dorms

COMPLICATIONS AND PROGNOSIS
- Mortality higher for sepsis (25%) alone than meningitis (5%)

- Hearing loss:
  - ~7% of pts w/ meningitis
  - Monitor hearing for possible need for hearing/speech interventions
- Skin necrosis:
  - ~4%
  - May progress to require amputation or grafts

MITRAL VALVE PROLAPSE (MVP)

SHARON E. O'BRIEN, M.D.

HISTORY AND PHYSICAL
- Family history:
  - MVP
  - Connective tissue disorders (Marfan syndrome)
  - Skeletal disorders
- May be asymptomatic
- Fatigue, dyspnea, palpitations, chest pain, syncope
- Asthenic body habitus
- Scoliosis
- Pectus excavatum, carnitum
- Accentuated S1 if prolapse early in systole
- Click
  - Classic: mid-systolic click
  - May be multiple clicks, different times in systole
- Murmur
  - High-pitched mid to late systolic: mitral regurgitation at apex and radiates to L axilla
  - Murmur may be heard at L sternal border when posterior mitral leaflet prolapses
- Click & murmur occur:
  - Later in systole w/ squatting
  - Earlier in systole w/ standing

TESTS
- Echocardiogram: assess mitral valve & degree of regurgitation
- ECG: 1st degree heart block, arrhythmias, T-wave abnormalities

DIFFERENTIAL DIAGNOSIS
- Tricuspid valve prolapse
- Hypertrophic cardiomyopathy

MANAGEMENT
- Subacute bacterial endocarditis prophylaxis if mitral regurgitation present
- Medication
- Surgery

SPECIFIC THERAPY
- Varies w/ severity of disease
- Avoid catecholamines, diuretics, dehydration
- Beta-blocker therapy
- Afterload reduction (ACE inhibitors)
- Mitral valve surgery

FOLLOW-UP
- Generally q2–3 y
- More frequent w/ severe disease

COMPLICATIONS AND PROGNOSIS
- Mitral regurgitation
- Endocarditis
- Congestive heart failure
- Arrhythmia
- Syncope
- Sudden death

Prognosis
- Excellent in majority
- Increased morbidity/mortality increases w/ degree of mitral regurgitation

MOLLUSCUM CONTAGIOSUM

SEAN PALFREY, M.D.

HISTORY AND PHYSICAL

History
- Common viral skin disease caused by DNA pox virus
- Usually no symptoms
- Contact with person w/ molluscum or similar skin lesion
- Lesions develop slowly (weeks to months)
- Usually begin on trunk & extremities

Physical signs
- Tiny, hard, painless, white or pinkish papules
- Central umbilication of lesions when large
- Location:
  - Children:
    - Scattered over body, but most commonly on arms, legs, trunk, neck
    - Usually spares palms & soles
  - Adults:
    - Localized to genitalia
    - Transmitted as STD
  - Immunocompromised: diffuse, widespread disease
- May appear in crops or linear distribution due to scratching
- Signs of secondary infection
- If unroofed, waxy material found inside papules

TESTS
- Clinical diagnosis
- Biopsy:
  - If diagnosis uncertain
  - Intracytoplasmic inclusion bodies
- Consider HIV testing (extensive mucocutaneous disease)

DIFFERENTIAL DIAGNOSIS
- Insect bites: molluscum is slow to develop, nonpruritic
- Varicella: molluscum lesions are hard, not vesicular, and present for weeks
- Warts
- Herpesvirus if lesions in genital area; painful and often ulcerate

MANAGEMENT

General measures
- Avoid direct contact with lesions
- Avoid scratching to minimize autoinoculation and secondary infection
- Reassure pt that lesions will disappear on their own

SPECIFIC THERAPY
- Usually self-limiting; no specific therapy needed
- Curettage for lesion removal
- Cryotherapy with liquid nitrogen

- Cantharidin (7 mg/mL of collodion) applied directly to lesion, repeated PRN
- Topical mupirocin or oral antibiotic (secondary infection)

FOLLOW-UP
- Observe over time for resolution of lesions

COMPLICATIONS AND PROGNOSIS

Complications
- Scarring secondary to inflammation or surgical removal
- Secondary infection
- Local irritation to mucosal surface if lesion located near eye, for example

Prognosis
- Generally excellent with resolution of lesions, which may take weeks to months

---

MUMPS/PAROTITIS

JO-ANN S. HARRIS, M.D.

HISTORY AND PHYSICAL
- Swelling and pain of salivary glands (parotid); 1/3 of cases subclinical

History
- Mumps vaccine status
- One ear; progresses rapidly to other ear

Physical signs
- Mild fever with swelling
- Dysphagia and dysphonia
- Ear displaced upward and outward; obscures mandible ramus
- Inflammation of Stensen's duct
- Pain intensifies with tasting sour liquids (lemon juice)
- Tender, edematous testicle if orchitis
- Testicular pain and swelling 1 wk after parotid symptoms

TESTS
- CBC with differential
- Amylase and lipase (pancreatic enzymes)

- LP, if indicated: 50% have pleocytosis
- Viral culture:
  - Throat washings
  - Urine
  - CSF
- Serology:
  - Rise in mumps IgG titers
  - Positive IgM titer

DIFFERENTIAL DIAGNOSIS
- Bacterial parotitis (*S. aureus*)
- Other viruses:
  - Influenza
  - Coxsackie A
  - Echovirus
  - Parainfluenza
  - HIV
- Cervical or preauricular adenitis (EBV, cat-scratch disease)
- Parotid duct stone
- Parotid tumor
- Sjogren syndrome

MANAGEMENT
- Supportive therapy

SPECIFIC THERAPY
- Antistaphylococcal agents (suppurative parotitis)

FOLLOW-UP
- Parotid swelling resolves by 1 wk
- Orchitis: testicle swollen, tender for 3–7 d
- May return to school 9 d after onset of swelling
- Monitor elevated pancreatic enzymes

COMPLICATIONS AND PROGNOSIS
- Self-limited; complete recovery in 1–2 wks
- More severe in adults
- Neurotropic virus:
  - 50% CSF pleocytosis
  - 1–10% meningitis or encephalitis
  - Rare:
    - Cerebellar ataxia

- • Transverse myelitis
- • Hearing impairment
- ■ Orchitis:
  - ➤ Usually unilateral
  - ➤ Uncommon in prepubertal males
- ■ 50% with orchitis have some testicular atrophy, infertility rare
- ■ Rare:
  - ➤ Arthritis
  - ➤ Thyroiditis
  - ➤ Mastitis
  - ➤ Myocarditis
  - ➤ Glomerulonephritis
  - ➤ Thrombocytopenia
  - ➤ Pancreatitis

MURMURS

SHARON E. O'BRIEN, M.D.

HISTORY AND PHYSICAL

History
- ■ Maternal history:
  - ➤ Infections (rubella): PDA, pulmonary stenosis
  - ➤ Illnesses (diabetes, lupus): septal hypertrophy, VSD, congenital heart block
  - ➤ Drugs (lithium, anticonvulsants, insulin): Ebstein's anomaly
    - • Street drugs (alcohol, cocaine)
- ■ Neonatal history:
  - ➤ Gestational age
  - ➤ Congenital anomalies
  - ➤ Difficult delivery
  - ➤ Murmur
  - ➤ Respiratory distress
- ■ Infant/childhood:
  - ➤ Prolonged febrile illness
  - ➤ Joint swelling
  - ➤ Rashes
  - ➤ Laxity of joints
  - ➤ Stroke, rheumatic fever
  - ➤ Lyme disease

- ➣ Frequent infections
- ➣ Anemia
- Family history:
  - ➣ Birth defects
  - ➣ Congenital heart disease (CHD)
  - ➣ Seizures
  - ➣ Sudden death
  - ➣ Rheumatic heart disease
- May be asymptomatic
- Failure to thrive
- Tachypnea, orthopnea, dyspnea
- Feeding intolerance
- Diaphoresis with feeds
- Vomiting
- Lethargy
- Cyanosis
- Edema
- Exercise intolerance
- Joint pain
- Chest pain
- Palpitations
- Syncope
- Syndromes associated with CHD:
  - ➣ Trisomy 21
  - ➣ CHARGE
  - ➣ Marfan's
  - ➣ Fetal alcohol syndrome

Physical
- Active precordium
- Asymmetric chest wall
- Petechiae, cyanosis, clubbing, perfusion
- Palpation:
  - ➣ Precordium: pain, thrill, RV heave, or displaced LV apex
  - ➣ Abdomen: hepatosplenomegaly
  - ➣ Extremities: assess brachial & femoral pulses simultaneously:
  - ➣ Delayed femoral pulses: coarctation
  - ➣ Brisk pulses: diastolic runoff (PDA, aortic regurgitation, sepsis, aortic-pulmonary shunt)
  - ➣ Diminished pulses may indicate CHF

- Auscultate:
  - ➤ Rate, rhythm
  - ➤ Rubs
  - ➤ S1– normally single
  - ➤ S2– normally variably split with respiration, same intensity as S1
    - Loud single S2: pulmonary hypertension
    - Wide fixed split S2: ASD
  - ➤ Systole:
    - Click
    - Murmur:
    - Intensity (I–VI/VI)
    - Timing, location, transmission
    - Quality (harsh, blowing)
  - ➤ Diastole:
    - Snap: mitral stenosis
    - Murmur
    - Rumble: A-V valve stenosis
    - Decrescendo: semilunar valve regurgitation
    - Continuous: venous hum, PDA, aortic-pulmonary shunt, coronary artery fistula, AV malformation

TESTS
- 4 extremity blood pressure
- Pulse oximetry
- ECG
- CXR
- Echocardiogram

DIFFERENTIAL DIAGNOSIS
- Innocent murmur
- Cardiac defect:
  - ➤ Holosystolic: AV valve regurgitation or VSD
  - ➤ Ejection: innocent, ASD, VSD, semilunar valve obstruction, right or left ventricular outflow tract obstruction

MANAGEMENT
- Varies depending on etiology
- Medical therapy for CHF
- Increased caloric intake for volume overload & CHF
- SBE prophylaxis
- Cardiac catheterization
- Surgery

SPECIFIC THERAPY
- Varies depending on etiology

FOLLOW-UP
- Varies depending on etiology
- None necessary for innocent murmur

COMPLICATIONS AND PROGNOSIS
- Varies depending on etiology

MYCOBACTERIUM TUBERCULOSIS

STEPHEN I. PELTON, M.D.

HISTORY AND PHYSICAL
- Highest risk in US: foreign-born
- 40–50% of infected children age <5 develop symptoms, compared to <10% of older children
- Time from infection to development of + Tuberculin Skin Test (TST): 2–12 wks

History
- Contact w/ infected person (most identified by contact tracing from adults)
- Cough
- Dyspnea
- Fever
- Night sweats
- Anorexia

Physical signs
- Exam often normal

TESTS
- CXR if + Mantoux
- Mantoux (PPD):
  - 5 TU intradermally
  - Induration read at 48–72 h
  - Interpretation:
    - >=5 mm + if contact of person w/ TB, abnormal CXR, HIV or immunosuppression
    - >=10 mm + if foreign born, healthcare worker, IV drug user
    - Age <4: >=15 mm always +

> False-negative:
>   • Viral infection or vaccines
>   • Malnutrition
>   • Renal failure
>   • HIV
>   • Steroids
>   • Extremes of age
> False-positive:
>   • BCG vaccine (young children for up to 3 yrs after immunization)
>   • Adolescents immunized w/ BCG: induration after Mantoux may be seen for up to 10 yrs; rarely exceeds 10 mm
■ Culture: early-morning gastric washings + in 40%
■ Bronchoscopy specimens: + in 13–62%

DIFFERENTIAL DIAGNOSIS
■ Viral pneumonia
■ Bacterial pneumonia
■ Pulmonary abscess
■ Bronchiectasis

MANAGEMENT
■ Children usually not considered contagious in absence of cavitation because of ineffective cough & low inocula
■ Presence of acid-fast bacilli (*M. tuberculosis*) on sputum smear: marker of infectivity
■ Treatment depends on clinical syndrome & risk for drug resistance
■ Primary disease:
>   Hilar (regional) adenopathy & small parenchymal infiltrate
>   Often resolves w/o specific therapy, esp. in older children/adolescents
■ Progressive primary disease:
>   Fever & cough
>   May occur if cavitation develops
■ Reactivation disease:
>   Adolescents (similar to adult disease)
>   Involvement of upper lobe(s)
>   Weight loss, anorexia, sweating, cough, chest pain, & hemoptysis
■ Risk factors for disease due to drug-resistant TB:
>   Hx of prior treatment

➤ Contact w/ drug-resistant TB
➤ Foreign-born
➤ Remaining smear-positive after 2 mo of treatment
■ Primary resistance: assoc. w/ single-drug resistance; secondary resistance assoc. w/ multiple-drug resistance

SPECIFIC THERAPY
■ Positive TST w/o clinical or radiologic evidence of disease:
➤ 9 mo isoniazid
➤ 6 mo rifampin
■ Pulmonary disease:
■ Hilar adenopathy:
➤ 9 mo isoniazid & rifampin qd, or
➤ 1 mo isoniazid & rifampin qd followed by 8 mo isoniazid & rifampin 2×/wk
■ Parenchymal disease:
➤ 2 mo isoniazid, rifampin, & pyrazinamide qd followed by 4 mo isoniazid & rifampin qd
➤ If drug resistance a concern: additional drug (ethambutol or streptomycin) added until susceptibilities known
■ Extrapulmonary (CNS, miliary, bone or joint):
➤ 2 mo isoniazid, rifampin, pyrazinamide, & streptomycin qd followed by 7–10 mo isoniazid & rifampin, or
➤ 2 mo isoniazid, rifampin, pyrazinamide, & streptomycin qd followed by 7–10 mo isoniazid & rifampin 2×/wk
■ Cervical lymphadenopathy: same as for pulmonary disease

FOLLOW-UP
■ CXR 2–3 mo after initiating therapy (hilar adenopathy may take years to resolve)
■ Monitoring of LFTs unnecessary in healthy children
■ Monitor LFTs initially monthly, then q3 mo in pts w/ concurrent liver disease, INH in combination w/ rifampin & pyrazinamide, clinical signs of liver disease (anorexia, vomiting, jaundice)
■ Monitor visual acuity & color vision in pts on ethambutol

COMPLICATIONS AND PROGNOSIS
■ Pleural TB: fever, pain, shortness of breath
■ Cardiac (pericarditis): chest pain, tachypnea, shortness of breath
■ Extrathoracic:
➤ Hematogenous:
• Miliary (2 or more organ systems)

- Follows primary disease
- Fever, hepatosplenomegaly, lymphadenopathy, reticular parenchymal disease

➤ Lymph node:
  - Most common
  - Post-primary event 6–9 mo after initial infection
  - Most often unilateral

➤ CNS:
  - Meningitis characterized by involvement of base of brain, frequently cranial nerves
  - Most frequent in ages 6 mo to 4 yr

Prognosis
- ■ Generally good except for drug-resistant TB & meningitis

MYCOPLASMA PNEUMONIA

JEROME O. KLEIN, M.D.

HISTORY AND PHYSICAL
- ■ Symptoms and signs indistinguishable from viral respiratory tract infections

History
- ■ General malaise, myalgia, sore throat, headache, fever, rhinorrhea, pharyngitis, otitis media, or croup syndrome may occur in children
- ■ Dry, nonproductive cough may become mucopurulent after 3–5 d; coughing may persist for 2 or more wks after resolution of fever

Physical
- ■ Signs include: sinus tenderness; posterior pharyngeal erythema; rales, and/or wheezes
- ■ Unusual complications include:
  - ➤ Rashes that may accompany the respiratory infection
  - ➤ Stevens-Johnson syndrome has been uniquely identified in mycoplasma infections
  - ➤ Central nervous diseases including aseptic meningitis, Guillain-Barre, encephalitis, and transverse myelitis
  - ➤ Aseptic meningitis and pneumonia or prolonged cough or exposure should suggest possibility of mycoplasmal infection

TESTS
- Routine tests (WBC) not likely to distinguish virus from mycoplasma infection
- Chest x-ray may vary from diffuse interstitial pattern to unilateral, segmental consolidation. Small amounts of pleural fluid may be present.
- Isolation by culture requires special media and is unavailable in most hospital laboratories
- Cold agglutinins (Ca)
  - IgM autoantibodies that appear within 7 to 10 d of initial symptoms and drop after 2 to 3 wks
  - Usually positive when there is significant mycoplasma pneumonia but may be negative in lesser disease (false negatives)
  - May be positive also in other viral respiratory tract infections such as influenza and adenoviruses (false positives).
- Serology performed using complement fixation test usually demonstrates a fourfold rise in antibody; since titer rise occurs weeks later it provides only retrospective diagnosis

DIFFERENTIAL DIAGNOSIS
- Other viral causes of pharyngitis, croup, bronchitis, or pneumonia.

MANAGEMENT
- If diagnosis known or suspected, an appropriate antibiotic is warranted
- Nonspecific management for persistent cough may be warranted

SPECIFIC THERAPY
- Macrolides are the preferred drugs: erythromycin, azithromycin, or clarithromycin
- Tetracycline may be used in children > 8 y

FOLLOW-UP
- No specific follow-up necessary unless cough and anorexia are prolonged

COMPLICATIONS AND PROGNOSIS
- Skin and central nervous system complications are noted above
- Prognosis good, although cough and debilitation may persist for weeks to months

MYOCARDITIS

SUSAN FOERSTER, M.D.
SHARON O'BRIEN, M.D.

HISTORY AND PHYSICAL

History
- Neonates & infants:
  - ➤ Tachypnea
  - ➤ Decreased feeding, easy fatigability
  - ➤ Listlessness
  - ➤ Diaphoresis
- Older children & adolescents:
  - ➤ Exercise intolerance
  - ➤ Easy fatigability & malaise
  - ➤ Chronic cough
  - ➤ Chest or abdominal pain
  - ➤ Palpitations, syncope

Physical signs
- Pallor
- Jugulovenous distention (older children)
- Weak peripheral pulses, cool & mottled extremities
- Tachycardia, hypotension
- Mitral regurgitation, cardiac gallop
- Tachypnea, retractions, wheezing, or cyanosis
- Hepatomegaly, RUQ tenderness
- Peripheral edema less likely
- Signs of meningoencephalitis

TESTS
- CXR: cardiomegaly, edema, effusions
- EKG: tachycardia, low voltages, ST changes, dysrhythmias
- Echocardiography: function, effusion
- Cardiac catheterization: hemodynamics, biopsy

DIFFERENTIAL DIAGNOSIS

Cardiac
- Anomalous coronary artery
- Pericarditis

- Other cardiomyopathy (dilated, restrictive, hypertrophic)
- Chronic tachydysrhythmia
- Congenital structural heart disease

Noncardiac
- Sepsis
- Infection
- Drugs/antineoplastic
- Metabolic disease or disturbance
- AV malformation

Causes
- Virus: enterovirus, adenovirus, Herpesvirus, CMV, HIV, others
- Bacteria: *Meningococcus, Klebsiella*
- Parasites, protozoa, & fungi
- Drugs
- Collagen vascular disease
- Kawasaki disease

MANAGEMENT

General measures
- Assess hemodynamic status & oxygenation
- Conservative fluid management
- Early use of inotropic agents/IVIG
- Consult intensivist/cardiologist

SPECIFIC THERAPY
- Supportive measures: airway & ventilation control as necessary
- Diuresis: furosemide or thiazides caution with hypotension
- Inotropic agents
  - Dobutamine 5–15 mcg/kg/min
  - Dopamine 5–15 mcg/kg/min
  - Milrinone, load 10–50 mcg/kg IV over 10 min, infusion 0.25–1 mcg/kg/min; may cause hypotension
- Vasodilators
  - Nitroprusside: 0.3–5 mcg/kg/min; use with inotropes; need arterial line for monitoring, monitor serum thiocyanate level
  - ACE inhibitors: mild cases & chronic use
- Immunosuppression (steroids, cyclosporin): not proven effective; may be detrimental
- IV gamma-globulin

- Anticoagulation: risk of cardiac thrombi
  - Heparin: acute stage
  - Coumadin or aspirin: convalescent stage
- Treat dysrhythmias
- Not recommended:
  - Antiviral agents: unproven
  - Nonsteroidals: increase mortality
- Severe cases:
  - Mechanical ventricular-assist devices
  - Extracorporeal membrane oxygenation
  - Transplantation

FOLLOW-UP
- Determine with pediatric cardiologist

COMPLICATIONS AND PROGNOSIS
- Neonates & infants: up to 75% mortality
- Older children & adolescents:
  - 50–67% complete recovery
  - 10–25% mortality
- Chronic cardiomyopathy:
  - Long-term: digoxin, ACE inhibitors; beta-blockers–controversial
  - May progress & require transplantation

NARCOTIC ABSTINENCE SYNDROME

ELIZABETH BROWN, M.D.

HISTORY AND PHYSICAL

History
- In utero narcotic exposure
- Mother receiving methadone maintenance
- Infant w/ prolonged need for narcotic analgesia
- Onset of symptoms depends on drug half-life:
  - Heroin: first day of life
  - Methadone: 3–10 d
- Other important factors:
  - Type of drug dose
  - Frequency of use
  - Timing of last dose
  - Exposure to other drugs

- Tremors, irritability, seizures
- Vomiting & diarrhea

Physical signs
- Increased muscle tone
- GI dysfunction:
  - Poor feeding
  - Uncoordinated, constant sucking
  - Poor weight gain
- Autonomic signs:
  - Increased sweating
  - Nasal stuffiness
  - Fever
  - Mottling
  - Temperature instability

TESTS
- CBC, platelets, blood culture
- Serum glucose, Ca
- Urine drug screen (baby & mother)
- Maternal HIV, hepatitis B/C
- Congenital viral disease

DIFFERENTIAL DIAGNOSIS
- Metabolic disorders:
  - Hypoglycemia
  - Hypocalcemia
  - Hypomagnesemia
- Sepsis/meningitis
- Primary seizure disorder
- Inborn errors of metabolism

MANAGEMENT
General measures
- Decrease sensory stimulation
- Hold, rock, swaddle infant
- Frequent feedings
- Increase caloric density of formula PRN for adequate weight gain
- Monitor using standardized Narcotic Abstinence Scoring (Finnegan system)
- Social service eval.

SPECIFIC THERAPY
- Finnegan system: Rx if 3 consecutive scores >8 or 2 scores >12
- Goals: normalize behavior, sleep pattern, feeding
- Avoid oversedation
- Pharmacotherapy:
- If exposed only to narcotics, use denatured tincture of opium (DTO), morphine, methadone to prevent withdrawal
- DTO schedule:
  - Dilute to 0.4 mg/mL morphine equivalent
  - Dose depends on NAS scores:

NAS Score

Dose

8–10	0.8 mL/kg/d divided q4h
11–13	1.2 mL/kg/d divided q4h
14–16	1.6 mL/kg/d divided q4h
>= 17	2.0 mL/kg/d divided q4h

- May use phenobarbital: initial loading dose, 10 mg/kg/dose up to 3 doses, then maintenance of 5–10 mg/kg/d
- Maintain on stable dose 2–3 d, NAS scores in range 6–8
- Begin slow detox by decreasing dose 10% of original dose/day as tolerated
- Exposure to multiple classes of psychotropics:
  - Often need two drugs
  - Begin w/ phenobarbital; add a narcotic as withdrawal symptoms worsen
- Never use narcotic treatment for withdrawal from other, non-narcotic drugs

FOLLOW-UP
- Early follow-up with primary care provider
- Consider newborn follow-up program
- Development screening, if appropriate

COMPLICATIONS AND PROGNOSIS

Complications
- Seizures, if drug withdrawal inadequately treated

Prognosis
- Most families require home health care services & social service intervention

- Parent/foster parent educ.: infants may have some symptoms for several months
- May need long-term development assessment and follow-up care

NEAR DROWNING

SCOT BATEMAN, M.D.

HISTORY AND PHYSICAL

History
- Length of time submerged
- Water temperature
- Length of time until return of spontaneous circulation
- Aspiration of gastric contents, coughing
- Salt water vs. fresh water

Physical signs
- Core body temperature
- Glasgow Coma Scale
- Pulmonary assessment:
  - ➤ Respiratory rate
  - ➤ Cyanosis, retractions
  - ➤ Grunting, wheezing, or rales
- Mental status: alert vs. CNS compromise
- Head or neck trauma

TESTS
- CBC
- Electrolytes, BUN/Cr
- CK, urinalysis for electrical injury
- ABG
- Chest x-ray
- Head CT, cervical spine films
- Toxicology screen, ethanol level (if toxin suspected)

DIFFERENTIAL DIAGNOSIS
- Hypothermia
- Electric shock
- Head trauma
- Drug ingestion
- Seizure

- Cardiac arrhythmia
- Child abuse

MANAGEMENT
- Aggressive CPR at scene
- Neck immobilization
- 100% oxygen
- Careful monitoring for CNS or pulmonary deterioration

SPECIFIC THERAPY
- Warm to core temperature of 33–34 °C, then slowly to 37 °C (warm humidified oxygen, warm IV fluids)
- Reversal of hypoxemia and metabolic acidosis needed for effective therapy
- Mechanical ventilation for ARDS
- Consider fluid restriction & diuretics for fluid overload in lungs
- No prophylactic antibiotics
- Treat fevers aggressively to avoid hyperthermia
- Treat increased ICP, if indicated

FOLLOW-UP
- Awake, alert pt:
  - ➤ Presume to have survived without CNS damage
  - ➤ Observe for 24 h
- Obtunded but arousable pt:
  - ➤ Certain but potentially reversible CNS damage
  - ➤ Vigilant treatment & follow-up for first 48–72 h
- Poor neurologic presentation (fixed dilated pupils, decorticate posturing): likely permanent neurologic injury

COMPLICATIONS AND PROGNOSIS
- Hypothermia (core temp <35°C) and young age appear to be protective
- Severe neurologic complications increase with depth of coma on presentation & victim's hemodynamic status at initial evaluation
- Other poor prognosis indicators:
  - ➤ pH < 7.1
  - ➤ Glasgow Coma Scale < 5
  - ➤ Fixed and dilated pupils
- Patients requiring PICU care:
  - ➤ Mortality rate 30%
  - ➤ Another 10–30% with severe brain damage
- 92% of near-drowning survivors recover completely

NEPHROTIC SYNDROME

MELANIE S. KIM, M.D.

HISTORY AND PHYSICAL

Syndrome consists of:
- Edema
- Hypoalbuminemia
- Proteinuria
- Hyperlipidemia

History
- Swelling/edema:
    - Periorbital
    - Boys: scrotal
    - Girls: labial
    - Lower extremity
- Decreased urine output
- Foamy urine
- History of preceding upper respiratory infection

Physical signs
- Weight
- Blood pressure
- Assessment of lungs, abdomen, & heart
- Sites & extent of edema

TESTS
- Urine protein:
    - Urinalysis
    - Timed urine collection
    - Protein excretion >40 mg/m^2/h or 50 mg/kg/d or 3g/d
    - Urine protein to creatine ratio: >=2.5
- Serum albumin: <=2.5 g/dL
- Serum cholesterol: usually elevated
- Creatinine, BUN
- Serum electrolytes
- Consider other etiologies:
    - Complement levels
    - ASLO or streptozyme titers
    - Antinuclear antibody
    - VDRL, HIV, or hepatitis B
- Renal biopsy

DIFFERENTIAL DIAGNOSIS

- Primary nephrotic syndrome:
  - Minimal change disease
  - Focal segmental sclerosis
  - Membranoproliferative glomerulonephritis
  - Membranous glomerulonephritis
- Secondary nephrotic syndrome:
  - Lupus (SLE)
  - Henoch-Schonlein purpura
  - Poststreptococcal nephritis
  - HBV, HIV, malaria
- Liver failure w/ hypoalbuminemia
- Protein-losing enteropathy

MANAGEMENT

What to do first

- Assess for hypovolemia

General measures

- No added salt diet $(1–2 \text{ g/m}^2)$
- Fluid restriction while proteinuric

SPECIFIC THERAPY

- Corticosteroid Rx if high probability of minimal change disease
  - Tuberculin skin test before Rx
  - Two options:
    - 2 mg/kg/d (60 mg/kg/m^2) divided BID or TID (max, 80 mg/d) for 4 wks; switch to alternate-day therapy 2 mg/kg/qod (60 mg/kg/m^2) as a single dose for additional 4–8 wks. Taper & discontinue over 2–3 mo
    - 2 mg/kg/d (60 mg/kg/m^2) divided BID or TID until protein-free for 5–7 d; switch to alternate-day therapy at 2 mg/kg/qod (60 mg/kg/m^2) as single dose, tapered over 4–8 wks
- Pneumococcal vaccine
- Use of diuretics alone not recommended; may predispose to circulatory collapse or hypercoagulability
- Active diuresis (see complications) 25% albumin $(0.5–1.0 \text{ g/kg})$ slow IV over 2–4 h with IV furosemide (1 mg/kg). Repeat q12–24h as needed.
- Consider renal biopsy if:
  - Age <1 y or >10 y

➤ Gross hematuria, hypertension, low serum C3 levels, or impaired renal function

FOLLOW-UP
- Avoid paracentesis & thoracentesis; may precipitate circulatory collapse
- Monitor urine
- Teach how to test urine for protein & to do daily weights
- Relapse in pt who has been steroid-responsive in the past: reinitiate steroid Rx
- Proteinuria despite 8 wks of steroids: refer to pediatric nephrologist
- Immunosuppressive therapy if steroid Rx fails

COMPLICATIONS AND PROGNOSIS

Complications
- Peritonitis w/ pneumococcus, gram-negative, & anaerobic bacteria:
  ➤ Broad-spectrum antibiotics
  ➤ Active diuresis
- Pleural effusion: active diuresis
- Pulmonary edema
- Thromboembolism: anticoagulants
- Skin breakdown

Prognosis
- Excellent for minimal change disease
- Other causes: may progress to ESRD

NEUROBLASTOMA

JANE E. MINTURN, M.D., PH.D.

HISTORY AND PHYSICAL
- Most cases:
  ➤ Age <4 y
  ➤ Metastatic at presentation
- Abdominal mass:
  ➤ Distention
  ➤ Palpable mass (fixed/firm/nontender)
  ➤ Bowel obstruction
  ➤ Lower extremity edema
  ➤ Hypertension

- Cervical/thoracic mass:
  - Supraclavicular node
  - Horner's
  - Anisocoria
  - Stridor
  - Respiratory distress
  - Superior vena cava syndrome
- Paraspinal mass:
  - Cord compression
  - Bladder & bowel dysfunction
  - Back pain
  - Paraplegia
- Metastatic disease:
  - Bone pain
  - Hepatomegaly
  - Cytopenia: marrow involvement
  - Periorbital ecchymosis
  - Nonspecific:
    - Fever
    - Irritability
    - Failure to thrive
- Paraneoplastic syndromes:
  - VIP syndrome:
    - Watery diarrhea
    - Abdominal distention
    - Electrolyte imbalance
  - Opsoclonus-myoclonus:
    - Chaotic eye movement
    - Myoclonic jerks
  - Catecholamine excess:
    - Flushing
    - Sweating
    - Tachycardia
    - Headache
    - Hypertension

TESTS
- CBC, electrolytes, LFTs
- CXR, KUB (calcification), CT, MRI, ultrasound
- Ferritin
- Urine catecholamines: VMA/HVA
- Bone scan

- Bone marrow aspirate/biopsy
- MIBG (nuclear) scan
- Tumor histology, biologic staging (*MYCN* copy number, DNA index)

DIFFERENTIAL DIAGNOSIS
- Abdominal mass:
  - Wilms tumor
  - Burkitt lymphoma
  - Germ cell tumor
- Thoracic mass:
  - Non-Hodgkin lymphoma
  - T-cell leukemia
  - Germ cell tumor
- "Small round blue cell" tumor:
  - Lymphoma
  - Ewing sarcoma
  - Rhabdomyosarcoma

MANAGEMENT
- Supportive care for emergencies:
  - Fluids
  - Electrolyte correction
  - Antihypertensives
  - Respiratory support
- Emergencies due to tumor bulk:
  - Surgery: cord or bowel compression
  - Chemotherapy: "non-life-threatening" emergencies (post-biopsy)
  - Radiation therapy (not first-line)

SPECIFIC THERAPY
- Based on risk strata:
  - Staging by International Neuroblastoma Staging System:
    - Local
    - Infiltrating (cross midline)
    - Disseminated
    - Metastatic
  - Age: <12 mo favorable
  - *MYCN* copy number; DNA index
- Low-risk: surgery alone (if complete resection safe)
- Intermediate-risk:
  - Chemotherapy
  - Surgical resection after tumor reduction

- High-risk:
  - Induction chemotherapy
  - Surgical resection
  - High-dose chemotherapy w/ autologous stem cell rescue (current protocol)
- Stage 4S:
  - Patients <12 mo, localized primary tumor, dissemination limited to skin, liver, and/or bone marrow
  - Often regress spontaneously
  - May not require treatment
- Radiation:
  - Local control (total resection not attained)
  - Total body irradiation: transplant regimen
  - Pain control for palliation
- Adjuvants: 13-*cis*-retinoic acid (cellular differentiation agent) given post-transplant to improve survival

FOLLOW-UP
- Monitor response:
  - CT of primary site
  - Bone scan
  - MIBG scan
  - Urine catecholamines
- Off-therapy:
  - MRI or CT of primary site
  - Bone scan/MIBG scan
  - Urine catecholamines

COMPLICATIONS AND PROGNOSIS
- Related to tumor size, location, & treatment

Prognosis
- Low-risk: 90% survival
- Intermediate-risk: 30–50% survival
- High-risk: <30% survival

NEUROFBROMATOSIS (NF)

HOWARD BAUCHNER, M.D.

HISTORY AND PHYSICAL
- NF1 (von Recklinghausen; 1/4000) and NF2 (1/40,000)
- Autosomal dominant

- 50% of cases occur spontaneously
- Diagnosis of NF1 requires at least two of the following:
  - 6 or more café-au-lait macules (prepubertal >5mm, postpubertal >15mm)
  - Freckling in axillary or inguinal region
  - Optic glioma
  - 2 or more Lisch nodules (iris hamartomas)
  - Distinctive osseous lesions
  - First-degree relative with NF1 by above criteria
- NF2: at least one of the following:
  - Bilateral acoustic neuromas
  - First-degree relative with NF2 and either unilateral acoustic neuroma or two of the following:
    - Meningioma
    - Schwannoma
    - Neurofibroma
    - Presenile lens opacity

TESTS
- No routine tests necessary
- Genetic testing possible for NF1: detection rates of 65–70%
- Consider imaging to confirm diagnosis or complications of disease:
  - CT/MRI in NF1 to exclude optic gliomas or other neoplasms
  - CT in NF2 to detect acoustic neuroma

DIFFERENTIAL DIAGNOSIS
- Multiple café-au-lait spots
- Tuberous sclerosis
- Noonan
- Multiple lipomatosis
- McCune-Albright

MANAGEMENT
- Early identification and treatment of complications
- Educate family to identify symptoms that require prompt medical attention:
  - Strabismus
  - Severe headaches
  - Precocious puberty

SPECIFIC THERAPY
- Tailored to specific complication

FOLLOW-UP
- Yearly routine healthcare:
  - ➤ Blood pressure measurement
  - ➤ Scoliosis screening
  - ➤ Ophthalmologic exam with vision screening
- NF2: yearly audiogram
- Consider referral to neurologist/geneticist/ophthalmologist

COMPLICATIONS AND PROGNOSIS
- Cutaneous or plexiform neurofibromas
- NF1:
  - ➤ 40% learning disabilities
  - ➤ Tumors: 15% optic glioma, pheochromocytoma
  - ➤ Disturbance of growth and sexual development
  - ➤ Hypertension from renal artery stenosis
  - ➤ Other non-CNS malignancies
  - ➤ Orthopedic problems: cortical thinning and intramedullary fibrosis

Prognosis
- Variable, generally better for NF2 than NF1
- Major causes of morbidity and mortality are hypertension and cancer
- Early detection of medical problems may reduce morbidity and mortality

NEUTROPENIA

ANDREW KOH, M.D.

HISTORY AND PHYSICAL
- Absolute neutrophil count $<1,500mm^3$; $<1,000mm^3$ ages 1 wk to 2 y

History
- Increased frequency of acute severe bacterial or fungal infections:
  - ➤ Sepsis
  - ➤ Cellulitis
  - ➤ Skin abscess
  - ➤ Pneumonia
  - ➤ Perirectal abscess
- Aphthous ulcers, gingivitis, periodontal disease
- Chills

- Malaise
- Fever

TESTS
- CBC:
  - Neutrophils: absent or markedly reduced
  - Monocytes & lymphocytes normal
  - Red cells & platelets usually not affected, except marrow infiltrative malignancies
- Bone marrow biopsy:
  - Normal erythroid series & megakaryocytes
  - Reduction in myeloid cells

DIFFERENTIAL DIAGNOSIS
- Congenital neutropenia:
  - Reticular dysgenesis (congenital aleukocytosis)
  - Kostmann: maturation defect in marrow progenitor cells
  - Shwachman (pancreatic insufficiency)
  - Cyclic neutropenia
- Metabolic & storage diseases
- Infection
- Drug or toxin:
  - Phenothiazines
  - Sulfonamides
  - Anticonvulsants
  - Penicillin
- Immune:
  - Neonatal alloimmune or autoimmune
  - Autoimmune or chronic benign neutropenia of childhood
- Ineffective granulopoiesis: vitamin B12, folate, or copper deficiency
- Malignancies: leukemia, lymphoma
- Bone marrow failure:
  - Aplastic anemia
  - Osteopetrosis

MANAGEMENT
What to do first
- Eliminate identifiable toxic agents, drugs
- Treat infection & underlying conditions

SPECIFIC THERAPY
- Recombinant G-CSF and GM-CSF: may increase neutrophil counts

- Prophylactic antibiotics not indicated
- Fever often harbinger of infection:
  - CBC & blood culture, empiric antibiotics
  - If cause not found, continue antibiotics until fever & neutropenia resolve

FOLLOW-UP
- Monitor neutrophil count

COMPLICATIONS AND PROGNOSIS
- Infection:
  - Acute severe bacterial:
    - *Staphylococcus aureus*, gram-negative bacteremia
    - Pneumonia, meningitis, sepsis
    - Cellulitis, skin abscess, perirectal abscess
  - Fungal

Prognosis
- Varies with cause & severity:
  - Severe cases w/ persistent neutropenia: prognosis often poor despite antibiotic treatment
  - Milder forms (ie, cyclic neutropenia): symptoms may be minimal; life expectancy may approach normal

NONTUBERCULOUS MYCOBACTERIA (NTM)

KATHERINE HSU, M.D.

HISTORY AND PHYSICAL
- Most common manifestation: subacute or chronic lymphadenitis
  - Cervical or submandibular
  - Unilateral
  - Firm
  - Painless
  - Mobile
  - Nonerythematous
  - Suppurates after weeks
  - No systemic symptoms
- Cutaneous infection, osteomyelitis, otitis media, & pulmonary disease (rare)
  - Acute or subacute onset
  - Lung disease more common in patients w/ chronic lung disease

- Disseminated disease (fever, night sweats, fatigue, prominent abdominal symptoms, anemia) almost always assoc. w/ deficient cell-mediated immunity (HIV, CD4+ counts <100/mcL)

History
- Organisms ubiquitous (soil, food, water, animals); specific risks:
  - *M. marinum* cellulitis: abrasion in fish tank or swimming pool
  - *M. chelonae* or *M. abscessus* cellulitis or otitis: contaminated multidose vaccine vials or improperly sterilized medical equipment
  - *M. ulcerans*: chronic tropical skin infections

Physical signs
- Size, shape, location of swollen nodes
- Assoc. disease

TESTS
- Diagnosis requires isolation of organism from sterile body site (blood, CSF, pleural fluid, bone marrow, tissue):
  - Blood cultures 90–95% sensitive in AIDS pts w/ disseminated infection
  - Culture from sputum, gastric washing, draining sinus tract, or urine difficult to interpret (contamination, colonization vs true disease?)
  - Repeated isolation of many colonies of single species likely to indicate disease

DIFFERENTIAL DIAGNOSIS
- Tuberculosis:
  - False-positive PPD w/ NTM but induration <10 mm & lack Hx of TB exposure
  - NTM adenitis unilateral w/ normal CXR vs. tuberculous adenitis bilateral w/ abnormal CXR
- Cat-scratch disease
- Mononucleosis
- Toxoplasmosis
- Brucellosis
- Tularemia
- Malignancy

MANAGEMENT
- Dictated by location of infection, species isolated, & results of drug-susceptibility testing

SPECIFIC THERAPY
- Consult expert for details about antibiotics
- Isolated lymphadenitis in otherwise healthy child: complete surgical excision
- Osteomyelitis: debridement & prolonged nonempiric antibiotic therapy
- Suspected *M. tuberculosis* adenitis or pulmonary disease: isoniazid, rifampin, & pyrazinamide until cultures confirm another cause
- *M. chelonae* cutaneous infections: clarithromycin + at least 1 other agent
- *M. marinum* cutaneous infection:
  - May self-resolve if minor or may require rifampin, co-trimoxazole, clarithromycin, or doxycycline
  - Consider surgical debridement
- *M. kansasii* pulmonary infection:
  - Isoniazid & rifampin
  - Consider ethambutol
- *M. avium* complex pulmonary infection: clarithromycin or azithromycin + another drug
- Disseminated *M. avium* complex:
  - Multidrug therapy for disease in immunocompromised pts
  - Consult expert (lack of consensus on optimal regimen)
  - Offer prophylaxis w/ azithromycin, clarithromycin against *M. avium* complex disease to HIV-infected patients who meet CD4+ T-lymphocyte count criteria

FOLLOW-UP
- Lymphadenitis cured by surgery alone
- Cutaneous lesions:
  - Can heal spontaneously after incision & drainage
  - May require months of antibiotic therapy
- Disseminated *M. avium* complex
  - Monitor clinical & microbiologic response to treatment closely
  - Substantial clinical improvement w/in 4–6 wk of therapy
  - Clearance of blood cultures may take longer (up to 4–12 wks)
  - Immune reconstitution may be necessary for cure
- Monitor all pts on therapy for drug adverse effects

COMPLICATIONS AND PROGNOSIS
- Incomplete excision of lymphadenitis:
  - May result in chronic draining sinus tracts
  - 6 mo of clarithromycin & rifabutin may be curative

Prognosis
- Good for cure of localized disease if excised or treated before caseation or extension
- Poor for disseminated *M. avium* complex disease unless immune system reconstitutes

NURSEMAID'S ELBOW

DAVID H. DORFMAN, M.D.

HISTORY AND PHYSICAL

History
- Most common age 1 to 5 y
- Hx of arm being pulled or child falling while hand is being held
- Occasionally Hx of falling
- Hx of recurrent event

Physical
- Child appears comfortable
- Arm held at side with slight elbow flexion, forearm pronated
- Minimal soft-tissue swelling
- Mild tenderness, especially with pronation/supination
- Minimal spontaneous arm movement

TESTS
- If history and physical are consistent with radial head subluxation, no tests required
- Consider x-ray if injury from fall or elbow tender
- X-ray if reduction maneuvers fail

DIFFERENTIAL DIAGNOSIS
- Fracture
- Dislocation
- Contusion

MANAGEMENT

General measures
- Examine child in guardian's lap
- Use distraction
- Try to coax child to move arm

SPECIFIC THERAPY
- Reduction of radial head subluxation

- Supination and flexion method
  - Examiner places hand on pt's radial head
  - Supinate forearm fully; flex at elbow until hand touches ipsilateral shoulder
  - May feel click as reduction accomplished
- Hyperpronation method
  - Grip pt's elbow in one hand while forcefully pronating the wrist
- Avoid all maneuvers if suspicious of fracture

FOLLOW-UP
- 90% have voluntary use of arm within minutes
- Counsel caretakers to avoid repetitive traction on arm
- If reduction is successful, no follow-up needed
- If no improvement after 15 min, repeat reduction; may use same or different maneuver
- If no improvement after 3 attempts, obtain radiograph
- If radiograph negative but pt not improved, place arm in sling or posterior splint
- Repeat assessment in 24 h

COMPLICATIONS AND PROGNOSIS
- Outcome uniformly excellent
- Recurrence possible (1/3 of patients)

OBSTRUCTIVE SLEEP APNEA (OSA)

MICHAEL J. CORWIN, M.D.
JEAN M. SILVESTRI, M.D.
DEBRA E. WEESE-MAYER, M.D.

HISTORY AND PHYSICAL

History
- Usually presents between ages 3 & 7
- During sleep:
  - Loud snoring interrupted by periods of silence but continued respiratory effort
  - Snorting
  - Struggling to breathe
  - Paradoxical inward movement of chest on inspiration
  - Sweating
  - Restlessness

- ➤ Periodic awakening
- ➤ Enuresis
- ■ Unusual sleeping position to allow neck hyperextension
- ■ Excessive daytime somnolence
- ■ Mouth breathing
- ■ Recurrent middle ear disease
- ■ Chronic rhinorrhea
- ■ Family Hx of OSA
- ■ Assoc. conditions:
  - ➤ Obesity
  - ➤ Trisomy 21
  - ➤ Craniofacial malformation
  - ➤ Macroglossia
  - ➤ Micrognathia
  - ➤ Neuromuscular weakness
  - ➤ Severe mental retardation
  - ➤ Hindbrain malformation or tumor
  - ➤ Severe laryngomalacia
  - ➤ Sedation, esp. chloral hydrate
  - ➤ Vocal cord paralysis

Physical signs
- ■ Height, weight, head circumference
- ■ Vital signs, particularly BP
- ■ Exam performed while awake & asleep
- ■ Nasal & oral airflow
- ■ Muscle tone, phonation, inspiratory stridor, hoarseness
- ■ Craniofacial structure, tongue size relative to oral airway, adenoids, tonsils, palatal mucosa & length
- ■ Auscultation of lungs
- ■ Cardiac exam; assess for pulmonary hypertension
- ■ Clubbing of extremities
- ■ Neurodevelopment

TESTS
- ■ Questionnaire to assess frequency of symptoms/signs
- ■ Growth curve (serial measurements of weight, height, head circumference)
- ■ Lateral neck x-ray
- ■ ECG
- ■ Multichannel polygraphic recording of sleep & wakefulness

- Airway fluoroscopy during sleep to localize site of obstruction (if enlarged adenoids/tonsils NOT likely cause)
- Video/audio taping

DIFFERENTIAL DIAGNOSIS
- Central apnea
- Mixed apnea: obstructive apnea temporally linked w/ central apnea
- Causes of obstructive sleep apnea:
  - Adenotonsillar hypertrophy
  - Assoc. conditions listed under History

MANAGEMENT
- Determine underlying cause & focus management directly:
  - Adenotonsillectomy
  - Weight loss (obese child)
  - Surgical repair of redundant or aberrant tissue
- Continuous positive airway pressure or bi-level positive airway pressure
- Tracheostomy

SPECIFIC THERAPY
See Management section

FOLLOW-UP
- Depends on specific etiology

COMPLICATIONS AND PROGNOSIS
- Failure to thrive
- Neurobehavioral symptoms due to sleep disruption and/or recurrent hypoxemia
- Pulmonary hypertension
- Cor pulmonale & CHF
- Respiratory arrest & sudden death
- Rare:
  - Seizures
  - Asphyxial brain damage
  - Coma

Prognosis
- Resolves dramatically w/ definitive procedure
- Central apnea often observed after resolution of OSA
- If treated, excellent catch-up growth

OSGOOD-SCHLATTER DISEASE

ILAN SCHWARTZ, M.D.

HISTORY AND PHYSICAL

History
- Most common age 10–15 y
- Young athletes and adolescents
- Gradually increasing pain and swelling in area of tibial tubercle
- Symptoms exacerbated by:
  - Vigorous physical activity
  - Running, jumping, climbing stairs
  - Squatting, kneeling, crawling

Physical signs
- Point tenderness at tibial tubercle
- Mild soft-tissue swelling
- Normal knee joint; some may have limitation of knee flexion

TESTS
- Diagnosis can be made clinically
- Lateral x-ray:
  - May be normal
  - May reveal prominent & irregular tibial tubercle with or without fragmentation

DIFFERENTIAL DIAGNOSIS
- Peripatellar pain syndrome
- Osteochondritis dissecans
- Jumper's knee

MANAGEMENT
- Limit activity to point of pain tolerance

SPECIFIC THERAPY
- Pain control with NSAIDs
- Physical therapy, esp. swimming
- Decrease flexion/extension at knee
- Immobilization for 4–6 wks: for extremely severe symptoms

FOLLOW-UP
COMPLICATIONS AND PROGNOSIS
- Generally no long-term complications
- Self-limited; subsides with fusion of tubercle at about age 15

OSTEOMYELITIS

KRIS REHM, M.D.

HISTORY AND PHYSICAL
- An infectious process primarily involving bone
- Signs/symptoms:
  - Fever
  - Local signs of inflammation or pain
  - Limited movement of affected limb
  - Local warmth, tenderness, or soft-tissue swelling
  - Older children can localize pain
  - Younger children show decreased voluntary movement
- In neonates: often result of iatrogenic procedures (i.e., heel sticks, fetal scalp monitoring)
- In patients w/ sickle cell disease:
  - Difficult to diagnose
  - Similar clinical presentation to vaso-occlusive pain crisis
  - Consider Salmonella, other gram-negative bacilli, *S. aureus*
- Vertebral osteomyelitis: most often in children age >8; result of hematogenous infection:
  - Often presents with fever, back pain, abdominal pain, or gait alterations
  - Examine for point tenderness on percussion over spinous process
  - Can lead to paraspinous abscess
- Pelvic osteomyelitis:
  - Pain in buttocks, hip, or knee
  - Gait disturbance
  - Often staph or salmonella; consider mycobacteria
- After puncture wound of foot: usually caused by *Pseudomonas*, esp. in children age >9 wearing sneakers

TESTS
- Microbiologic diagnoses: blood culture positive in 50–60% of cases
- Bone aspiration or biopsy

- Consider urine bacterial antigen for *S. pneumoniae* or *H. influenzae*
- X-ray: may be negative early in infection, periosteal reaction takes 10–14 d to become evident
- Bone scan: uptake of isotope affected by osteoblastic activity & increased vascularity
- CT: useful in osteomyelitis of pelvis & vertebrae
- MRI: most sensitive in detecting inflammation
- Serum markers of inflammation: CRP, ESR

DIFFERENTIAL DIAGNOSIS
- Pyomyositis
- Cellulitis
- Bursitis
- Abscess
- Septic arthritis
- Diskitis
- Bony malignancy:
  - Neuroblastoma
  - Ewing sarcoma
  - Leukemia
  - Lymphoma
- Toxic synovitis of hip
- Vaso-occlusive crisis in sickle cell anemia

MANAGEMENT
- Antimicrobial therapy
- Additional therapy: pain relief, nutrition, hydration, immobilization
- Physical therapy depending on joint involved

SPECIFIC THERAPY
- Neonates: anti-staph empiric antibiotics (nafcillin, oxacillin), as well as group B strep coverage (aminoglycoside)
- Children age <5: cover staph & *Haemophilus* (cephalosporins: cefuroxime, ceftriaxone)
- Children age >5: antistaphylococcal penicillin
- Sickle cell: aminoglycoside + anti-staph penicillin
- Antibiotic failure: consider surgical intervention

FOLLOW-UP
- Initial response to treatment:
  - Improvement in local signs of inflammation and infection
  - Decreased fever

- Monitor for decline in WBC, ESR, CRP
- Follow growth of involved limb

COMPLICATIONS AND PROGNOSIS
- Septic arthritis
- Bony deformity
- Altered growth
- Pathologic fractures
- Chronic osteomyelitis

Prognosis
- Good for uncomplicated osteomyelitis diagnosed early

OSTEOSARCOMA

KIMBERLY STEGMAIER, M.D.

HISTORY AND PHYSICAL

History
- Pain
- Soft-tissue swelling
- Rare: fever, weight loss
- Peak incidence: 2nd decade

Physical signs
- Palpable mass
- Tenderness over involved area
- Frequent site:
  - ➤ Femur
  - ➤ Proximal tibia
  - ➤ Humerus

TESTS
- Plain x-ray:
  - ➤ Sclerotic, mixed, rarely lytic lesion
  - ➤ Soft-tissue mass
  - ➤ Intense periosteal new bone formation, lifting of bone w/ Codman's triangle
  - ➤ Eccentric location in metaphyseal portion of long bones
  - ➤ Soft-tissue ossification in radial or sunburst pattern
- MRI:
  - ➤ Define tumor extent

➤ Assess joint space & adjacent structures (neurovascular bundle)
➤ Plan surgery
■ Chest CT
■ Bone scan:
➤ Define tumor extent
➤ Evaluate metastases to other bones & skip lesions in involved bone
■ Biopsy:
➤ Diagnostic
➤ Histology: pleomorphic, spindle-shaped tumor forming extracellular osteoid matrix

DIFFERENTIAL DIAGNOSIS
■ Osteomyelitis
■ Ewing's sarcoma
■ Aneurysmal bone cyst
■ Chondrosarcoma
■ Bony metastasis from other tumor

MANAGEMENT
■ Confirm diagnosis w/ biopsy
■ Metastatic workup: chest CT, bone scan
■ Consult orthopedic surgeon, pediatric oncologist
■ Central venous access for chemotherapy
■ Baseline organ function:
➤ Echocardiogram
➤ Creatinine clearance
➤ Audiogram
➤ Sperm banking for males
■ Psychosocial support
■ Transfusion support during chemotherapy

SPECIFIC THERAPY
■ Nonmetastatic:
➤ Combination therapy:
 • Agents
 • Doxorubicin
 • Cisplatin
 • Ifosfamide
 • Methotrexate
 • Cyclophosphamide
➤ Induction chemotherapy prior to surgical resection

➤ Post-surgical resection: Chemotherapy for several months
➤ Surgery:
  • Wide en bloc resection
  • Prosthesis replacement
  • If compromise of neurovascular bundle, amputation possibly
■ Metastatic:
  ➤ Intensive combination chemo
  ➤ Detectable disease not cured by chemo; needs resection (if possible)
  ➤ Not usually radiation-sensitive; radiation used as adjunct to surgery if complete resection not possible

FOLLOW-UP
■ Monitor CBC, LFTs, electrolytes, BUN/Cr, echocardiogram, audiogram
■ Monitor for surgical & long-term chemo complications
■ Evaluate febrile episodes
■ Physical therapy

COMPLICATIONS AND PROGNOSIS
■ Tumor: pathologic fracture
■ Surgery:
  ➤ Fracture
  ➤ Nonunion
  ➤ Infection of allograft or metal prosthesis
■ Chemo:
  ➤ Infection:
    • Risk factors: neutropenia, mucosal breakdown, central venous catheter
    • Bacterial, viral (HSV/zoster), fungal, parasitic
  ➤ Hemorrhagic cystitis/bladder scarring (ifosfamide, cyclophosphamide)
  ➤ Renal injury (cisplatin, methotrexate, ifosfamide)
  ➤ Deafness (cisplatin)
  ➤ Cardiomyopathy (anthracyclines)
  ➤ Infertility (ifosfamide, cyclophosphamide)

Prognosis
■ Nonmetastatic: 60–70% long-term disease-free survivors
  ➤ Good initial response to chemo: favorable
■ Metastatic disease:
  ➤ Poorer prognosis

➤ Cure only if complete resection of all visible disease & chemotherapy

OTITIS MEDIA WITH EFFUSION (CHRONIC OTITIS)

KENNETH GRUNDFAST, M.D., F.A.C.S., F.A.A.P.

HISTORY AND PHYSICAL

History
■ Usually follows acute otitis media
■ May or may not be accompanied by ear discomfort
■ Parent may notice child pulling at affected ear(s)
■ Usually accompanied by mild conductive hearing loss in affected
ear(s)

Physical signs
■ Eardrum appears dull, retracted, possibly has amber hue
■ Eardrum has poor mobility as tested with pneumatic otoscopy

TESTS
■ Tympanogram: flat
■ Hearing test: mild conductive hearing loss
■ Otoacoustic emission absent

DIFFERENTIAL DIAGNOSIS
■ End-stage adhesive otitis media
■ Myringosclerosis
■ Congenital cholesteatoma

MANAGEMENT
■ Repeated courses of antimicrobial therapy NOT indicated
■ Watchful waiting acceptable if child's hearing is adequate in at least
one ear
■ Speech development:
➤ If delay in speech development: need to be more aggressive in
considering insertion of tubes in ears

SPECIFIC THERAPY
■ Surgery:
➤ Myringotomy with insertion of tympanostomy tubes

➤ Adenoidectomy or adenotonsillectomy with insertion of tubes may help diminish likelihood that persistent otitis media will be problem in future

FOLLOW-UP
■ Repeat office exam q30 d to observe for resolution of effusion
■ Hearing test q2–3 mo as long as effusion persists

COMPLICATIONS AND PROGNOSIS
■ Adhesive otitis media
■ Ossicle erosion
■ Impaired speech development

Prognosis
■ Good if no significant hearing loss

PANCREATITIS

JAIME BELKIND-GERSON, M.D.

HISTORY AND PHYSICAL

History
■ Severe abdominal pain (often constant) with vomiting
■ Lack of oral tolerance (often includes fluids)
■ Blunt abdominal trauma
■ History of chronic disease, esp. lupus & cystic fibrosis (CF)
■ Preceding viral illness, esp. mumps
■ Obstruction in pancreatobiliary system (cholelithiasis)
■ Drug-induced:
  ➤ Steroids
  ➤ Alcohol
  ➤ Valproic acid
  ➤ Antibiotics
■ Previous bout of pancreatitis

Physical signs
■ Tachycardia
■ Mild jaundice possible
■ Fever common
■ Pain and tenderness:
  ➤ Continuous

- Mid-epigastric; may radiate to back
- Some degree of peritoneal irritation common
- Restless; often knee-chest position
- Bowel sounds decreased or absent
- Hemorrhagic pancreatitis:
  - Ascites
  - Pleural effusion
  - Cullen's sign (bluish periumbilical discoloration)
  - Grey Turner's sign (bluish flank discoloration)

TESTS
- Amylase: rises within hours, stays so 4–5 d
- Lipase (more sensitive than amylase): rises within hours, stays so 8–14 d
- CBC
- Electrolytes, glucose
- Liver function tests
- CXR for pleural effusions
- Abdominal ultrasound:
  - Edematous pancreas
  - Pseudocyst
  - To R/O cholelithiasis
- CT (in severe disease or equivocal ultrasound)
- ERCP:
  - Biliary stone
  - Chronic recurrent pancreatitis

DIFFERENTIAL DIAGNOSIS
- Peptic ulcer disease
- Intestinal obstruction w/ or w/o perforation
- Gastroenteritis
- Appendicitis
- Diabetic ketoacidosis
- Mumps (salivary hyperamylasemia)

MANAGEMENT
General measures
- Remove cause if possible
- NPO with IV fluids
- NG tube (persistent emesis)
- Pain relief

SPECIFIC THERAPY
- Pain control: meperidine; avoid morphine and codeine
- ERCP to remove stone(s) in biliary pancreatitis
- Severe pancreatitis: correct anemia, hypocalcemia, hypoalbuminemia, electrolyte imbalances, hypoxemia
- TPN or jejunostomy feeding
- Surgery:
  - Ductal rupture
  - Abscess formation
  - Pancreatic necrosis

FOLLOW-UP
- Improvement w/in 2–4 d
- Restart feeding when symptoms resolve & amylase near normal (not necessary to wait until lipase has normalized)
- Ultrasound 2–4 wks after resolution to R/O pseudocyst formation

COMPLICATIONS AND PROGNOSIS
Complications
- Severe hemorrhagic pancreatitis: 15% of cases
- Pseudocyst formation: suspect when failure of resolution, w/ recurrence or abdominal mass
- Pseudocysts <4 cm usually resolve spontaneously, larger ones may require drainage
- Chronic pancreatitis (rare in children, more common in hereditary pancreatitis or CF)
- Pancreatic abscess: high fever

Prognosis
- Usually single episodes that spontaneously resolve and have good outcome
- Severe pancreatitis: 20% mortality in children

PELVIC INFLAMMATORY DISEASE (PID)

MARISA BRETT, M.D.

HISTORY AND PHYSICAL
History
- Sexual history
- Assess risk for PID:

- ➤ Prior history of STD/PID
- ➤ Multiple sexual partners
- ➤ Partner w/ GU symptoms
- ➤ Pregnancy history, incl. ectopic
- Contraception, incl. oral contraceptives and IUD use
- Vaginal discharge
- Urinary tract symptoms
- Fever, abdominal pain
- Arthralgia, arthritis, rash

Physical signs

- Fever, systemic symptoms
- Lower abdominal pain, usually bilateral
- Vaginal discharge
- Cervical motion tenderness
- Adnexal tenderness

TESTS

- Vaginal discharge analysis
- Cervical swabs for gonorrhea & chlamydia
- CBC, ESR
- Urine hCG
- Urinalysis, urine culture
- Ultrasound (transabdominal/transvaginal) for:
  - ➤ Pelvic mass or severe pain (R/O torsion, tubo-ovarian abscess [TOA], ectopic pregnancy), or to verify intrauterine pregnancy (IUP) with positive hCG
  - ➤ Inability to perform adequate pelvic exam
- HIV testing

DIFFERENTIAL DIAGNOSIS

- PID:
  - ➤ Lower abdominal pain, adnexal tenderness, cervical motion tenderness
  - ➤ Also one of the following: temp >38.3 °C, elevated WBC, vaginal/cervical discharge, ESR >20 (or elevated C-reactive protein), documented gonorrhea or chlamydia assay
- Gynecologic:
  - ➤ TOA
  - ➤ Endometritis, peritonitis
  - ➤ IUP or ectopic pregnancy
  - ➤ Spontaneous abortion

➤ Ovarian torsion
➤ Endometriosis
➤ Ovarian cyst (rupture/bleed)
➤ Ovarian tumor
➤ Mittelschmerz, dysmenorrhea
■ GU:
  ➤ UTI
  ➤ Nephrolithiasis
  ➤ Pyelonephritis
■ GI:
  ➤ Appendicitis
  ➤ Pancreatitis
  ➤ Inflammatory bowel disease
  ➤ Abdominal catastrophe
  ➤ Constipation

MANAGEMENT

General measures
■ Hydration
■ Hospitalization:
  ➤ Unclear diagnosis
  ➤ Pregnancy
  ➤ Failure of outpatient regimen, severe illness, or TOA
  ➤ HIV or other immune compromise

SPECIFIC THERAPY
■ Antibiotics:
  ➤ Outpatient:
    • Ofloxacin 400 mg po bid ×14 d + metronidazole 500 mg po bid ×14 d
    • Alternative: ceftriaxone 250 mg IM ×1 or cefoxitin 2 g IM with probenecid 1 g po ×1 + doxycycline 100 mg po bid ×14 d
  ➤ Inpatient:
    • Cefoxitin 2 g IV q6h or cefotetan 2 g IV q12h + doxycycline 100 mg IV/po q12h
    • Alternative: clindamycin 900 mg IV q8h + gentamicin 2 mg/kg IV load followed by 1.5 mg/kg IV q8h; latter preferable for TOAs for better anaerobic coverage

FOLLOW-UP
■ 24–48 h after IV meds: change to oral doxycycline 100 mg po bid to complete 14 d; may use erythromycin if pregnant

- Education & preventive measures
- Contraceptive counseling
- Treat sexual partners
- Abstention from intercourse for 7 d after completion of therapy

COMPLICATIONS AND PROGNOSIS
- Ectopic pregnancy (3–7 fold greater risk)
- Infertility: 20% after 1 episode, >60% after 3 episodes
- Chronic abdominal pain
- Recurrent PID
- Dyspareunia
- Pelvic adhesions
- TOA

Prognosis
- Therapy effective for individual episodes
- Education & preventive measures critical but challenging in adolescent population

---

PEPTIC ULCER DISEASE

ROBERT VINCI, M.D.

HISTORY AND PHYSICAL

History
- Epigastric abdominal pain; may radiate to the back
- Often described as burning
- Pain may be relieved by eating
- Pain often awakens child at night
- Non-bilious vomiting; may be blood-tinged
- Heartburn or chest discomfort
- History of frequent burping
- Medication use: aspirin, NSAIDs, steroids
- Recent alcohol consumption
- Family history

Physical signs
- Usually well appearing
- Epigastric tenderness to palpation

TESTS
- Stool for guaiac may be positive

- CBC to evaluate for anemia
- Serum amylase/lipase
- Endoscopy with biopsy and urease breath test for *H. pylori*
- Serum *Helicobacter pylori* antibody assay

DIFFERENTIAL DIAGNOSIS
- Gastroesophageal reflux
- Esophagitis
- Gastritis
- Cholelithiasis
- Pancreatitis
- *Giardia* infection
- Inflammatory bowel disease
- Recurrent abdominal pain
- Irritable bowel syndrome

MANAGEMENT
General measures
- Stop aspirin and NSAIDs
- Avoid alcohol
- Antacids at bedtime and 2 h after meals
- IV fluids if dehydrated
- GI referral:
  - Endoscopy
  - Intractable symptoms

SPECIFIC THERAPY
- Antacids
- H2-receptor antagonist
- Proton pump inhibitor
- *H. pylori* infection:
  - Proton pump inhibitor + amoxicillin/metronidazole or clarithromycin/amoxicillin
  - Bismuth subsalicylate + amoxicillin/metronidazole
- Surgery (rarely indicated)

FOLLOW-UP
- Rx *H. pylori* infection for 2 wk
- Monitor for resolution of symptoms

COMPLICATIONS AND PROGNOSIS
Complications
- GI bleeding

- Gastric outlet obstruction
- Rarely gastric perforation

Prognosis
- Generally good with optimal medical management and avoidance of precipitating agents; recurrence rates as high as 35% have been reported

PERITONSILLAR AND PHARYNGEAL ABSCESSES

MUNISH GUPTA, M.D.

HISTORY AND PHYSICAL

History
- Peritonsillar abscess/cellulitis:
  - Infection of tonsillar fossa
  - Older children, adolescents
  - Etiology:
    - *S. pyogenes*
    - Anaerobes
    - *S. aureus*
  - Usually preceded by pharyngitis
  - Common symptoms:
    - Asymmetric throat pain
    - Trismus
    - Dysphagia
    - Drooling
    - Muffled "hot-potato" voice
  - Can see torticollis
- Retropharyngeal abscess:
  - Infection of potential space
  - Mostly in children age <4
  - Etiology:
    - *S. pyogenes*
    - Anaerobes
    - *S. aureus*
  - Common symptoms:
    - Preceding URI or pharyngitis
    - High fever
    - Sore throat
    - Dysphagia

- Stridor
- Drooling
➤ Can produce meningismus
➤ Most children appear acutely ill
➤ Head often kept extended
■ Lateral pharyngeal abscess:
➤ Infection of deep tissues of neck
➤ Usually infants, young children
➤ Common symptoms:
  - High fever
  - Trismus
➤ Usually have torticollis

Physical signs
■ Pharyngeal exam
■ Peritonsillar abscess/cellulitis:
➤ Asymmetric red large tonsils
➤ Bulge in soft palate
➤ Uvula deviation
➤ Fluctuance of peritonsillar tissue:
  - Yes: peritonsillar abscess
  - No: peritonsillar cellulitis
➤ Cellulitis can be bilateral
➤ Significant trismus
■ Retropharyngeal abscess:
➤ May see only erythema
➤ May see asymmetric swelling
■ Lateral pharyngeal abscess:
➤ Pharyngeal exam may be normal
➤ Can see submandibular swelling

TESTS
■ Peritonsillar abscess: clinical diagnosis
■ Retropharyngeal abscess:
➤ CT diagnostic
➤ Lateral x-ray of neck; inspiratory w/ full neck extension
➤ X-ray suggestive of abscess if:
  - Wide retropharyngeal space
  - At C2 >7 mm wide
  - At C4 >14 mm wide
  - >1/2 width of vertebral body
■ Lateral pharyngeal abscess:
➤ CT diagnostic

➤ CBC
➤ Blood culture if appears toxic

DIFFERENTIAL DIAGNOSIS
■ Viral or bacterial pharyngitis
■ Foreign body
■ Epiglottitis
■ Croup
■ Mononucleosis
■ Lymphadenitis
■ Lymphoma
■ Vertebral osteomyelitis

MANAGEMENT
■ Assess airway, respiratory status
■ Prompt consultation with ENT airway or respiratory compromise
■ Peritonsillar abscess:
  ➤ Drain, culture of material
  ➤ Nontoxic: oral antibiotics
  ➤ If ill-appearing: IV antibiotics
■ Peritonsillar cellulitis: hospitalize (IV antibiotics)
■ Retropharyngeal abscess:
  ➤ Hospitalize (IV antibiotics)
  ➤ Most require drainage
■ Lateral pharyngeal abscess:
  ➤ Hospitalize (IV antibiotics)
  ➤ Requires drainage

SPECIFIC THERAPY
■ Antibiotics:
  ➤ Polymicrobial coverage
  ➤ 1st-line:
    • Clindamycin
    • Penicillin
  ➤ Alternatives:
    • Macrolides
    • 1st-generation cephalosporin
    • Ampicillin/sulbactam
  ➤ Maintain hydration w/ IVF
■ Pain control
■ Drainage by ENT as necessary

FOLLOW-UP
- Recurrent peritonsillar disease occurs in 10–50%
- If frequent recurrence: tonsillectomy

COMPLICATIONS AND PROGNOSIS
- Airway/respiratory compromise
- Spontaneous rupture, aspiration
- Local spread of infection to:
  - Central vein thrombophlebitis
  - Septic embolization
  - Cellulitis
  - Ludwig angina
  - Mediastinitis

Prognosis
- Generally excellent

PERTUSSIS (WHOOPING COUGH)

COLIN MARCHANT, M.D.

HISTORY AND PHYSICAL
- Infants, unimmunized children
- Rare in immunized children
- More frequent in previously immunized adolescents and adults

History
- Household member or other close contact with pertussis

Physical signs
- Course:
  - Coryza & cough for 1–2 wks
  - Then paroxysmal coughing ± vomiting
  - Apnea and cyanosis in infants
  - Often lasts for weeks or months

TESTS
- WBC: absolute lymphocytosis typical but should not be relied upon for diagnosis or exclusion of the diagnosis
- Nasopharyngeal swab for culture of *Bordetella pertussis*:
  - Most useful in early weeks of disease

- Slow-growing bacterium; needs special culture media & may take 7–10 d to grow
- Some pts w/ typical pertussis may be culture negative
- PCR of nasopharyngeal secretions:
  - May be + in a few culture-negative patients
  - Limited availability
  - Serology available for diagnosis in some areas
- Report confirmed cases to local health authorities

DIFFERENTIAL DIAGNOSIS
- Vomiting infants:
  - Gastroesophageal reflux
  - Pyloric stenosis
- Coughing infants:
  - Pneumonia
  - Sepsis
- Severe/chronic cough in adolescents:
  - Sinusitis
  - *Mycoplasma pneumoniae*

MANAGEMENT
- Hospitalize and monitor young infant with history of apnea and/or cyanosis
- Intubation sometimes required
- Albuterol inhalations and corticosteroids of unproven value

SPECIFIC THERAPY
- Antibiotics:
  - Reduces transmission to others
  - Shortens disease duration if started in 1st 2 wks of illness
- Erythromycin:
  - For 14 days
  - Unproven alternatives that are probably effective:
    - Clarithromycin for 7 d
    - Azithromycin for 5 d
- Patients allergic to macrolides: consider co-trimoxazole
- Antimicrobial prophylaxis:
  - Household contacts
  - Close contacts in schools, day care
- Consult with local health authorities
- Sedatives, cough suppressants: not indicated

FOLLOW-UP
COMPLICATIONS AND PROGNOSIS
- Pneumonia rare; usually requires no treatment other than antibiotics
- Encephalopathy (presumably anoxic):
  - Rare complication of severe disease in infants
  - Prevented by mechanical ventilation of infants w/ significant apnea and/or cyanosis

Prognosis
- Generally excellent

PHARYNGITIS

JACK MAYPOLE, M.D.

HISTORY AND PHYSICAL

History
- Fever
- Sore throat
- Headache
- Abdominal pain
- Anorexia
- Chills
- Malaise
- History of contact with carrier

Physical
- No single finding differentiates bacterial from viral etiology
- Bacterial:
  - Group A beta-hemolytic streptococci (GABHS)
  - *N. gonorrhoeae*
  - *C. diphtheriae*
  - *H. influenzae*
  - *M. catarrhalis*
  - Group C & G streptococci
- Scarlet fever (GABHS):
  - "Sandpaper" rash
  - Erythematous macules
  - Pastia lines in antecubital fossa
- Mononucleosis: exudate, false membranes
- Diphtheria: thick, gray membranous exudate

- Chronic:
  - ➤ Postnasal drip/sinus infection
  - ➤ Chemical irritation
  - ➤ Neoplasm

TESTS
- Throat culture: GABHS
- Rapid strep test: 90% sensitive & 95–100% specific compared to throat culture
- Positive rapid strep test: throat culture not necessary
- Appropriate cultures (other etiologies suspected)
- Viral cultural (rarely)

DIFFERENTIAL DIAGNOSIS
- GABHS
- Viral pharyngitis
- Bacterial pharyngitis
- Mononucleosis
- Diphtheria
- Gonorrhea
- Peritonsillar abscess
- Epiglottitis
- Tracheitis

MANAGEMENT
- Culture before treatment for GABHS
- Antibiotics: GABHS
- Supportive care for pain, fever

SPECIFIC THERAPY
- Penicillin (first-line)
- Amoxicillin: superior for taste & compliance in young children
- Early treatment (w/in 48 h) may decrease duration of symptoms, but cause failure to develop immune response to GABHS
- Erythromycin (second-line if PCN allergic): poor compliance/taste
- Other: clarithromycin, azithromycin
- Cephalosporins:
  - ➤ Generally effective
  - ➤ Risk of PCN allergy
  - ➤ Cefuroxime, cefixime, cefpodoxime, loracarbef

FOLLOW-UP
- Monitor for dehydration in younger children; supportive care as necessary
- Most better w/in 24 h; return for reevaluation if no better by 48 h
- ENT referral (recurrent/severe infection)
- No clear role of antibiotics for family prophylaxis

COMPLICATIONS AND PROGNOSIS
- Symptoms usually resolve w/in 5–7 d
- Treatment of GABHS prevents development of acute rheumatic fever
- Rare:
  - Peritonsillar abscess
  - Sepsis
  - Mastoiditis
  - Sinusitis

PINWORMS

ELIZABETH BARNETT, M.D.

HISTORY AND PHYSICAL

History
- Perianal pruritus, usually occurring at night

Physical signs
- Small white worms from anus or found in stool

TESTS
- Visualization of worms
- Scotch tape test:
  - Apply sticky side of tape to anus in a.m.
  - Place on microscope slide
  - Identification of eggs makes diagnosis
- Eggs of *Enterobius vermicularis* in stool

DIFFERENTIAL DIAGNOSIS
- Anal fissure
- Perianal group A streptococcal infection
- Fungal vulvovaginitis
- Diaper or chemical dermatitis

MANAGEMENT
- Treat all affected family members

- Wash sheets, towels, clothing
- Vacuum house

SPECIFIC THERAPY
- Mebendazole
- Pyrantel pamoate
- Albendazole

Side effects of treatment
- Mebendazole:
  - ➤ Diarrhea
  - ➤ Abdominal pain
- Pyrantel pamoate:
  - ➤ GI disturbance
  - ➤ Headache
  - ➤ Dizziness
  - ➤ Rash
  - ➤ Fever
- Albendazole:
  - ➤ Abdominal pain
  - ➤ Reversible alopecia
  - ➤ Increased serum transaminase activity

FOLLOW-UP
- Symptoms should improve in several days
- Reinfection may occur

COMPLICATIONS AND PROGNOSIS
- No complications
- Prognosis excellent

PITYRIASIS ROSEA

SEAN PALFREY, M.D.

HISTORY AND PHYSICAL

History
- Common skin disorder of unknown etiology
- Often history of preceding viral infection
- Single macule at onset of rash (herald plaque), usually on trunk
- New lesions appear over next days to weeks
- Generally noncontagious

- No systemic symptoms
- Mild pruritus

Physical signs
- Generally well appearing
- Lesions usually oval, 2 mm–2 cm long
- Lesions salmon-colored or slightly darker than normal skin
- Raised, flaky edge; wrinkled center; mild excoriation
- "Christmas tree" pattern: slants from highest point near the midline, down across back & abdomen
- May also occur on face

TESTS
- Clinical diagnosis; diagnostic testing usually not indicated
- Skin biopsy (in uncertain cases)
- Syphilis testing (possible secondary syphilis)

DIFFERENTIAL DIAGNOSIS
- Nummular eczema:
  - Lesions more circular
  - Lesions not oriented in specific direction
- Secondary syphilis:
  - Lesions not oriented in specific direction
  - Lesions not as flaky or pruritic
- Tinea corporis:
  - Lesions more ringlike
  - Lesions scattered more randomly
- Tinea versicolor:
  - Lesions not as flaky or raised
  - May fluoresce under Wood's lamp

MANAGEMENT

General measures
- Usually no therapy necessary
- Lesions usually resolve in 2–3 mo
- Moderate sun exposure: speeds resolution
- Oatmeal baths, lubricants, mild topical steroids: to decrease itching
- Oral antihistamines: to decrease itching

SPECIFIC THERAPY
- No specific therapy

FOLLOW-UP
- Follow up management of symptoms
- Lesions often increase in number and size for 4–6 wks

COMPLICATIONS AND PROGNOSIS
- Often resolves over 4–8 wks with no long-term complications

PNEUMONIA

MUNISH GUPTA, M.D.

HISTORY AND PHYSICAL
- Common etiologies:
  - RSV: infants/toddlers
  - *Streptococcus pneumoniae*: all ages
  - Mycoplasma and chlamydia: generally age 4
- Less common etiologies:
  - Adenovirus, parainfluenza
  - Nontypeable *H. influenzae*
  - *Moraxella catarrhalis*
  - *S. aureus*: rare but serious
  - *S. pyogenes*: rare but serious
  - Tuberculosis
  - Pneumocystis
- Uncommon etiologies:
  - Rickettsiae
  - Fungi
  - Enteric bacteria
  - Pertussis
- Neonatal:
  - *E. coli*
  - Group B streptococci
  - Listeria
  - *Chlamydia trachomatis*

History
- Fever
- Cough
- Chills
- Often preceding/concurrent URI

- Fussiness, poor feeding (infants)
- Can mimic:
  - Meningismus (upper lobe)
  - Acute abdomen (lower lobe)

Physical signs
- Tachypnea: most sensitive sign
- Increased work of breathing
- Hypoxia
- Rales (can be absent)
- Wheeze: viral or mycoplasma
- Decreased breath sounds
- Dullness to percussion
- Can be occult in infants, with only fever and elevated WBC

TESTS
- CXR:
  - Indications:
    - Uncertain diagnosis
    - Acutely ill or toxic
    - Assist in determining etiology
    - Assess for complications
  - Interstitial: viral, atypical
  - Lobar: pneumococcus
  - Diffuse, patchy: any etiology
  - Pneumatoceles: *S. aureus*
  - Can be clear if dehydrated
- WBC:
  - Indications:
    - Aid in determining etiology
    - Predicts bacteremia in infants
  - Mildly elevated: viral
  - Elevated (<15–20,000): bacterial
- Blood culture: + in >5%
- Other tests:
  - Urine pneumococcal antigen
  - Cold agglutinins: mycoplasma
  - Bronchoscopy (if unresponsive to therapy)
  - Thoracentesis (if effusion present)
- Sputum unhelpful in young children
- NP swab generally unhelpful

DIFFERENTIAL DIAGNOSIS
- Bronchiolitis
- Asthma
- Aspiration
- Foreign body
- Hydrocarbon exposure
- Hypersensitivity reaction
- Pneumonitis
- Atelectasis
- Congenital malformation
- Tuberculosis
- Cystic fibrosis

MANAGEMENT
- Hospitalization:
  - Young age (suspected sepsis)
  - Hypoxia
  - Significant work of breathing
  - Assoc. effusion or empyema
  - Significant dehydration
  - Poor response to oral therapy

SPECIFIC THERAPY
- Antibiotics (outpatient):
  - 1st line: amoxicillin, cefuroxime
  - Age >4–5 yrs: azithromycin, clarithromycin
- Antibiotics (inpatient):
  - Ampicillin
  - Cefuroxime
  - Cefotaxime, ceftriaxone
- Penicillin-resistant pneumococcus suspected:
  - Cefotaxime, ceftriaxone
  - Vancomycin (if seriously ill)
- *S. aureus* suspected: add vancomycin or clindamycin
- IVF & oxygen if necessary
- Ribavirin (severe RSV)

FOLLOW-UP
- Usually no specific follow-up necessary
- Follow-up CXR for effusions
- Repeated bacterial pneumonia: evaluate for immunodeficiency

COMPLICATIONS AND PROGNOSIS

Complications
- Bacterial: effusion, empyema
- Viral: bronchiolitis obliterans

Prognosis
- Generally excellent
- Can have long course in infants
- Empyema can resolve slowly

PROTEINURIA

MICHELLE A. BAUM, M.D.

HISTORY AND PHYSICAL

History
- Recent illness
- Fever
- Rash
- Joint swelling
- Edema
- Systemic diseases
- Discolored urine
- Decreased urine output
- Hx of urinary tract infections (UTI)
- Family Hx of renal disease

Physical signs
- Blood pressure
- Growth
- Edema:
  - Periorbital
  - Pretibial
  - Sacral
- Rash
- Joint swelling
- Hepatosplenomegaly

TESTS

Phase 1
- Reconfirm: Dipstick first AM urine specimen

- Microscopic exam: fresh urine
- Urine protein/creatinine (Cr) ratio: normal <0.2

Phase 2
- Serum Cr
- If indicated:
  - Electrolytes
  - Albumin
  - Cholesterol
  - C3
  - ASLO
  - ANA
  - Syphilis
  - Hepatitis screen
  - HIV
- Renal imaging:
  - Ultrasound (UTI)
  - VCUG: if US suggestive of reflux or Hx of reflux

Phase 3
- Renal biopsy:
  - Active urine sediment
  - Constant proteinuria >600 mg/m^2
  - Exacerbating proteinuria
  - Hematuria, hypertension, renal insufficiency, systemic disease, or family history of ESRD

DIFFERENTIAL DIAGNOSIS
Transient:
- Dipstick <=2+
- Resolves spontaneously
- Causes:
  - Exercise
  - Stress, cold
  - Fever
  - Seizures
  - CHF
  - Epinephrine

Persistent
- Orthostatic:
  - Normal protein excretion when lying, increases on standing
  - Etiology unclear

➤ First AM urine (–), ambulatory urine >=2+
➤ <1 g/24 h
■ Persistent low-grade:
  ➤ Pro/Cr <1, >600 mg/m^2/d
  ➤ Workup negative; proteinuria persistent & not increasing
■ Persistent higher-grade:
  ➤ Pro/Cr >1, >600 mg/m^2/d
  ➤ Glomerular:
    • Minimal change disease
    • Focal segmental glomerulosclerosis
    • Chronic glomerulonephritis: postinfectious, membranoproliferative, membranous, IgA, HSP, Alport/hereditary nephritis, lupus
  ➤ Tubular: <2 g/d
    • Toxins: drugs or heavy metals
    • Ischemia
    • Fanconi
    • Lowe
    • Tyrosinemia
    • Cystinosis

MANAGEMENT
■ Transient/orthostatic:
  ➤ Reassure, yearly follow-up
■ Persistent asymptomatic:
  ➤ Renal biopsy to guide treatment
  ➤ Consider ACE inhibitor
  ➤ Quantify proteinuria 3 times/y
  ➤ Monitor Cr yearly
  ➤ BP
■ Persistent higher-grade:
  ➤ Renal biopsy to guide treatment
  ➤ Consider ACE inhibitor
  ➤ Steroids if disease responsive

SPECIFIC THERAPY
See Management section

FOLLOW-UP
■ Transient/orthostatic:
  ➤ Yearly BP & first AM urinalysis

➤ Phase 2 or 3 eval. if first AM urine becomes + or if active urine sediment
■ Persistent: depends on underlying cause

COMPLICATIONS AND PROGNOSIS
■ Transient/orthostatic: no evidence of progressive renal disease
■ Persistent low-grade: most have normal biopsies & no evidence of progressive renal disease
■ Persistent high-grade: depends on underlying cause

PSORIASIS

ALBERT C. YAN, M.D., F.A.A.P.

HISTORY AND PHYSICAL

History
■ May begin during childhood or adolescence
■ Chronic rash; waxing & waning course
■ May improve during warm, sunny weather and worsen in fall & winter
■ Associated arthritis (5%)

Physical signs
■ Papules/plaques w/ silvery scale
■ Auspitz sign: removal of scale reveals punctate bleeding
■ Nails: pitting, thickening, & oil spot
■ Koebner phenomenon: traumatized areas may develop psoriasis
■ Forms:
➤ Plaque-type: elbows, knees, dorsal hands
➤ Inverse: axillae, inguinal & genital areas
➤ Guttate: droplike papules on torso & extremities
➤ Pustular:
• Lakes of pustules on hands, feet, other body areas
• Can rapidly progress
➤ Erythrodermic: generalized scaly red skin over 90% of body
■ Examine joints

TESTS
■ Usually clinical diagnosis
■ Testing for group A strep infection (guttate)
■ Skin biopsy (rarely)

DIFFERENTIAL DIAGNOSIS
- Plaque-type:
  - Parapsoriasis
  - Cutaneous T-cell lymphoma
- Inverse:
  - Seborrheic dermatitis
  - Contact dermatitis
  - Tinea cruris
  - Reiter's
- Guttate:
  - Parapsoriasis
  - Pityriasis rosea
  - Pityriasis lichenoides
- Pustular:
  - Impetigo
  - Pustular drug eruption
  - Bullous tinea
  - Dishydrotic eczema
- Erythrodermic:
  - Atopic dermatitis
  - Drug eruption
  - Cutaneous T-cell lymphoma
  - Seborrheic dermatitis
  - Generalized contact dermatitis

MANAGEMENT
General measures
- Rheumatology consult (psoriatic arthritis)
- Avoid systemic steroids; severe flares can occur while tapering
- Gradually increase natural sunlight before 10 am, after 3 pm
- Avoid sunburn

SPECIFIC THERAPY
- Topical steroids:
  - Ointments better than creams
  - Limit potent topical steroids to bid up to 4 wks; 1-wk break & repeat
  - Face & genital areas:
    - Hydrocortisone ointment/cream
    - Desonide ointment/cream

- Scalp:
  - Fluocinolone solution (mild)
  - Mometasone lotion (moderate)
  - Clobetasol solution (severe)
- Hands and feet:
  - Fluocinolone ointment/cream (mild)
  - Betamethasone ointment/cream (moderate–severe)
  - Clobetasol ointment/cream (severe)
- Body areas:
  - Hydrocortisone ointment/cream (mild)
  - Fluocinolone 0.025% ointment/cream (mild-moderate)
  - Triamcinolone 0.1% ointment/cream (moderate-severe)
  - Fluocinonide ointment/cream (severe)
- Tar preparations:
  - Useful but photosensitizing
  - Tar shampoos daily PRN
  - Tar baths daily PRN
- Anthralin: short-contact therapy on resistant plaques
- Retinoids:
  - Mildly to moderately irritating
  - Tazarotene gel 0.05%, 0.1% qd to bid for body plaques
- Phototherapy: may provide remission
- Systemic immunosuppressives: severe flares

FOLLOW-UP
- Monitor for side effects of topical steroids
- Educate on steroid use
- Monitor for toxicity to vitamin D & A analogs

COMPLICATIONS AND PROGNOSIS
- Chronic arthritis
- Steroid side effects
- Hypercalcemia (systemic absorption of calcipotriene)
- Acute flares of pustular or erythrodermic; evaluate for:
  - Thermal instability
  - Fluid & electrolyte imbalances
  - Secondary infection & sepsis
- Psychological stress from intermittent flares
- Treatment controls signs & symptoms; occasionally results in re-mission

PSYCHOSIS

IRENE TIEN, M.D.

HISTORY AND PHYSICAL
- Psychiatric psychosis: often presents insidiously w/ prior psychiatric Hx (self or family)
- Organic psychosis:
  - Due to chronic illness, medication, or drug ingestion
  - May manifest visual and/or tactile hallucinations; rarely auditory hallucinations
- Pt often presents in agitated/confused state
- Orientation to time & place often disturbed
- May be highly distractible w/ significant disturbance of recent memory
- May persist in activities that place at risk
- Intellectual functioning may also be impaired

Physical signs
- Psychiatric: normal vital signs, neurologic, & mental status exams
- Organic: may be assoc. w/:
  - Fever (infection)
  - Tachycardia (assoc, w/ chronic illness or intoxication)
  - Evidence of pulmonary, cardiac, liver, or autoimmune disease
  - Neurologic exam: signs of CNS disease, esp. increased ICP
  - Signs of autonomic dysfunction (intoxication)

TESTS
- Suspected organic psychosis:
  - CBC
  - Urinalysis
  - Serum electrolytes
  - Calcium
  - BUN/Cr
  - Blood glucose
  - Complete drug & alcohol screens
  - Consider head CT, LP, LFTs, TFTs

DIFFERENTIAL DIAGNOSIS
- Psychiatric:
  - Autism: onset before age 30 mo

- Other pervasive developmental disorders: onset age 30 mo to 12 yr
- Adult-type schizophrenia: onset in adolescence
- Acute reactive psychosis
- Bipolar or manic-depressive illness

■ Organic:
  - CNS lesions:
    - Tumor
    - Brain abscess
    - Cerebral hemorrhage
    - Meningitis or encephalitis
    - Temporal lobe epilepsy
  - Cerebral hypoxia:
    - Pulmonary insufficiency
    - Severe anemia
    - Cardiac failure
    - Carbon monoxide poisoning
  - Metabolic & endocrine disorders:
    - Electrolyte imbalance
    - Hypoglycemia
    - Hypocalcemia
    - Thyroid disease
    - Adrenal disease
    - Uremia
    - Hepatic failure
    - Diabetes mellitus
    - Porphyria
  - Rheumatic diseases:
    - SLE
    - Polyarteritis nodosa
  - Infections:
    - Malaria
    - Typhoid fever
    - Subacute bacterial endocarditis
  - Miscellaneous:
    - Wilson
    - Reye

MANAGEMENT
■ Psychiatric:
  - Immediate psychiatric consult

- Quiet room, family & friends if appropriate, constant medical supervision
- No antipsychotic medication in ED when possible
- Use restraints if necessary for safety of pt, others
- Look for clinical variations of extrapyramidal reactions to antipsychotics
- Organic:
  - Diagnose underlying cause
  - Hospitalize for further evaluation & treatment
  - Consider psychiatric consult for drug ingestion-associated psychosis
  - Ensure pt & staff safety w/ chemical or physical restraints if necessary

SPECIFIC THERAPY
- Psychiatric: psychiatric consult & evaluation
- Organic: identify & treat underlying disorder

FOLLOW-UP
- Depends on underlying cause

COMPLICATIONS AND PROGNOSIS
- Psychiatric: often limited response to treatment w/ medication
- Organic:
  - Often respond dramatically to medical support & medication
  - Transient; prognosis depends on rapid identification & treatment of underlying illness

---

PULMONARY EMBOLISM (PE)

IRENE TIEN, M.D.

HISTORY AND PHYSICAL

History
- Ascertain risk factors:
  - Immobilization for >1wk
  - Hx of PE or DVT
  - Recent trauma, incl. femoral venous cannulation
  - Surgery in past month (esp. of lower extremities)
  - Recent long-distance air travel
  - Clotting disorder

➤ Female smoker on oral contraceptives
➤ Cardiorespiratory disorder
■ Classic presentation:
➤ Acute-onset pleuritic chest pain
➤ Shortness of breath
➤ Hemoptysis
➤ Other symptoms:
• Dyspnea
• Cough
• Syncope
• Cyanosis
• Cardiac arrest
• CHF
• Signs/Sx of DVT

Physical signs
■ Tachypnea
■ Tachycardia
■ Hypoxia
■ Hypotension

TESTS
■ ECG: T-wave inversion V1–V4; S1Q3T3: S-wave in lead 1, Q-wave in lead III, inverted T-wave in lead III
■ CXR:
➤ Focal oligemia
➤ Peripheral wedge-shaped density
➤ Enlarged right descending pulmonary artery
➤ Elevated hemidiaphragm
■ D-dimer (ELISA method): negative predictive value 90% but poor specificity; elevated if >500 mg/mL
■ ABG: normal A-a gradient in 50%
■ Duplex of legs
■ V/Q scan:
➤ Normal or low/intermediate/high probability
➤ Normal rules out, high probability rules in, low or intermediate probability is indeterminate
■ Spiral chest CT: may miss peripheral emboli
■ Echocardiogram: evidence of RV dysfunction secondary to larger PEs
■ Pulmonary angiogram:
➤ Gold standard
➤ Consider if other tests indeterminate but high clinical suspicion

DIFFERENTIAL DIAGNOSIS
- Pneumonia/bronchitis/asthma
- Myocardial infarction
- Pulmonary edema
- Costochondritis
- Anxiety
- Pneumothorax
- Chest trauma

MANAGEMENT
- Establish airway, breathing, circulation
- Supportive care
- May require blood pressure support

SPECIFIC THERAPY
- Initiate if high clinical suspicion regardless of diagnostic workup
- Unfractionated heparin:
  - 80 U/kg bolus, then 18 U/kg/h IV
  - Goal: PTT 60–80 sec
- Warfarin:
  - Start after therapeutic on heparin
  - Goal: INR 3.0 (3.5 if on heparin)
  - Not used in pregnancy
- Other potential therapy:
  - Low-molecular-weight heparin
  - Thrombolysis:
    - Used for massive PE and failure to respond to conventional therapy
    - Contraindicated in recent major trauma, surgery w/in past 10 d, CVA w/in 2 mo, bleeding diathesis, active internal hemorrhage
    - Local administration of thrombolytics
    - Surgical thrombectomy

FOLLOW-UP
- Admit for anticoagulation
- Discharge once therapeutic on warfarin and stable
- Warfarin:
  - 6 mo if first PE
  - Longer if recurrent PE or coagulation disorder
- Evaluate for coagulation disorder

COMPLICATIONS AND PROGNOSIS
- Most arise from failure to identify PE
- Massive emboli are often fatal; present as cardiorespiratory arrest
- Recurrence depends on etiology
- Worse prognosis: RV dysfunction on initial evaluation
- Prevention of recurrence: consider IVC filter if anticoagulation is contraindicated

---

PUNCTURE WOUNDS OF THE FOOT

ERIC FLEEGLER, M.D.

HISTORY AND PHYSICAL

History
- Determine time, mechanism, degree of contamination
- Identify penetrating object & history of foreign body (FB) in wound
- Occurred indoors or outdoors? Type of footwear?
- History of fever, local infection, or lymphangitis
- >50% plantar surface of foot
- Common causes: by nails (>90%), wood, metal, plastic, glass

Physical signs
- Fever
- Examine wound area; assess circulation & motor function distal to wound
- FB identified using good light, magnifying device
- Erythema, swelling, persistent pain (wound infection or retained FB)
- Pain and swelling >5 d after injury (suggest osteomyelitis)

Tests
- Radiograph (high suspicion for retained FB)
    - Glass and most metal 100% visible
    - May see filling defects of soft tissue or air in radiolucent FB
- Check for osteochondritis with periosteal reaction or bone/cartilage destruction
- Ultrasound or CT for wood splinters, shoes, socks, or debris
- Bone scan or MRI for presumed osteomyelitis

DIFFERENTIAL DIAGNOSIS
- Cellulitis
- Septic arthritis
- Abscess

- Osteomyelitis
- Osteochondritis

MANAGEMENT
- Blind wound exploration not recommended
- High-pressure irrigation using sterile saline with 18G angiocatheter
- Surgical referral for deep imbedded FB
- Organisms:
  - *Staphylococcus aureus*
  - Beta-hemolytic streptococci
  - Anaerobic bacteria
  - *Pseudomonas* (puncture wound through sneaker)
  - *Pasteurella multocida* (animal bite/claw puncture wounds)
- Rest, elevation, and intermittent warm-water soaks

SPECIFIC THERAPY
- Remove FB to avoid permanent tattooing; may use local anesthesia or nerve block to facilitate removal
- Leave surface open & bandaged
- If <24 h: antibiotics usually not needed except w/ animal-inflicted wounds
- If 24–72 h: oral anti-staphylococcal antibiotic (cephalexin, dicloxacillin, erythromycin)
- Possible *P. aeruginosa* or osteochondritis:
  - Orthopedic referral
  - IV antibiotics
  - Consider ciprofloxacin
  - May need surgical debridement
- Tetanus: determine immunization status

FOLLOW-UP
- See primary doctor w/in 48 h
- If pain persists >4 d: immediate evaluation needed; can be limb-threatening

COMPLICATIONS AND PROGNOSIS
Complications
- Low risk of infection <24 h after injury
- Osteochondritis of foot (of articular and physis cartilage)
  - 90% caused by *P. aeruginosa*
  - Most common if wound in forefoot, especially if wearing sneakers

- Toxic shock syndrome or streptococcal toxic shock-like syndrome
- Higher rate of infection in diabetic patients

Prognosis
- Most do well if managed with careful local wound care & judicious antibiotic use

PYLORIC STENOSIS

STEVE MOULTON, M.D.

HISTORY AND PHYSICAL

History
- Nonbilious, forceful ("projectile") vomiting
- Vomiting 30–60 min after feeding
- Infant hungry/active after vomiting
- Most common age 3–5 wks
- Male to female ratio: 4:1
- Common in first-born males
- Familial tendency

Physical signs
- Dehydration
- Gastric peristaltic waves in LUQ
- Palpable pyloric muscle ("olive")
- Lethargy (late finding)
- Cachexia

TESTS
- Electrolytes
- Ultrasound:
  - Channel length >16 mm
  - Muscle thickness >4 mm
- Upper GI study (if ultrasound nondiagnostic):
  - Enlarged stomach
  - Poor gastric emptying
  - Narrow pyloric channel (string sign)

DIFFERENTIAL DIAGNOSIS
- Overfeeding
- Pylorospasm: evident on ultrasound
- Gastroesophageal reflux
- Chalasia
- Malrotation

- Antral or duodenal web
- Pyloric duplication cyst
- Sepsis
- CNS or metabolic disorder
- Inborn error of metabolism

MANAGEMENT
What to do first
- Fluid management:
- IV hydration to correct electrolyte & fluid abnormalities
- ± Nasogastric tube

SPECIFIC THERAPY
- Operative approach:
  - ➤ Perioperative IV antibiotic
  - ➤ Pyloromyotomy:
    - Laparoscopy
    - Open procedure: incise serosa longitudinally over pylorus & split pyloric muscle
  - ➤ Postoperative feeds when fully awake/alert
  - ➤ Pedialyte to start & advance as tolerated in volume; then to normal diet of either breast milk or formula
  - ➤ Adjust IV fluids accordingly

FOLLOW-UP
- Routine post-op follow-up

COMPLICATIONS AND PROGNOSIS
- Wound infection (0.2–15%)
- Wound dehiscence/incisional hernia
- Inadequate myotomy (prolonged vomiting):
  - ➤ If no clinical signs of perforation, wait 1–2 wks before re-operating
  - ➤ R/O other causes

RABIES

EILEEN A. KENECK, M.D.

HISTORY AND PHYSICAL
History
- Bite or exposure to rabid animal's saliva via open wound
- History of being in enclosed space w/ bat

- Cave exploration
- Laboratory exposure to rabies virus
- High risk:
  - Raccoons, bats
  - Skunks, foxes
  - Woodchucks
  - Dogs in developing countries
  - Unprovoked attack by dog
- Lower risk:
  - Unimmunized dogs and cats in developed countries
  - Livestock
- Low risk:
  - Rodents
  - Rabbits

Physical signs
- Early symptoms:
  - May be nonspecific:
    - Pain at site of bite
    - umbness
    - Tingling
- Furious rabies (encephalitic form):
  - Agitation
  - Hydrophobia
  - Irritability
- Paralytic rabies ("dumb" form): resembles Guillain-Barre
- Rapidly progresses to death

TESTS
- Euthanize suspected animals; test brain tissue for fluorescent antigen
- Most human Dx made postmortem
- Antemortem Dx:
  - Skin biopsy from nape of neck (fluorescent microscopy)
  - Virus isolation in saliva
  - CSF or serum antibody detection

DIFFERENTIAL DIAGNOSIS
- Encephalitis
- Guillain-Barre

MANAGEMENT
- Prevention best: avoid bites
- Irrigate wound thoroughly

- Assess need for tetanus booster
- Don't suture wound if possible
- Assess need for rabies postexposure prophylaxis (PEP)
- Contact public health department
- Once symptomatic, almost all die

SPECIFIC THERAPY
- Test animal if possible
- Dogs, cats, and ferrets may be observed for 10 d; if still healthy, presumed not rabid
- If animal high risk or unavailable for testing: begin rabies PEP
- Rabies vaccine: 1.0 mL IM (deltoid) days 0, 3, 7, 14, and 28
- Rabies immune globulin (RIG):
  - 20 IU/kg (no max), as much as possible to infiltrate wound; remainder IM (gluteus)
  - Given day 0
  - If small volume needed to infiltrate, dilute with saline
- NEVER give vaccine and RIG at same site
- Side effects (rare in children):
  - Local reaction to immunization
  - Headache
  - Muscle aches
  - Dizziness
  - Reports of Guillain-Barre and other transient neurologic syndromes after immunization; causation unclear
- Those at high risk may be prophylactically immunized; do not require RIG if later exposed

FOLLOW-UP
- Potential rabies exposure: follow-up for subsequent vaccines
- Usual wound care

COMPLICATIONS AND PROGNOSIS
- Rare problems with rabies PEP
- Rabies disease fatal

RECURRENT ABDOMINAL PAIN

Joshua Sharfstein, M.D.

HISTORY AND PHYSICAL
- Defined as at least 3 paroxysmal episodes of pain between age 4 and 16 that affect day-to-day activities and occurs over 3 mo

- Key: differentiate functional pain (90% of cases) from specific disorder (10% of cases)
- Warning signs and symptoms requiring more extensive evaluation:
  - Onset < age 4
  - Pain awakens child
  - Pain not localized to umbilicus
  - Weight loss
  - Abnormal laboratory evaluation
  - Blood in stool
  - Perianal skin tags
  - Fissures
  - Rash or joint symptoms
  - Family history of significant GI disease
- Assess possible psychosocial stresses and triggers (e.g., pain began as soon as younger sibling was born)

TESTS
- Weight trend over time
- Stool for culture and ova and parasites
- Urinalysis, urine culture
- CBC, differential
- ESR
- Amylase, lipase, liver function tests, BUN, creatinine
- Rectal exam with stool guaiac
- More extensive lab and imaging evaluation if abnormal results or warning signs from history or family history

DIFFERENTIAL DIAGNOSIS
- Anatomic problems (i.e., obstruction)
- Infectious diseases (parasites, *H. pylori* gastritis)
- GI pathology:
  - Ulcers
  - Hepatitis
  - Pancreatitis
- Metabolic problems (lactose intolerance)
- Renal pathology (ureteropelvic junction obstruction)
- Gynecologic pathology:
  - Endometriosis
  - Imperforate hymen

MANAGEMENT
- Try to avoid "shotgun" approach of all possible diagnostic tests; may traumatize child & reinforce behaviors

■ Screening tests plus specific investigation based on abnormal results or specific symptoms

SPECIFIC THERAPY
■ If believed functional: reassure parents and encourage child to continue with normal routine
■ Consider psychologist consult

FOLLOW-UP
■ Inform parents of warning signs of severe disease
■ Frequent visits to monitor symptoms

COMPLICATIONS AND PROGNOSIS
■ Only 1/3 of children resolve pain w/in 5 yr

RESPIRATORY SYNCYTIAL VIRUS (RSV)

ELLEN COOPER, M.D.

HISTORY AND PHYSICAL
■ Older children have antibodies that neutralize RSV in vitro
■ Immunity incomplete, but protects against lower respiratory infections
■ Peak age for bronchiolitis: 2–8 mo (transplacentally acquired antibodies wane)
■ Premature infants miss major transplacental transfer of maternal antibody
■ Transmission:
  ➤ Hand-to-hand and/or fomites
  ➤ Aerosolized secretions less important
■ Incubation period: 3–5 d
■ Season: November–March
■ High risk for severe disease:
  ➤ Premature infants (<35 wks)
  ➤ Chronic lung disease
  ➤ Congenital heart disease
  ➤ T-cell defects
  ➤ Neuromuscular disease
  ➤ Metabolic disorders
■ Signs and Symptoms:
  ➤ URI

> Progression to cough
> Coryza
> Wheezing
> Rales
- Low-grade fever (10–20% have high fevers)
- Oral intake (hydration status critical)
- Retractions and cyanosis
- Apnea

TESTS
- Lab tests not routinely indicated
- Based on history and physical:
  > CBC, serum electrolytes
  > U/A
  > Oxygen saturation; ABGs if concern about oxygen retention
  > CXR: hyperinflated lung fields w/ increase in interstitial markings (20–25% have focal atelectasis)

Specific diagnostic test
- Nasal wash for antigen detection (rapid test) or culture

DIFFERENTIAL DIAGNOSIS
- Parainfluenza
- Adenovirus
- Influenza
- Mycoplasma

MANAGEMENT
- Admission criteria:
  > History of prematurity or other high-risk factor (e.g., BPD)
  > Age <3 mo
  > Atelectasis/pneumonitis on CXR
  > Oxygen sat <95% on room air

SPECIFIC THERAPY
- Hydration
- Monitor respiratory status
- Oxygen if necessary
- Beta-agonists suggested; supporting data conflicting
- Vaporized epinephrine
- Aerosolized ribavirin: use controversial, but consider for severe disease

FOLLOW-UP
- If admitted, monitor for hypoxia/respiratory distress
- If discharged, early follow up with PMD

COMPLICATIONS AND PROGNOSIS
- RSV bronchiolitis assoc. w/ subsequent wheezing & abnormal pulmonary function for up to 10 yrs
- Prevention:
  - RSVIG
  - Monoclonal antibody (palivizumab): better tolerated, easier to administer
  - Both given monthly during RSV season
  - Candidates in 1st year of life:
    - Infants born <28 wks gestation
    - Infants born at 29–32 wks and age <6 mo at onset of RSV season
    - Infants born at 33–35 wks w/ additional risk factors

RETINOBLASTOMA

JENNIFER MACK, M.D.

HISTORY AND PHYSICAL
- Leukokoria
- Strabismus: poor vision due to macular involvement
- Red, painful eye:
  - Intraocular inflammation
  - Uveitis
  - Vitreous hemorrhage
- Fixed pupil

TESTS
- Evaluate extent of intraocular tumor:
  - Dilated funduscopic exam under general anesthesia
  - Orbital ultrasound
- Evaluate orbital extension: CT of brain & orbit
- Metastatic disease evaluation:
  - MRI of brain & orbit
  - CSF cytology
  - Bone marrow aspirate/biopsy
  - Abdominal CT

DIFFERENTIAL DIAGNOSIS
- Coats disease

- Retinopathy of prematurity
- Persistent hyperplastic primary vitreous
- Severe uveitis

MANAGEMENT
- Ophthalmologist, oncologist referrals
- Options based on likelihood of maintaining useful vision & whether orbital extension & distant metastasis

SPECIFIC THERAPY
- Stage I (localized intraocular disease, normal intraocular pressure):
  - Small primary tumors:
    - Anterior retina: cryotherapy
    - Posterior retina: photocoagulation
  - Larger solitary tumors:
    - Plaque brachytherapy
    - Vitreous seeding: external beam radiation w/ adjunct cryotherapy
  - Extensive retinal involvement w/ no chance of preserving vision: enucleate
  - Alternative: chemotherapy to cytoreduce & avoid enucleation
- Stage II (orbital disease):
  - Disease beyond globe but not to lamina cribrosa: enucleate
  - Residual optic nerve involvement after enucleation: orbital irradiation, systemic & intrathecal chemotherapy
- Stage III (intracranial extension):
  - Enucleate
  - Orbital & whole-brain irradiation
  - Systemic & intrathecal chemotherapy
- Stage IV (distant metastases):
  - Enucleate
  - Orbital irradiation
  - Systemic & intrathecal chemotherapy
  - Alternative: high-dose chemotherapy w/ autologous marrow rescue

FOLLOW-UP
- Ongoing evaluation:
  - Recurrent disease (most w/in 3 y)
  - Second malignancies:
    - Osteogenic sarcoma
    - Soft-tissue sarcoma

- Brain tumor
- Leukemia
- Epithelial tumor
■ Ophthalmologic exam under general anesthesia: q4–6 wk first year; decrease frequency, yearly after 5 y
■ Consider head CT, CSF cytology, bone scan q3 mo (extraocular disease)
■ Children/siblings of pts w/ hereditary retinoblastoma: ophthalmologic exam under general anesthesia q3–4 mo for first 2 yr of life

COMPLICATIONS AND PROGNOSIS
■ Enucleation:
➤ Stunted growth of orbit with sunken appearance
➤ Loss of vision
■ Radiation:
➤ Stunted growth of orbit with sunken appearance
➤ Radiation vasculitis of choroid & retina
➤ Secondary glaucoma
➤ Cataracts
➤ Increased risk of second tumors
■ Photocoagulation:
➤ Retinal detachment
➤ Hemorrhage & dissemination of tumor into choroid & sclera
➤ Vision loss if used on optic disk or fovea
■ Cryotherapy:
➤ Localized vitreous hemorrhage
➤ Focal retinal detachment
■ Side effects of chemotherapy (cyclophosphamide, doxorubicin, vincristine, cisplatin, etoposide)

Prognosis
■ >85% survival
■ ~80% survival w/ useful vision
■ 30–50% w/ hereditary disease: second malignant tumors

RICKETS

KEVIN STRAUSS, M.D.

HISTORY AND PHYSICAL
History
■ Dietary Hx: Ca, phosphate, vitamin D
■ Sun exposure

- Growth delay
- Muscle weakness, hypotonia
- Tooth eruption delay
- May be seen in:
  - Fat malabsorption: flatulence, frequent bulky foul-smelling oily stools
  - Renal insufficiency
  - Liver disease
- Tetany, seizures

Physical signs
- Wide sutures/fontanel, parietal flattening, frontal bossing
- Rachitic rosary: prominent costochondral junctions
- Harrison's groove: indentation of ribs at diaphragmatic insertion
- Long bones:
  - Wide epiphyseal plates
  - Bowing
  - Fractures
- Tetany: Chvostek sign
- Tachycardia
- Weakness, hypotonia
- Seizure
- Teeth:
  - Enamel defects
  - Delayed eruption

TESTS
- Electrolytes, BUN, Cr, Ca, phosphate, Mg, ionized Ca
- Albumin
- X-rays:
  - Long bones:
    - Thin cortices
    - Bowing
    - Fractures
    - Metaphyseal flaring
  - Chest: rachitic rosary
- Serum ALP
- 25-hydroxy & 1,25-dihydroxy-vitamin D
- PTH
- ECG:
  - Long QTc AV block
  - Sinus tachycardia

- As clinically indicated:
  - Renal disease:
    - Urinalysis
    - Urine phosphate
  - Liver disease:
    - LFTs
    - Clotting studies
  - Malabsorption:
    - Other fat-soluble vitamins (A, E)
    - Fecal fat
    - Test for cystic fibrosis

DIFFERENTIAL DIAGNOSIS
- Vit D deficiency:
  - Dietary insufficiency
  - Malabsorption
  - Inadequate sunlight exposure
- 25-hydroxy-vit D deficiency: liver disease
- 1,25-dihydroxy-vit D deficiency: renal disease
- Vit D-dependent: defective Vit D receptor
- Hypophosphatemia:
  - Dietary insufficiency
  - Impaired renal tubular resorption:
    - Fanconi
    - X-linked vit D-resistant
- Hypoparathyroidism

MANAGEMENT
What to do first
- Correct cardiac arrhythmia, respiratory distress, seizure
- IV calcium:
  - CaCl 10%:
    - 0.2 mL/kg/dose, infuse over 2 min, repeat q10 min, max infusion rate 90 mg/kg/h
    - Immediate bioavailability
    - Use for cardiac arrhythmia
    - Side effect: vein sclerosis
  - Ca gluconate 10%: 1 mL/kg/dose, infuse over 2 min, repeat q10 min, max infusion rate 240 mg/kg/h
  - Avoid bicarbonate in same line: Ca carbonate precipitation in IV line/vein
- Hypocalcemia refractory to treatment: check Mg

SPECIFIC THERAPY
- Vit D deficiency:
  - Multivitamins
  - Ergocalciferol (25-hydroxy-vit D)
  - Calcitriol (1,25-dihydroxy-vit D)
- Hypophosphatemia:
  - IV route w/ severe symptomatic hypophosphatemia
  - Phosphate 5–10 mg/kg/dose IV q6–10 h, max infusion rate, 3 mg/kg/h
  - Oral: 30–90 mg/kg/d, dose greater w/ renal tubular defects
  - Monitor Ca: increasing phosphate too quickly could lead to hypocalcemia
- Diet: adequate Ca, phosphate

FOLLOW-UP
- Frequently assess skeletal growth
- Limit activity until bone strength restored
- Monitor Ca, phosphate, & Vit D metabolites during therapy
- Other F/U depends on underlying condition
- Genetic counseling & testing

COMPLICATIONS AND PROGNOSIS
- Seizure
- Fracture
- Arrhythmia
- Respiratory failure
- Overtreatment: hypercalcemia

Prognosis
- Dietary cause:
  - Generally good prognosis
  - Advanced case: permanent bone deformity and/or stunted growth
- Hereditary and systemic causes: variable

ROCKY MOUNTAIN SPOTTED FEVER (RMSF)

ELLEN COOPER, M.D.

HISTORY AND PHYSICAL
- Etiologic agent: *Rickettsia rickettsii*
- Carried by ticks, generally from Maryland to Georgia and west to Oklahoma

- Rare in Rocky Mountains (except in Bitter Root Valley)
- Peak incidence: correlates with tick activity (April–September)
- Children at greater risk than adults

History
- Nonspecific initial symptoms:
  - Severe headache (less often ataxia, delirium, stupor)
  - Myalgia
  - Nausea, vomiting
  - Photophobia

Physical signs
- Classic triad: fever, rash, and history of tick bite (1/3 conjunctival hyperemia)
- Rash:
  - Develops later and in only 80–90%
  - Starts 3–5 d after onset of fever
  - Blanching maculopapular eruption on ankles & wrists, spreading centripetally over 2–3 d, sparing face, but involving palms & soles
  - 50% progress to petechiae/purpura
- Severe vasculitis w/ occlusion of vessels, coagulopathy, & hypotension: can result in focal necrosis and (rarely) gangrene
- BP abnormalities: common secondary to abnormal fluid balance
- Periorbital edema

TESTS
- CBC:
  - Left shift
  - Mild anemia, thrombocytopenia in 1/3
- Electrolytes: hyponatremia in 20%
- LFTs: may be elevated
- Low serum albumin
- High BUN
- CSF:
  - Usually normal
  - Pleocytosis can occur
- Serologic assays that detect IgG to *R. rickettsii*:
  - Appears in 2nd–3rd wk of illness
  - Acute & convalescent sera recommended to avoid misinterpretation
- Newer rapid PCR techniques in development
- Weil-Felix test no longer recommended

DIFFERENTIAL DIAGNOSIS
- Meningococcemia
- Rickettsial pox
- Streptococcus
- Staphylococcus
- Enterovirus
- *Ehrlichia* infection
- Q fever
- Typhus
- Noninfectious vasculitis

MANAGEMENT
- Early therapy correlates w/ improved survival
- Treatment begun empirically

SPECIFIC THERAPY
- Doxycycline (drug of choice)
- Therapy continued until patient afebrile for at least 2–3 d (usually 7–10 d)
- Severe cases: supportive care for DIC, including careful fluid administration
- Steroids: use controversial; unproven benefit

FOLLOW-UP
COMPLICATIONS AND PROGNOSIS
- DIC leading to renal failure
- Cardiovascular collapse
- SIADH
- Pulmonary edema
- Intra-alveolar hemorrhage
- Children at greater risk than adults
- Mortality preantibiotic era: 30%; now 2% in children, 9% in elderly

SALMONELLA INFECTIONS

THOMAS SANDORA, M.D.

HISTORY AND PHYSICAL
- Gram-negative rods
- Principal reservoirs for nontyphoidal *Salmonella*: animals (poultry, livestock, reptiles, pets)

History
- Modes of transmission:
  - ➣ Foods of animal origin (poultry, red meat, eggs, unpasteurized milk)
  - ➣ Contaminated water
  - ➣ Infected reptiles
  - ➣ Person-to-person (fecal-oral route)
- *S. typhi*: found only in humans; contracted during travel to developing countries or by consumption of food contaminated by chronic carrier
- Duration of fecal excretion:
  - ➣ Variable, can last beyond 1 yr
  - ➣ Younger children excrete longer than older children

Physical signs
- Asymptomatic carriage
- Gastroenteritis:
  - ➣ Incubation: 6–72 h
  - ➣ Symptoms:
    - Diarrhea (+/– blood)
    - Abdominal pain
    - Fever
- Enteric fever (caused by *S. typhi*):
  - ➣ Incubation: usually 7–14 d
  - ➣ Signs/symptoms:
    - Fever
    - Constitutional sx: headache, malaise, anorexia, lethargy
    - Abdominal pain
    - Hepatosplenomegaly
    - Rose spots
    - Changes in mental status
  - ➣ Can progress to stupor & shock
- Bacteremia
- Focal infections:
  - ➣ Meningitis
  - ➣ Osteomyelitis
  - ➣ Abscesses

TESTS
- Cultures (depending on suspected syndrome):
  - ➣ Stool (gastroenteritis)

> Blood, stool, urine, bone marrow (enteric fever)
> Material from foci of infection (abscess, osteomyelitis)
■ Serologic tests for *Salmonella* agglutinins: may suggest *S. typhi*, but not recommended; poor sensitivity & specificity

DIFFERENTIAL DIAGNOSIS
■ Bacterial infections:
> *Shigella*
> *Yersinia*
> *Campylobacter*
> *E. coli*
■ Viral gastroenteritis
■ IBD
■ Surgical emergencies:
> Appendicitis
> Intussusception

MANAGEMENT
■ Hydration (IV fluids if necessary)
■ Serial abdominal exams
■ Antimicrobial therapy when indicated
■ Isolation (incl. contact precautions for hospitalized patients)
■ Control measures:
> Sanitation for food preparation
> Avoidance of raw poultry & eggs
> Handwashing
> Prohibition of reptiles as pets in homes w/ children age <5
> Report, investigation of outbreaks

SPECIFIC THERAPY
■ Antimicrobial therapy: usually not indicated for immunocompetent pts w/ uncomplicated gastroenteritis caused by nontyphoidal *Salmonella*, can prolong excretion of organisms
■ Antibiotics: gastroenteritis in:
> Age <3 mo
> Malignancy, hemoglobinopathy, HIV, other immunosuppression
> Chronic GI disease or severe colitis
■ Invasive *Salmonella* disease (typhoid, nontyphoid bacteremia, osteomyelitis):
> Ampicillin, amoxicillin, trimethoprim-sulfamethoxazole, cefotaxime, or ceftriaxone (based on sensitivities)

- ➤ *S. typhi*: 14-d therapy recommended
- ➤ Invasive infections w/o localization (i.e., bacteremia): treat for 14 d (HIV pts w/ bacteremia: 4–6 wks treatment)
- ➤ Localized infections: longer treatment
  - Osteomyelitis: 4–6 wks
  - Meningitis: at least 4 wks w/ ceftriaxone or cefotaxime
- ■ Chronic *S. typhi* carriage: eradicated in some pts by high-dose ampicillin or amoxicillin + probenecid or cholecystectomy
- ■ Corticosteroids: may be beneficial in critically ill pts w/ severe enteric fever & shock
- ■ Vaccine:
  - ➤ Typhoid vaccine
  - ➤ Indicated for travelers to developing countries or those with intimate exposure to documented carrier
  - ➤ Oral, live-attenuated or IM Vi polysaccharide vaccine
  - ➤ Contraindications:
    - Hx of severe local or systemic reaction after previous dose
    - Immunocompromised pts or w/in 24 h of dose of mefloquine; inhibits growth of vaccine strain *in vitro* (oral vaccine)

FOLLOW-UP
- ■ Isolation:
  - ➤ Incontinent or diapered children: for duration of illness
  - ➤ Enteric fever: until (–) cultures of 3 consecutive stool specimens obtained at least 48 h after cessation of antimicrobial therapy
- ■ Notification of public health authorities: important in detection & investigation of outbreaks

COMPLICATIONS AND PROGNOSIS
- ■ Relapse frequent after treatment of *S. typhi*; retreatment indicated
- ■ *Salmonella* gastroenteritis: bacteremia
- ■ Recognizable focal infections (meningitis, osteomyelitis, abscesses) in up to 10% of pts w/ *Salmonella* bacteremia; higher complication rate in age <5

Prognosis
- ■ Good in immunocompetent patients
- ■ Mortality more frequent in infants & those w/ underlying diseases (esp. hemoglobinopathy, malignancy, and immune deficiency)

SCABIES

GEOFF CAPRARO, M.D.

HISTORY AND PHYSICAL

History
- Intense generalized pruritus
- Sleep disturbance
- Excoriation
- Burrows/papules
- Web spaces, wrists, axillae, areola, buttocks, genitals
- Days–weeks
- Other family members w/ symptoms
- Fomites, close contacts, incl. sexual
- Developing countries (high prevalence)

Physical signs
- Well appearing, often itching
- Preschool/older:
  - Intertriginous burrows +/– black fleck
  - Excoriation
  - Papules
  - Nodules
- Infants/toddlers:
  - Atypical patterns
  - Large, red-brown papules/nodules
  - Wide distribution, incl. face & scalp
  - May lack burrows
- Norwegian scabies
  - Diffuse hyperkeratosis
  - Immunocompromised

TESTS
- Usually clinical Dx
- Direct microscopy of scraping
  - Scabies mite
    - Pincers at mouth
    - 8 short legs (larvae 6)
    - void body
  - Eggs
  - Feces

DIFFERENTIAL DIAGNOSIS
- Rhus dermatitis (exposure history to plants, fields, yardwork)
  - Linear arrays
  - Not intertriginous
  - No black fleck
  - More vesicular
  - Shorter duration
- Dyshydrotic eczema (more diffuse, scaling)
- Contact dermatitis (history of sensitivity, exposure)

MANAGEMENT
What to do first
- Educate contagious
- Educate that even w/ treatment itching can persist for weeks; mite products, excrement under skin are pruritic

General measures
- Keep nails short, clean
- Treat household & intimate contacts
- Hot-water wash bedding, towels, night clothes, & reworn clothes or place in plastic bag 2–3 d
- Antihistamines for pruritus
- Oilated oatmeal baths, emollients

SPECIFIC THERAPY
Indications for treatment
- Microscopy-confirmed Dx
- Strong clinical suspicion

Treatment options
- Permethrin 5% cream
  - Head to toe, 12–14 h overnight
  - Bath in am
  - Clean clothes/bedding
- Older children/adults: neck down
- Crotamiton cream/lotion: q24h ×2, bathe day 4
- Lindane 1%
  - 3rd line
  - Not for infants

Side effects and complications
- Occasional burning/stinging
- Permethrin: neurotoxicity (rare/theoretical)

■ Lindane (usually if misused):
  ➤ Possible seizures
  ➤ Vertigo
  ➤ Headache
■ Treatment failure: permethrin (<1/10)

Contraindications to treatment

Absolute
■ Allergy

Relative
■ Other Dx item more likely
  ➤ Empirically treat other Dx
  ➤ Perform scraping
■ Ragweed allergy (caution with pyrethrins)

FOLLOW-UP

During treatment
■ Pruritus
■ Contacts adequately treated
■ No new lesions
■ Failure/reinfestation only judged at 4 wks (healing course & life cycle)

Routine
■ If Dx uncertain

COMPLICATIONS AND PROGNOSIS
■ Recurrence
  ➤ Repeat permethrin
  ➤ Consider crotamiton
■ Superinfection common: mupirocin or cephalexin
■ STD evaluation if sexually active

Prognosis
■ Excellent

SCOLIOSIS

DONNA PACICCA, M.D.

HISTORY AND PHYSICAL

History
■ Present from birth (congenital scoliosis)
■ Chronic neurologic or paralytic disease may lead to scoliosis

- Most no etiology; age at onset is classified as follows:
  - Infantile: birth to 3 y
  - Juvenile: 4 y to onset of puberty
  - Adolescent: postpubescent
- Back pain (may indicate associated pathology)
- May worsen during adolescent growth spurt
- Family history of scoliosis (30%)
- Bowel/bladder incontinence and radicular symptoms (spinal cord pathology)

Physical signs
- Note posture and alignment of spine
- Evaluate for leg length discrepancy
- Evaluate flank crease symmetry
- Difference in height of shoulder may suggest scoliosis
- Adam's test: have patient bend forward at the waist to determine degree and direction of vertebrae rotation
- Measure degree of deformity with a Scoliometer™
- Foot deformity (e.g., cavus feet): suggests spinal cord pathology
- Hemiatrophy/hypertrophy
- Thorough neurologic exam, incl. abdominal reflexes (spinal cord pathology)

TESTS
- Plain radiographs with long cassette
- Need to equalize leg length difference with a lift
- Cobb angle: to measure angle of scoliosis; 10° requires referral
- Evaluate vertebral rotation based on asymmetry of pedicles
- Ossification of iliac apophysis correlates with spinal growth remaining
- MRI:
  - Atypical scoliosis
  - Possible spinal cord pathology
  - Left thoracic curve
  - Rapid curve progression

DIFFERENTIAL DIAGNOSIS
- Neuromuscular disease
- Spinal tumors
- Vertebral body anomalies
- Marfan's syndrome
- Neurofibromatosis

MANAGEMENT

General measures
- Orthopedic consult:
  - Scoliometer™ measurement >7°
  - Neurologic abnormality
- Observation for curves <7° measured with Scoliometer™

SPECIFIC THERAPY
- Bracing to prevent progression of curve in skeletally immature patient with further growth potential and progressive curve
- Surgical fusion and instrumentation: correct curve and prevent progression
- Ineffective treatments:
  - Chiropractic manipulation
  - Physical therapy
  - Electrical stimulation

FOLLOW-UP
- Depends on age of patient and degree of curvature
- Careful re-evaluation during periods of rapid growth
- May require repeat films
- Brace until skeletal maturity

COMPLICATIONS AND PROGNOSIS
- If progression is prevented, most do well
- Progression after skeletal maturity:
  - Curves <30°: unlikely to progress
  - Curves >50°: likely to progress
  - >30° in lumbar spine: likely to progress
- Cardiopulmonary compromise
- Restrictive lung disease
- Cor pulmonale in thoracic curves >90°
- Chronic back pain

SEIZURES/EPILEPSY

LAURIE DOUGLAS, M.D.

HISTORY AND PHYSICAL
- Epilepsy: 2 or more seizures

- Generalized seizures:
  - Generalized tonic-clonic (GTC):
    - Loss of consciousness (LOC)
    - Stiffening
    - Then entire body may jerk
  - Atonic: quick loss of body tone
  - Typical absence:
    - Usually 3–10 sec
    - LOC
    - Staring
    - Possibly eye fluttering
    - Ends abruptly
  - Atypical absence:
    - Usually 5–30 sec
    - Pt often delayed
    - Variable LOC
    - Staring
    - May involve eye fluttering
  - Myoclonus: shocklike jerks
- Simple partial seizures (no LOC):
  - Motor: focal twitching
  - Sensory: abnormal sensations
  - Autonomic: rare
  - Psychic phenomena
- Complex partial seizures:
  - Often <2 min
  - Stare
  - Decreased responsiveness
  - Automatisms
  - Drowsy afterward
- Common seizure syndromes:
  - Benign rolandic epilepsy (BRE):
    - Onset age 4–10
    - Nocturnal GTC seizures & morning facial twitching w/ speech arrest
    - EEG: centrotemporal spikes
  - Childhood absence epilepsy (CAE):
    - Family Hx often significant
    - Onset age 4–8
    - Several dozen absence seizures/day
    - Rare GTC seizures

  - Normal intellect
  - EEG: 3-Hz generalized spike waves
- Juvenile myoclonic epilepsy (JME):
  - Often positive family Hx
  - Peak onset age 12–18
  - Myoclonic & GTC seizures
  - 1/3 have absence seizures
  - Seizures often in a.m.
  - Triggers: lights, alcohol, sleep deprivation
- Lennox-Gastaut (LGS):
  - Childhood onset
  - Delayed development
  - Multiple seizure types
  - EEG: refractory, slow spike wave
- West:
  - Mental retardation
  - Infantile spasms
  - EEG: hypsarrhythmia
- Status epilepticus: any seizure lasting >30 min or 2 seizures with no recovery between

History
- Triggers, timing
- Warnings
- Focal features
- Incontinence
- Injuries
- Postictal period
- Family Hx

Physical signs
- Note any stigmata consistent w/ syndromes that include seizures

TESTS
- Electrolytes, glucose, Mg, phosphate, Ca, toxicology screen
- Anticonvulsant levels
- CT (suspected intracranial bleed)
- MRI: not for idiopathic epilepsy (CAE, JME, BRE) or simple febrile seizures
- EEG: not helpful for simple febrile seizures
- LP (suspected meningoencephalitis)
- Hyperventilation for 3 min: test for absence seizures

DIFFERENTIAL DIAGNOSIS
- Syncope or syncopal convulsion:
  - Preceded by dizziness or visual graying
  - Postictal state: tired but not confused
- Breath-holding spells
- Pseudoseizures
- Staring spells:
  - Daydreaming
  - Depression
  - ADHD
- Myoclonus:
  - Non-epileptiform myoclonus
  - Tics
  - Chorea

MANAGEMENT
- Status epilepticus:
  - Support respiratory effort & circulation
  - Secure IV access, obtain labs noted above
  - Glucose if hypoglycemic
- Treatment depends on seizure type, epilepsy syndrome, & cause
- Often do not treat initial seizure; do not treat febrile seizure or BRE unless upsetting to child/family

SPECIFIC THERAPY
- Status epilepticus:
  - Lorazepam initial drug of choice; may be repeated
  - Phenytoin, phenobarbital if lorazepam ineffective
  - Persists >60 min: anesthetic doses of barbiturates, benzodiazepines, or propofol
  - IV access difficult: consider rectal diazepam or IM fosphenytoin
- 1st-line:
  - GTC:
    - Carbamazepine
    - Oxcarbazepine
    - Phenytoin
    - Valproic acid
  - Absence:
    - Ethosuximide
    - Valproic acid
    - Avoid carbamazepine & phenytoin

➤ Simple partial, complex partial, & partial seizures w/ secondary generalization:
  • Carbamazepine
  • Oxcarbazepine
  • Phenytoin
➤ Myoclonic seizures:
  • Valproic acid
  • Benzodiazepines
■ Gabapentin (partial seizures)
■ Lamotrigine (broad-spectrum)
■ Topiramate (broad-spectrum)
■ Carbamazepine (partial; some GTC)
■ Zonisamide (broad-spectrum) Tiagabine (partial seizures)
■ Felbamate (broad-spectrum)
■ ACTH (infantile spasms)

FOLLOW-UP
■ Depends on cause of seizure, seizure type, response, & type of treatment

COMPLICATIONS AND PROGNOSIS
■ Risk of second seizure after first unprovoked seizure: ~40% (excludes absence or myoclonus; rarely occurs once)
■ Risk of third seizure after second: >80%
■ CAE & BRE: usually remit in puberty
■ JME: easy to control w/ modest dosages of medication but requires lifelong treatment
■ LGS:
  ➤ Refractory to treatment
  ➤ Possible progressive cognitive decline
■ Infantile spasms:
  ➤ Small percentage have normal development & remain seizure-free
  ➤ Most have moderate to severe developmental delays & refractory epilepsy

SEPTIC ARTHRITIS

KRIS REHM, M.D.

HISTORY AND PHYSICAL
■ Acute inflammation localized to a joint

- Pain, tenderness, swelling, erythema, decreased range of motion
- Early septic arthritis may have high fever & toxic-appearing pt
- Neonates
  - ➤ Poor feeding, irritability
  - ➤ "Pseudoparalysis" common, may present as sepsis
  - ➤ May be polyarticular, polymicrobial
- Young children (3 mo to 15 yr)
  - ➤ Fever, joint symptoms, limp
  - ➤ Osteomyelitis in children <1 yr, pain may be referred to a site other than the joint itself
- Older children & adolescents: fever, joint symptoms, limp

Physical
- Joint may be kept in position to maximize articular volume & decrease pressure in the joint (antalgic position)
- Hip: flexion, abduction, external rotation
- Knee/ankle: partial flexion
- Shoulder: adduction & internal rotation
- Elbow: midflexion

TESTS
- Laboratory tests: elevated ESR, CRP, WBC
- Blood culture positive in 30–40%
- Gold standard is arthrocentesis
- Appearance of synovial fluid may be purulent with WBC count >100,000
- Joint fluid culture positive in 70–80% of cases
- Gram stain joint fluid + in 50%
- Use antigen detection tests in patients pretreated with antibiotics
- Imaging tests: plain films, ultrasound, & nuclear scanning
- Plain films: swelling with widening of the joint space & soft tissue swelling
- Ultrasound: useful in evaluating hip joint for effusions & intra-articular bone disease
- Technetium bone scans: increased uptake in joint
- MRI most useful
- Synovial biopsy useful to diagnose Mycobacterium, fungi, or rheumatologic conditions

DIFFERENTIAL DIAGNOSIS
- Osteomyelitis
- Deep cellulitis

- Pyomyositis
- Psoas/retroperitoneal abscess
- Synovitis
- Septic bursitis
- Reactive arthritis
- Systemic vasculitis

MANAGEMENT
- Antibiotics, irrigation of joint space, & immobilization
- NSAIDs found to limit joint destruction in animals
- Early mobilization limits joint destruction – although no weight bearing

SPECIFIC THERAPY

Specific treatment
- Empiric antibiotics based on age, host-specific pathogens, Gram stain
- Initially given IV
- Longer duration in infections caused by *S. aureus* & Gram-negative rods
- *S. aureus* requires 4–6 wks
- *H. influenzae* & *S. pneumoniae* 10–14 d of therapy
- Open surgical drainage in all cases of hip infections, most in the shoulder, & those in which frank pus is obtained
- Supportive therapy includes splinting the joint initially
- Passive range of motion after 72 h

FOLLOW-UP
- Acutely, fever lasts 72 h-persistence suggests possibility of abscess, loculations, or osteomyelitis
- Joint inflammation resolves within 5–7 d
- Close monitoring required once pt has been transitioned to oral antibiotics

COMPLICATIONS AND PROGNOSIS
- Most important prognostic indicator is early diagnosis & treatment
- Poor prognostic indicators: age <6 mo, delayed treatment, *S. aureus*, Gram-negative, or fungal infections, hip or shoulderjoint involvement, & associated osteomyelitis
- Long-term complications include effects of epiphyseal damage, angular deformity, limb length shortening, early degenerative changes, & limited range of motion

SERUM SICKNESS

AMY L. WOODWARD, M.D.

HISTORY AND PHYSICAL

- Antigen-antibody immune complex deposition causes inflammation & tissue damage

History

- Occurs 7–10 d after exposure to causative agent
- Onset more rapid if prior exposure
- Can also see delayed symptoms
- Classic serum sickness: IV injection of heterologous serum protein:
  - Uncommon; decreased use of heterologous serum
  - Seen with antitoxin, antivenom, antithymocyte globulin
- Serum sickness-like reaction: similar to classical serum sickness:
  - Non-protein medication
    - Antibiotics: penicillin, sulfonamide, cephalosporin, streptomycin
    - Hydantoins
    - Thiouracil
  - Allergy immunotherapy
  - Insect sting (*Hymenoptera*)
  - Infectious agent

Physical signs

Classical 5 features:

- Fever (usually present): 10–20%, precedes rash
- Rash (95%)
  - Urticaria: 90% of rashes
  - Maculopapular, petechial, or purpuric lesions also seen
- Angioedema: (esp. face/neck)
- Lymphadenopathy: 10–20%
- Arthralgia/arthritis: 10–50%
- Less common features:
  - Nephritis
  - Carditis, pericarditis
  - Wheezing
  - Abdominal pain
  - Hepatosplenomegaly
  - Neuritis (central or peripheral)

TESTS
- None diagnostic
- CBC:
  - ➤ Leukopenia or slight leukocytosis
  - ➤ Possible eosinophilia
- ESR: often elevated
- C3, C4, CH50: may be decreased
- Cryoglobulins: may be elevated
- Hepatitis B screen
- Urinalysis: possible proteinuria, hematuria, hyaline casts
- Stool guaiac (abdominal pain)
- ECG (cardiac symptoms)

DIFFERENTIAL DIAGNOSIS
- Infection (esp. hepatitis B)
- Autoimmune disease: SLE, systemic JRA
- Drug reaction

MANAGEMENT
- Discontinue exposure to causative agent
- Supportive care

SPECIFIC THERAPY
- Antihistamines: urticaria, angioedema
- NSAIDs: arthritis, fever
- Corticosteroid: severe, refractory cases; short course, taper 10–14 d

FOLLOW-UP
- Majority: manage as outpatient
- Severe case: hospitalization may be beneficial
- Avoid causative agent in future
- Consider desensitization if future avoidance not possible

COMPLICATIONS AND PROGNOSIS
- Generally excellent; gradual resolution over 1–2 wks

SEVERE COMBINED IMMUNODEFICIENCY DISORDERS (SCID)

ANDREW KOH, M.D.

HISTORY AND PHYSICAL
- Severe impairment/absence of antibody-mediated (B cell) and cell-mediated (T cell) immunity from birth

- Genetic heterogeneity
- Variants:
  1. X-linked SCID
  2. Adenosine deaminase deficiency
  3. SCID with leukopenia: reticular dysgenesis
  4. SCID with defective expression of HLA antigens
  5. T-cell kinase deficiencies
  6. SCID with reticuloendotheliosis:

History
- Diarrhea, vomiting within first few mos after birth
- Recurrent infection:
  - Otitis media
  - Pneumonia
  - Sepsis
  - Skin infection
- Persistent infection w/ opportunistic pathogens:
  - *Candida albicans*
  - *Pneumocystis carinii*
  - Cytomegalovirus
  - Epstein-Barr
  - Varicella
  - Respiratory syncytial virus
  - Parainfluenza
  - Adenovirus
- FTT due to diarrhea/infection
- Rashes secondary to infection or GVHD
- Absent tonsils or palpable lymph nodes
- Small thymus

TESTS
- Immunoglobulin (Ig) levels: very low or absent
- CBC:
  - Lymphopenia (some variants)
  - All lymphocyte subsets low in ADA-deficient SCID
  - Very low or absent T cells
- Absence of lymphocyte proliferative responses to mitogens, antigens, & allogeneic cells in vitro
- NK cells & function: very low in X-linked SCID pts
- Genetic/molecular tests: for diagnosis

DIFFERENTIAL DIAGNOSIS
- Secondary immunodeficiencies:

> HIV infection
> GI protein-losing enteropathy

MANAGEMENT

What to do first
- Tests and genetic/molecular confirmation
- Treat infections w/ antibiotics
- Consider IgG replacement

General measures
- Transfuse w/ irradiated blood products only (avoid GVHD)
- *Pneumocystis* prophylaxis: co-trimoxazole
- Future pregnancies:
  > Antenatal diagnosis of X-linked SCID by molecular methods
  > All other SCID syndromes: 15 wk gestation fetal blood lymphocyte phenotyping

SPECIFIC THERAPY
- Bone marrow transplantation with matched sibling marrow (best chance for survival & correction)

FOLLOW-UP
- Monitor Ig levels, T cell function, growth
- Watch for possible infection

COMPLICATIONS AND PROGNOSIS
- Opportunistic infections

Prognosis
- Morbidity and mortality depend on particular SCID syndrome
- Unless bone marrow transplantation, high fatality rate

SHIGELLA INFECTIONS

THOMAS SANDORA, M.D.

HISTORY AND PHYSICAL
- Gram-negative rods of 4 species (*S. sonnei* & *S. flexneri* most common in U.S.)
- Source: feces of infected humans (no known animal reservoirs)

History
- Predisposing factors:
  > Crowded living conditions

> Poor hygiene
> Travel to developing countries
- Transmission: by fecal-oral route; ingestion of contaminated food or water
- Most common in children age 1–4 yr; frequent in child care centers
- Incubation period: 1–7 d; carrier state usually ceases w/in 4 wk of onset of illness

Physical signs
- Diarrhea (+/– blood or mucus)
- Fever
- Abdominal pain
- Headache
- Seizures

TESTS
- Cultures of feces or rectal swab specimens
- Bacteremia rare; blood cultures necessary only in severely ill or immunocompromised pts
- Stool smear stained w/ methylene blue may reveal leukocytes (indicative of enterocolitis but not specific for *Shigella*)

DIFFERENTIAL DIAGNOSIS
- Bacterial infections:
  > *Salmonella*
  > *Yersinia*
  > *Campylobacter*
  > *E. coli*
- Viral gastroenteritis
- Inflammatory bowel disease
- Surgical emergencies:
  > Appendicitis
  > Intussusception

MANAGEMENT
- Hydration (IV fluids if necessary)
- Serial abdominal exams
- Antimicrobial therapy
- Isolation (incl. contact precautions for hospitalized pts)
- Control measures:
  > Handwashing (most important)

> Sanitation for food preparation & water supplies
> Prevention of contamination of food by flies
> Report & investigation of outbreaks

SPECIFIC THERAPY

■ Antimicrobial therapy for all pts w/ *Shigella* (shortens duration of diarrhea and eliminates organisms from feces, which prevents spread)
■ Antibiotic susceptibility testing indicated; resistance is common
■ Ceftriaxone (initial drug of choice when sensitivities unknown)
■ Ampicillin and trimethoprim-sulfamethoxazole: effective for sensitive strains
■ Consider fluoroquinolones for resistant strains
■ Oral therapy acceptable except in seriously ill pts; treatment course is 5 d
■ Contraindications: antidiarrheal compounds that inhibit intestinal peristalsis (prolong clinical & bacteriologic course of disease)

FOLLOW-UP

■ When *Shigella* identified in child care attendee or staff member, stool specimens from other symptomatic persons should be cultured; household contacts w/ diarrhea should also be cultured
■ Pts should not be permitted to re-enter programs until diarrhea has ceased and stool cultures are negative
■ If several persons are infected, consider cohort system until stool cultures negative
■ Notification of public health authorities

COMPLICATIONS AND PROGNOSIS

■ Rare sequelae:
■ Bacteremia
■ Reiter *syndrome* (after *S. flexneri* infection)
■ HUS (from *S. dysenteriae* type 1 infection)
■ Colonic perforation
■ Fulminant toxic encephalopathy (which can be lethal w/in 4–48 h of onset)

Prognosis

■ Generally good in absence of CNS involvement or other complications

SHORT STATURE

SULEIMAN NJELAWUNI MUSTAFA-KUTANA, M.D.

HISTORY AND PHYSICAL

Defined by:

- Height <2 SDs below mean
- Height <2 SDs below mean parental height (MPH), calculated by:
  - Boy = [mother's ht + father's ht +5″ (13 cm)]/2
  - Girl = [mother's ht + father's ht −5″ (13 cm)]/2
    - Find MPH percentile at 18–20-y point; extrapolate back to current age on growth chart
- "Falling off" usual growth curve

History

- Measurements:
  - Supine stadiometer for age <3 y or child unable to stand
  - Sturdy "against the wall" stadiometer for age >3 y
  - Average of 3 measurements
  - Measure at same time of day for each pt: up to a 0.5-cm difference between am & pm
- Plot heights on growth chart for age (closest month)
- Pregnancy/fetal history (intrauterine infection or growth delay)
- Chronic illness & drugs:
  - Asthma
  - Diabetes
  - Failure to thrive
  - Renal
  - Cardiac
  - Steroids
- Weight
- Diet, appetite
- Malabsorption:
  - Foul-smelling oily frequent stools
  - Flatulence
- Trauma/injuries, esp. to head
- Size of siblings & parents
- Dysmorphisms, height/weight ratio
- Previous growth points: crossing 2 percentiles usually means pathology
- Pubertal developmental stage, Hx in parents

TESTS
- CBC, electrolytes
- BUN/creatinine
- Liver function tests
- Thyroid function studies
- Urinalysis
- Bone-age x-ray:
- As clinically indicated:
  - IGF-1 & IGFBP-3
  - Chromosome analysis

DIFFERENTIAL DIAGNOSIS
- Major organ system disease:
  - CNS
  - Cardiac
  - Pulmonary
  - Hematologic
  - Renal
  - GI or nutritional
- Chromosomal disorder (e.g., Turner)
- Inborn errors of metabolism
- IUGR
- Familial or genetic short stature
- Constitutional delay of growth & adolescence
- Endocrine disorders:
  - Hypothyroidism
  - Poorly controlled diabetes
  - Cortisol excess
  - Growth hormone (GH) deficiency
  - Rickets
- Deprivation or psychosocial

MANAGEMENT
- Treat underlying cause
- Endocrinology consult for unclear cases

SPECIFIC THERAPY
- GH replacement:
  - Approved for GH deficiency, Turner, chronic renal insufficiency
  - Currently being studied: constitutional delay, familial short stature, idiopathic short stature

FOLLOW-UP
- Endocrinology visits q3–4 mo while on GH therapy
- Treat until puberty is fully established and/or response is minimal

COMPLICATIONS AND PROGNOSIS
- No major complications w/ recombinant GH
- Side effects:
  - Insulin resistance
  - Mild water/sodium retention
  - Joint pains
  - Discomfort at injection site
  - No evidence for increased risk of malignancies in those w/o risk factors; may be <2-fold increase

Prognosis
- Usually excellent w/ GH therapy in approved diagnosis & effective monitoring:
  - Improved self-image & self-confidence
  - No reported disadvantage in 20 y follow-up

SHOULDER INJURIES

ELIZABETH CALMAR, M.D.

HISTORY AND PHYSICAL

History
- Mechanism of injury
- Previous injury or surgery
- Acute vs. chronic (attrition)
- Radicular pain to elbow or hand
- Paresthesias to lower extremity
- Sports (overuse; stress fracture)
- Does shoulder lock or grind during movement (bone fragment or labral tear)?
- Pain at rest: bursitis vs. infection or malignancy
- Pain at night (osteoid osteoma)
- History of minor trauma w/ pain & swelling: always R/O malignancy

Physical
- Key points on exam:
  - Active ROM
  - Passive ROM

➤ Impingement sign: pain on forward flexion past 90°
➤ Palpate clavicle, AC joint, biceps tendon, rotator cuff
➤ Apprehension sign:
  • Guarding against passive positioning of arm in abduction/ external rotation suggests chronic dislocator
■ Drop arm test for rotator cuff tear:
➤ Passively bring arm to 90° abduction
➤ Unable to hold against gravity = full tear
➤ Unable to hold against resistance = partial tear
■ Crossover arm test:
➤ Abduct arm 90° & reach for opposite shoulder
➤ Pain = AC joint injury

TESTS
■ Routine x-rays:
➤ AP internal rotation
➤ Axillary lateral
➤ AP external rotation
■ Trauma series:
➤ True neutral AP
➤ Y-lateral
➤ Axillary lateral

DIFFERENTIAL DIAGNOSIS
■ Bursitis:
➤ Inflammation of lining over rotator cuff
➤ Pain at rest & all ROMs
■ Tendinitis:
➤ Inflammation of biceps or rotator cuff tendons
➤ Pain on palpation
➤ Impingement sign
■ Rotator cuff tear:
➤ Weakness
➤ + drop arm test
■ Chronic dislocator:
➤ Anterior instability
➤ Apprehension sign
■ Separation: AC joint injury
■ Dislocation (glenohumeral joint)
■ Fracture
■ Infection

MANAGEMENT

What to do first
- Assess for neurovascular compromise
- Emergency reduction of dislocation
- Make certain no Salter fractures:
    - Reduction maneuvers:
        1. Traction-countertraction
        2. Adduction/gentle external rotation
        3. Gentle forward elevation

General measures
- Sling & swathe immobilization
- Ice
- Anti-inflammatory drugs
- Orthopedic consult:
    - Salter fracture
    - Fracture dislocation
    - Pathologic lesion

SPECIFIC THERAPY
- Depends on extent of initial injury
- Operative repair for chronic dislocator
- Physical therapy
- IV antibiotics for septic joint

FOLLOW-UP
- Fracture/dislocation: depends on extent of initial injury

COMPLICATIONS AND PROGNOSIS

Complications
- Nerve impingement w/ acute dislocation

Prognosis
- Most do well w/ proper care & appropriate physical therapy

SICKLE CELL DISEASE

SHARON SPACE, M.D.

HISTORY AND PHYSICAL
- Hereditary hemoglobinopathy with abnormal beta-globin chain
- Recurrent vaso-occlusive crises (VOC) & hemolytic anemia

History
- Frequency & severity of crises varies
- Severity of anemia varies; symptoms reflect severity

Physical signs
- Pallor
- Scleral icterus
- Systolic ejection murmur
- Delayed puberty

TESTS
- Newborn screening confirmed by Hb electrophoresis
- CBC w/ differential, reticulocyte

DIFFERENTIAL DIAGNOSIS
- Variants:
  - Hb SS, Hb S-B°thal: more severe disease
  - Hb SC, Hb S-B+thal: milder disease

MANAGEMENT
- Education: importance of infection, fever, & pain management

SPECIFIC THERAPY
- Chronic hemolytic anemia: folic acid 1 mg po qd
- Increased risk of infection:
  - Penicillin prophylaxis: 125 mg po bid age <3 yr, 250 mg po bid age >3 yr (until at least age 5)
  - Standard immunizations, incl. PCV, meningococcal vaccine (age 2), influenza vaccine annually
- Hydroxyurea:
  - Increases HbF production
  - Decreases frequency & severity of VOC
  - Indicated in severe disease:
    - Multiple acute chest syndrome (ACS)
    - Frequent hospitalization
  - Monitor CBC q2–4 wk for toxicity; neutropenia most common sign
- PRBC transfusions:
  - Simple transfusion:
    - To increase oxygen-carrying capacity
    - May be indicated for severe or worsening anemia or ACS

➤ Exchange transfusion:
  • To decrease % Hb S <30
  • Indicated for CVA, severe ACS
➤ Chronic monthly transfusion: pts w/ CVA

FOLLOW-UP
■ Annual/biannual visits at sickle cell center
■ Annual labs:
  ➤ CBC & reticulocyte count
  ➤ LFTs
  ➤ Bilirubin
  ➤ Urinalysis
  ➤ BUN/Cr
■ Cardiology evaluation in early adolescence
■ Ophthalmology follow-up annually after age 10: screen for sickle retinopathy
■ Transcranial Doppler ultrasound: screening for CVA risk in children w/ Hb SS and Hb Sb°-thal

COMPLICATIONS AND PROGNOSIS
■ VOC pain/painful crisis:
  ➤ Any organ system; commonly musculoskeletal or abdominal
  ➤ Hydration at maintenance (avoid overhydration; can precipitate ACS)
  ➤ Pain medication:
    • Start w/ acetaminophen or NSAID
    • Increase as needed to oral or IV narcotics
■ ACS:
  ➤ New infiltrate on CXR w/ fever >101°F, cough, chest pain, hypoxia (oxygen saturation 3–5% below baseline), or shortness of breath
  ➤ Hospitalize for treatment:
    • Broad-spectrum antibiotic (ceftriaxone or ceftazidine) for 48 h
    • Erythromycin to cover mycoplasma if age >2 yr
    • Oxygen as indicated
  ➤ Bronchodilator, esp if Hx of reactive airway disease
  ➤ Incentive spirometry
  ➤ Consider PRBC transfusion for worsening or severe disease
■ Fever:
  ➤ >101°F: immediate medical evaluation:
    • CBC with differential & reticulocyte

- Blood cultures
- CXR
- Type and screen
- Urinalysis for males age <6 mo & females age <2 yr
- ➤ Parenteral broad-spectrum antibiotic for encapsulated organisms for at least 48 h
- ➤ Admit if age <9 mo, fever >103°F, toxic appearance, unable to maintain oral hydration, new neurologic findings, Hb/Hct below or above baseline, concern regarding noncompliance with follow-up
- ➤ Others managed as outpatient w/ second evaluation & parenteral antibiotics 24 h later
- ▪ Splenic sequestration:
  - ➤ Acute increase in spleen size w/ decrease in Hb >1g ± thrombocytopenia
  - ➤ Most common in children w/ Hb SS age <3 yr
  - ➤ Treatment:
    - Evaluate for shock; treat accordingly
    - Monitor Hb/Hct & spleen size frequently until stable
    - onsider PRBC transfusion as indicated for worsening anemia or clinical deterioration
  - ➤ High risk of recurrence
  - ➤ Consider splenectomy for pts w/ 1 severe life-threatening or recurrent sequestration
- ▪ Stroke:
  - ➤ 10%
  - ➤ Acute treatment: exchange transfusion immediately to decrease % Hb S <30
  - ➤ Long-term treatment:
    - 90% recurrence w/o intervention
    - Chronic monthly PRBC transfusion to maintain Hb S <30% w/ iron chelation
- ▪ Complications due to chronic hemolysis: >50% develop gallstones
- ▪ Aplastic crisis: parvoviral infection stops bone marrow RBC production, temporarily causing severe anemia & often requiring transfusion
- ▪ Recurrent VOC & tissue infarction: significant morbidity in adults:
  - ➤ Chronic restrictive lung disease
  - ➤ Renal failure

➤ Liver dysfunction
➤ Pulmonary hypertension
■ Average life expectancy: 40–50 y

SINUSITIS

LISE NIGROVIC, M.D.

HISTORY AND PHYSICAL

History
■ Predisposition:
  ➤ Medical conditions:
    • Allergic rhinitis
    • Asthma
    • Immunologic defects
    • Dental infections
    • Cystic fibrosis
  ➤ Anatomic factors:
    • Adenoid hypertrophy
    • Septal deviation
    • Nasal trauma
  ➤ Environmental factors:
    • Day care attendance
    • Tobacco smoke exposure
■ Sinus development:
  ➤ Ethmoid sinuses developed at birth
  ➤ Maxillary sinuses: age 18 mo
  ➤ Sphenoid sinuses: age 3–5 yr
  ➤ Frontal sinuses: age >6 yr
■ Complicates 0.5–5% of URI
■ Blocked sinus ostia:
  ➤ Inflammation or anatomic abnormalities
  ➤ Leads to retained secretions & sinusitis
  ➤ Symptoms:
    • Fever
    • Headache
    • Purulent nasal discharge
    • Nighttime cough
  ➤ Must persist 7–10 d for diagnosis
  ➤ Chronic sinusitis: symptoms persisting >3 mo

Physical signs
- Localized tenderness to pressure, malodorous breath, or periorbital swelling
- Sinus opacity w/ transillumination (not diagnostic in young children)

TESTS
- Typically clinical diagnosis
- Sinus x-rays:
  - Often misleading, esp. in young children
  - Positive findings:
    - Sinus opacification
    - Air-fluid levels
    - Mucosal thickening (>4 mm)
- Sinus CT:
  - Most sensitive to visualize sinus disease
  - May show early changes of URI, leading to overdiagnosis
- Sinus aspiration identifies organism for persistent cases or immuno-compromised host
- Gram stain:
  - Polynuclear cells (infection)
  - Eosinophils (allergic disease)
  - Most common:
    - *Streptococcus pneumoniae*
    - Nontypeable *Haemophilus influenzae*
    - *Moraxella catarrhalis*
  - Viral:
    - Rhinovirus
    - Influenza
    - Parainfluenzae
  - Less common:
    - *Staphylococcus aureus*
    - Group A & C streptococci
    - Anaerobes

DIFFERENTIAL DIAGNOSIS
- Viral URI
- Allergic rhinitis
- Periorbital cellulitis

MANAGEMENT
- Nasal saline drops

- Humidified warm air
- Decongestants not helpful

SPECIFIC THERAPY
- Acute sinusitis:
  - Antimicrobials (10–14 d):
    - Amoxicillin
    - Co-trimoxazole
    - Amoxicillin/clavulanate
    - Cefuroxime
    - Azithromycin
- Chronic sinusitis:
  - Nasal corticosteroids: to block mucosal hyperactivity & edema
  - Antibiotics: 6 wks
- Surgical options: for antibiotic treatment failures or for intraorbital or intracranial complications

FOLLOW-UP
- Return to physician after completing treatment course
- Consider retreating for persistent symptoms

COMPLICATIONS AND PROGNOSIS
- Infectious:
  - Periorbital or orbital cellulitis
  - Meningitis
  - Epidural, subdural, or brain abscess
  - Cranial osteomyelitis
- Thrombotic: cavernous vein thrombosis
- Neurologic:
  - Optic neuritis
  - Ophthalmic migraine
  - Trigeminal neuralgia (sphenoid sinusitis)

Prognosis
- 70% spontaneous resolution
- 85% resolution w/ first course of antibiotics

SLIPPED CAPITAL FEMORAL EPIPHYSIS (SCFE)

DONNA PACICCA, M.D.

HISTORY AND PHYSICAL
- Adolescent
- Males > females

History
- Limp, usually in the absence of trauma
- Hip or knee pain, usually lateral thigh:
  - May affect both legs in 1/3 of cases
  - Pain may occur in thigh
- Pain may be intermittent
- Chronic SCFE: insidious onset of pain
- Acute SCFE: usually abrupt onset of pain
- Unstable SCFE: inability to bear weight
- Family history of SCFE
- Endocrinopathy

Physical signs
- Obesity common
- Examine those hips!
- Patient prefers position of obligate external rotation w/ hip flexion
- Pain with motion of hip, especially with internal rotation & hip flexion
- Limp with Trendelenburg gait (abductor lurch) or external rotation of affected side

TESTS
- X-ray:
  - AP and frog-leg lateral of both hips
  - May have asymptomatic slip on other side
  - Apparent loss of height of epiphysis
  - Irregularity and widening of the physis
  - Line tangential to superior femoral neck (Klein's line) does not intersect epiphysis
  - Frog-leg lateral view will show posterior slip of epiphysis

DIFFERENTIAL DIAGNOSIS
- Acute fracture through physis: usually high-energy injury in young child
- Musculoskeletal injury to hip/thigh
- Legg-Calve-Perthes

MANAGEMENT

What to do first
- Prevent progression by making non-weight bearing

General measures
- Pain control

- Hospitalization
- Orthopedic consult

SPECIFIC THERAPY
- Operative treatment
- Postoperative physical therapy

FOLLOW-UP
- Standard postoperative care
- Return promptly for pain in either hip
- Hardware not routinely removed

COMPLICATIONS AND PROGNOSIS
- Osteonecrosis:
  - Associated with unstable slips, multiple (>2) screws, aggressive reduction may occur in absence of treatment
- Chondrolysis: loss of articular cartilage

STREET DRUGS

ROBERT VINCI, M.D.

HISTORY AND PHYSICAL

History
- Recent "rave" party attendance
- Previous street drug use; may develop tolerance to drugs & their effects
- Amount & type of drug use
- Co-ingestion of alcohol
- Euphoria, confusion, or agitation

Physical signs
- Respiratory depression
- Fluid loss, dehydration
- Skin exam for IV drug use
- Dilated pupils (sympathomimetics)
- Excessive catecholamine state (cocaine, amphetamines, Ecstasy):
  - Tachycardia
  - Hypertension
  - Hyperthermia
  - Seizures
  - Arrhythmia

- Muscle spasms (Ecstasy)
- Nystagmus (gamma-hydroxybutyric acid & ketamine)

TESTS
- Serum alcohol level
- Specific drug levels
- Serum electrolytes, BUN, creatinine
- EKG, CK, troponin
- Urine for myoglobin
- Contact crime lab: assay for "date rape" drugs, esp. Rohypnol (short-acting benzodiazepine not detected in routine urine screens)

DIFFERENTIAL DIAGNOSIS
- Cocaine
- Amphetamines
- Ecstasy
- Gamma-hydroxybutyric acid
- Ketamine
- Rohypnol
- Head trauma
- Metabolic abnormality
- Heat stroke

MANAGEMENT
What to do first
- Assess for respiratory depression
- Emergency airway support

General measures
- Contact local Poison Control Center
- IV fluids
- Gastric lavage (minimal benefit)
- Rapid cooling
- Benzodiazepines for anxiety
- Monitor for arrhythmias

SPECIFIC THERAPY
- Benzodiazepines for seizures
- Antihypertensives for malignant hypertension
- Consider flumazenil for benzodiazepine overdose:
    - 0.02 mg/kg (max, 0.2 mg)

➤ Contraindications: mixed overdoses w/ seizure potential, esp. TCA
- Treat serotonin syndrome:
  - ➤ Rapid cooling
  - ➤ Serotonergic antagonists: chlorpromazine, cyproheptadine
  - ➤ Beta-blockers; may block serotonin receptors
  - ➤ Dantrolene for hyperthermia

FOLLOW-UP
- Admit for severe symptoms
- Monitor for complications

COMPLICATIONS AND PROGNOSIS
- Depends on degree of overdose
- HIV and hepatitis with IV drug use
- Thrombophlebitis
- Sympathomimetic overdose:
  - ➤ Heat stroke
  - ➤ Fluid/electrolyte abnormalities
  - ➤ Cardiac arrhythmias
  - ➤ DIC
  - ➤ Rhabdomyolysis (marathon dancing)
  - ➤ Multisystem organ failure
  - ➤ Myocardial ischemia
- Long-term neurologic sequelae with Ecstasy use:
  - ➤ Cognitive deficits
  - ➤ Long-term memory loss
  - ➤ Parkinsonism

STRIDOR

KENNETH GRUNDFAST, M.D., F.A.C.S., F.A.A.P.

HISTORY AND PHYSICAL
- NOT a diagnosis, but a symptom
- Stridor is not asthma
- Must find site of lesion & make specific diagnosis

History
- Inspiratory stridor: site of airway obstruction cephalad to vocal cords
- Both inspiratory and expiratory: subglottic narrowing, such as sub-glottic stenosis or subglottic hemangioma

- Prodrome (e.g., URI): laryngotracheitis (croup) rather than epiglottitis
- Abnormal voice or cry: vocal cord paresis/paralysis or lesion of a vocal cord such as papilloma
- Stridor that worsens w/ feeding: vascular ring or mediastinal mass
- Stridor that is worse prone than supine: laryngomalacia
- Drooling: epiglottitis or retropharyngeal abscess
- Maternal history of "venereal warts": laryngeal papilloma

Physical signs
- Look for cutaneous hemangioma that might correlate w/ subglottic hemangioma

TESTS
- Flexible direct laryngoscopy
- Plain radiographs:
  - "Airway films"
  - Steeple sign (narrow subglottis)
  - AP/lateral: high kilovoltage to make airway more visible
- Video fluoroscopy
- Direct rigid bronchoscopy

DIFFERENTIAL DIAGNOSIS
- Croup = laryngotracheitis
- Epiglottitis
- Vocal cord paralysis
- Laryngeal papilloma
- Subglottic hemangioma
- Subglottic stenosis
- Foreign body
- Adenotonsillar hypertrophy
- Retropharyngeal abscess

MANAGEMENT
- Ensure airway is adequate!
- Don't risk airway compromise
- Need to make diagnosis
- Assess severity
- Monitor oxygen saturation
- Otolaryngology consult

SPECIFIC THERAPY
- Observe, monitor

- Significant airway compromise: secure IV access as soon as possible
- Nebulized racemic epinephrine and oral steroids
- Laryngoscopy and bronchoscopy (inadequate airway or nonspecific diagnosis)
- Endotracheal intubation: to treat severe croup & epiglottitis
- Tracheotomy if adequate airway cannot be secured w/ endotracheal intubation
- Laser removal (laryngeal papilloma)
- Surgical repair for subglottic stenosis

FOLLOW-UP
- Depends on lesion
- Recurrence not expected
- Recurring croup: underlying lesion
- Teach parents what to do if child develops signs of airway compromise (e.g., recurring stridor, cyanosis)

COMPLICATIONS AND PROGNOSIS
- Hypoxemia
- Respiratory distress
- Respiratory arrest
- Bradycardia/arrhythmia

Prognosis
- Depends on adequacy of treatment for underlying disorder or specific lesion

SUICIDE

HOWARD BAUCHNER, M.D.

HISTORY AND PHYSICAL
- Third leading cause of death in teenagers
- Completed suicide 5 times more common in boys than girls
- Attempted suicide 5 times more common in girls

History
- Previous suicide attempts
- Direct or indirect communication of intent
- Symptoms of depression
- History of life stresses, substance abuse

Physical signs
■ Consistent with depression or other psychiatric disorders

TESTS
■ Interview family members and child
■ Assess risk for suicide:
   ➤ Low risk:
     • No prior attempts
     • No substance abuse
     • No psychiatric disorder
     • Ambivalence about desire to die
   ➤ Moderate risk:
     • History of suicide attempts
     • Psychiatric history
     • Substance abuse
     • Plan vague
     • Limited feasibility
   ➤ High risk:
     • Psychotic thinking
     • Unremitting crisis
     • Clear plan
     • Lack or rejection of family support

DIFFERENTIAL DIAGNOSIS
■ Need to assess risk

MANAGEMENT
■ Low risk: enlist support of families or others
■ Moderate or high risk: psychiatric evaluation

SPECIFIC THERAPY
■ Consider hospitalization depending on psychiatric evaluation
■ Psychopharmacologic evaluation coupled with behavioral therapy

FOLLOW-UP
■ Low risk: mental health provider follow-up within 72 hr
■ Moderate to high risk: follow recommendations from psychiatric evaluation

COMPLICATIONS AND PROGNOSIS
■ Depends on associated co-morbidities and access to and success of psychiatric evaluation and treatment

SUNBURN

JENNIFER KASPER, M.D. MPH

HISTORY AND PHYSICAL
- Prolonged exposure to sun with minimal/no sun protection
- Risk factors for melanoma:
  - Blistering sunburns in childhood
  - Intermittent intense sun exposure

History
- Infants at increased risk because not ambulatory
- Caucasian, Celtic, Irish most at risk

Physical signs
- 1st degree:
  - Epidermis involved
  - Painful, erythematous
- 2nd degree:
  - Epidermis and less than half of dermis
  - Painful, blisters
- 3rd degree:
  - Full-thickness
  - Painless
  - Pale/charred color, leathery

TESTS
- None indicated

DIFFERENTIAL DIAGNOSIS
- Water, chemical, electrical burn
- Cold injury/frostbite

MANAGEMENT
- First aid: cool water
- No ice, grease, or butter

SPECIFIC THERAPY
- If sunburn extensive:
  - Debride edges, leave blisters intact
  - Apply silver sulfadiazine (bacitracin if sulfonamide sensitivity), loose gauze
  - Dressing changes bid
  - Ibuprofen 10 mg/kg for pain

- Consider IV fluids if dehydrated
- Prophylactic antibiotics not recommended

FOLLOW-UP
- If extensive, q1–2 d until healing well underway

COMPLICATIONS AND PROGNOSIS
- 1st degree: heals in 3–5 d without scarring
- 2nd degree: heals in 2 wks with minimal scarring
- 3rd degree: heals in weeks, skin grafting often necessary
- Nausea, malaise, headache, fever/chills, delirium, prostration
- Prevention:
  - Clothing with tightly woven fabrics, hats, sunglasses
  - Avoid sun between 10 am and 2 pm
  - Use waterproof sunscreens with at least 30 SPF with UVA and UVB protection, or zinc or titanium dioxide
  - Higher elevations need sunscreen with higher SPF
  - Reapply sunscreen q4 h
- Drugs that induce photosensitivity:
  - NSAIDs
  - Griseofulvin
  - Oral contraceptives
  - Phenothiazine
  - Psoralens
  - Sulfonylureas
  - Tretinoin
  - PABA-containing sunscreens
  - Tetracycline
  - Diuretics

SUPRAVENTRICULAR TACHYCARDIA (SVT)

STEVE SESLAR, M.D.
SHARON O'BRIEN, M.D.

HISTORY AND PHYSICAL
- Infants:
  - SVT short: asymptomatic
  - SVT >1–2 d: congestive heart failure (CHF)
  - Feeding intolerance
  - Irritabilitity
  - Diaphoresis

- Toddlers:
  - Sudden change in activity
  - Creative descriptions: "there's a woodpecker in my chest" or "my heart is beeping"
  - May perceive palpitations as pain
- Older children/adolescents:
  - Palpitations or racing heart
  - Often nausea or dizziness
- Precipitants: stimulants (e.g., caffeine, pseudoephedrine)
- History of congenital heart disease

Physical
- Assess for hemodynamic compromise:
  - Blood pressure
  - Pulses
  - Mentation
- Pulse rate, rhythm
- Evidence of congenital heart disease:
  - Cyanosis
  - Clubbing
  - Sternotomy scar
- Signs of CHF: see "Congestive heart failure" entry

TESTS
- EKG: 12-lead EKG & rhythm strip; narrow complex, regular tachyarrhythmia with 1:1 AV relationship (when P waves visible), retrograde P waves following QRS
- Continuously running rhythm strip during conversion
- EKG following termination: assess pre-excitation (i.e., Wolff-Parkinson-White syndrome) or other conduction abnormalities
- Echocardiogram: rule out structural heart disease, assess function

DIFFERENTIAL DIAGNOSIS
- Sinus tachycardia
- Primary atrial arrhythmia (ectopic atrial tachycardia, atrial flutter, or fibrillation)
- Junctional ectopic tachycardia
- Ventricular tachycardia: wide & fast

MANAGEMENT
What to do first:
- Synchronized DC cardioversion, 0.5–1 joules/kg if unstable or ventricular tachycardia cannot be excluded

- Vagal maneuvers: ice to face, gagging, Valsalva
- Adenosine:
  - Dose 0.1 mg/kg
  - Double if ineffective
  - Max dose 12 mg
  - Diltiazem in older children if adenosine not effective
- If available, temporary pacing may be used by experienced personnel

SPECIFIC THERAPY
- Prevent recurrence
- Consider no therapy for 1st time uncomplicated episode or for infrequent recurrences that spontaneously terminate
- Teach parent or pt how to check pulse rate & vagal maneuvers
- Medications: beta-blockers, digoxin, class IC antiarrhythmics (i.e., flecainide)
- Radiofrequency catheter ablation
- Assess for cardiac disease

FOLLOW-UP
- No symptoms w/ spontaneous or adenosine termination: follow as outpatient
- CHF, tachycardias refractory to cardioversion, or suspicion of structural heart disease: admit, observe, & further evaluate
- Long-term: depends on frequency of episodes & treatment strategy

COMPLICATIONS AND PROGNOSIS

Complications
- Conduction defect
  - Syncope
  - Need electrophysiology study & possible radiofrequency catheter ablation
- Cardiomyopathy from prolonged or incessant tachycardia
- Cardiac arrest & death

Prognosis
- Good without structural heart disease
  - 85% of infants "outgrow" SVT; of these 33% will have recurrence in adolescence
  - Beyond infancy, most will continue to have episodes of SVT
- Very young & very old tolerate SVT poorly

SYNCOPE

SHARON O'BRIEN, M.D.

HISTORY AND PHYSICAL

Neurocardiogenic syncope: most common cause of noncardiac syncope

History

- Sudden, brief loss of consciousness
- Prodrome of pallor, nausea, diaphoresis, lightheadedness, dizziness, hyperventilation
- Associated with fright, anxiety, fasting, heat, crowds, prolonged standing
- Falling usually without injury
- Brief (<1 min) duration
- History of the following increases risk of serious cause
  - Injury
  - Syncope with exercise
  - Lack of prodrome
  - Prolonged or frequent syncope
  - Chest pain
  - Palpitations
  - Loss of bowel/bladder control
  - Seizure
- Family history
  - Seizures
  - Syncope
  - Sudden death
  - Hearing loss: prolonged QTc syndrome

Physical

- May be normal
- Orthostatic hypotension: drop of 15 mmHg from supine to standing blood pressure consistent with vasovagal syncope
- Obvious injuries
- Cardiac murmurs (obstructive lesions)
- Abnormal neurologic exam
- Hyperventilation may reproduce episode

TESTS

- ECG

- Electrolytes/glucose
- CXR
- EEG
- Tilt table test
- Echocardiogram

DIFFERENTIAL DIAGNOSIS
- Autonomic: neurally mediated most common
- Cardiac
  - Prolonged QTc syndrome
  - Arrhythmia (see "Arrhythmia" entry)
  - Obstructive lesion (AS/IHSS)
- Neurologic
  - Seizures
  - Hyperventilation
  - Dysautonomia
- Metabolic
  - Hypoglycemia
  - Hypovolemia

MANAGEMENT
- Treat underlying cause
- Avoid triggers

SPECIFIC THERAPY
- Depends on cause
- Neurocardiogenic
  - Fluids
  - Normal eating habits
  - Increased salt intake
  - Beta blockade
  - Fluorocortisone
- Cardiac
  - Intervention for structural cardiac abnormalities
  - Drug treatment for arrhythmias
  - Device placement for cardiac pacing/defibrillation
- Neurological
  - Drug treatment for seizures

FOLLOW-UP
- Variable depending on etiology, response to treatment

COMPLICATIONS AND PROGNOSIS
- In general very good
- In neurocardiogenic syncope, as patients mature symptoms tend to diminish
- In patients with structural heart disease, prognosis dictated by the heart disease

SYNDROME OF INAPPROPRIATE ANTIDIURETIC HORMONE SECRETION (SIADH)

MELANIE S. KIM, M.D.

HISTORY AND PHYSICAL

History
- Lethargy
- Irritability, combativeness, confusion
- Nausea, vomiting
- Headache
- Seizure, coma
- Decreased urine output
- Associated CNS disease
- May be seen with malignancy
- Drug-induced: vincristine

Physical signs
- Weight gain; usually no edema noted
- Exam usually normal
- Severe cases: change in mental status

TESTS
- Simultaneous serum & urine tests for electrolytes, osmolality:
  - ➤ Low serum sodium & osmolality concomitant w/ urine that is inappropriately not maximally dilute (osmolality 250–1,200 mmol/L)

DIFFERENTIAL DIAGNOSIS
- CNS disorders:
  - ➤ Infection:
    - Meningitis
    - Encephalitis
  - ➤ Trauma, subarachnoid hemorrhage

> Tumors
> CNS leukemia
- Pulmonary:
  > Tuberculosis
  > Pneumonia
  > Positive-pressure ventilator
- Drugs:
  > Vincristine
  > Oxytocin
  > Cyclophosphamide
- Malignancy: Ewing's sarcoma

MANAGEMENT

What to do first

- Severe cases w/ seizure/coma, serum sodium <120 mEq/L: correct sodium level w/ use of hypertonic saline & furosemide

SPECIFIC THERAPY

- Diagnose & treat underlying cause
- Restrict fluid to insensible loss w/ appropriate sodium content (replace urine sodium loss) to allow slow excretion of excess free water:
  > Rate: 0.5 mEq/L/h until sodium is 120–125 mEq/L
- Monitor correction & readjustment of therapy:
  > Frequent monitoring of serum & urine electrolytes & osmolality
  > Frequent pt weights

FOLLOW-UP

- Depends on underlying cause
- Frequent monitoring of serum/urine electrolytes & osmolality

COMPLICATIONS AND PROGNOSIS

- Cerebral edema w/ sodium <120 mEq/L
- Central pontine myelinolysis w/ subsequent neurologic sequelae w/ too-rapid correction of hyponatremia

SYSTEMIC LUPUS ERYTHEMATOSUS (SLE)

AMY L. WOODWARD, M.D.

HISTORY AND PHYSICAL

- Signs and symptoms vary; can change over time

- Diagnostic criteria (4 of 11 for Dx)
  1. Malar (butterfly) rash
  2. Discoid rash:
     - Erythematous raised patches w/ adherent keratotic scaling & follicular plugging
     - Atrophic scarring may occur in older lesions
  3. Photosensitivity: rash from unusual reaction to sunlight
  4. Oral or nasopharyngeal ulcers: usually painless
  5. Arthritis: non-erosive arthritis involving 2 peripheral joints
  6. Serositis:
     - Pleuritis: pleuritic pain, rub or pleural effusion
       OR
     - Pericarditis: ECG, rub, or pericardial effusion
  7. Renal disorder
     - Persistent proteinuria: >3+ or 0.5 g/d
       OR
     - Casts: red cell, hemoglobin, granular, tubular, or mixed
  8. Neurologic disorder: absent other causes
     - Seizures
       OR
     - Psychosis
  9. Hematologic: 1 of following
     - Hemolytic anemia
     - Leukopenia: $<4,000/mm^3$ on 2 occasions
     - Lymphopenia: $<1,500/mm^3$ on 2 occasions
     - Platelets: $<100,000/mm^3$
  10. Immunologic: 1 of following:
      - Anti-DNA
      - Anti-Sm
      - Antiphospholipid antibodies based on:
        - IgG or IgM anticardiolipin antibodies
          OR
        - Positive lupus anticoagulant
          OR
        - False-positive serologic test for syphilis for at least 6 months
  11. ANA

TESTS

Blood:

- CBC
- ANA
- Anti-Sm antibodies

- Anti-DNA antibodies
- Lupus anticoagulant
- Anti-cardiolipin antibodies
- Immunoglobulins (IgG often high)
- Complement levels (often low)
- Electrolytes, BUN/creatinine, LFTs

Urine

- Urinalysis
- 24-h urine protein, creatinine clearance

Other tests (as clinically indicated)

- Renal biopsy
- PFTs
- Chest CT

DIFFERENTIAL DIAGNOSIS
- Mixed connective tissue disease
- Drug-induced lupus syndrome
- Infection/sepsis

MANAGEMENT
- Determine organ system involvement
- Tailor pharmacotherapy accordingly
- Treat until remission achieved, then taper meds as able

SPECIFIC THERAPY
- Based on severity/specific organ involvement:
  - NSAIDs: mild disease w/o nephritis, esp. if arthritis present
  - Hydroxychloroquine: may prolong remissions
  - Oral steroids: systemic disease
  - Immunosuppressives:
    - Life-threatening disease, esp. renal/CNS
    - Pulse IV steroid, azathioprine, cyclophosphamide, plasma-pheresis

FOLLOW-UP
- Frequent during initial workup & flares
- Remission: every few mo

COMPLICATIONS AND PROGNOSIS
- Infection:
  - Leading cause of death
  - Common & opportunistic organisms
- Renal:
  - Nephritis

- ➢ Renal failure
- ■ Hematologic:
  - ➢ Anemia
  - ➢ Cytopenias
  - ➢ Procoagulants
- ■ Neurologic:
  - ➢ Seizures
  - ➢ Cranial nerve palsies
  - ➢ Psychosis
  - ➢ Transverse myelitis
- ■ Pulmonary:
  - ➢ Pleural effusion
  - ➢ Embolus
  - ➢ Hemorrhage
  - ➢ Pulmonary hypertension
- ■ Cardiac:
  - ➢ Pericarditis
  - ➢ Myocarditis
- ■ GI:
  - ➢ Pancreatitis
  - ➢ Gut vasculitis
  - ➢ Peritonitis
  - ➢ Hepatomegaly
- ■ Hypertension: due to renal disease, primary vasculopathy, steroids
- ■ Vascular:
  - ➢ Vasculitis
  - ➢ Raynaud's phenomenon

Prognosis
- ■ Depends on severity/type of organ involvement

TESTICULAR TORSION

DAVID H. DORFMAN, M.D.

HISTORY AND PHYSICAL

History
- ■ Any age; most common in newborn and early puberty
- ■ Newborns present with scrotal swelling
- ■ Older pts present with acute onset of severe pain
- ■ Nausea and vomiting common

- Hx of trauma possible
- Hx of recurrent pain

Physical signs
- Swollen hemiscrotum
- High-riding testicle w/ horizontal lie
- Loss of cremasteric reflex common
- Testicular tenderness
- Scrotal edema, erythema

TESTS
- Urinalysis
- Doppler flow study of testicle: reduced or absent blood flow to symptomatic testicle
- Testicular nuclear medicine scan: reduced or absent blood flow to symptomatic testicle
- Gonorrhea and Chlamydia testing, if sexually active

DIFFERENTIAL DIAGNOSIS
- Epididymitis
- Torsion of appendix testes
- Orchitis
- Trauma
- Hydrocele:
  - Infants
  - Generally nontender swelling of testicle
- Henoch-Schonlein purpura
- Incarcerated hernia
- Testicular tumor with hemorrhage (rare)
- Adenitis
- Acute idiopathic scrotal edema:
  - Benign
  - Bilateral
  - Usually prepubertal boys

MANAGEMENT
- High clinical suspicion:
  - Immediate surgical consult for repair
  - Ischemia, testicular infarction if repair delayed >6 h
- Suspicion high despite normal or inconclusive imaging study: urologist/surgical consult

SPECIFIC THERAPY
- Orchiopexy: timely surgical correction to detorse affected testicle & anchor both testicles w/in scrotum
- Neonatal testicular torsion: nonoperative management; salvage rate low
- Manual detorsion:
  - ➤ May be attempted if delay in surgery
  - ➤ Left testes rotated clockwise, right testes counterclockwise until pain alleviated

Side effects of treatment
- Surgical and anesthesia risks
- Loss of testicle if found to be necrotic

FOLLOW-UP
- Monitor surgical healing
- Long-term follow-up: seemingly viable testes may become atrophic

COMPLICATIONS AND PROGNOSIS
- Depends on state of involved testicle at time of surgery
- Salvage rate:
  - ➤ >95% if surgery w/in 6 h
  - ➤ 70% if surgery 6–12 h
  - ➤ 20% if surgery delay >12 h
- Testicular ischemia
- Sterility
- Injury to uninvolved testicle and impaired spermatogenesis secondary to anti-sperm antibodies

---

TETRALOGY OF FALLOT

ALEJANDRO ITHURALDE, M.D.
SHARON E. O'BRIEN, M.D.

HISTORY AND PHYSICAL
- Large ventricular septal defect (VSD)
- Right ventricular (RV) outflow tract obstruction; severity of disease depends on degree of obstruction
- Aortic override
- RV hypertrophy

History
- Family history

- ➤ Congenital heart disease (CHD)
- ➤ Syndromes associated with CHD
- Cyanosis
- Tachypnea, dyspnea on exertion
- Squatting
- Hypoxic spells

Physical signs
- Increased RV impulse
- Single S2
- Murmur
  - ➤ Generally loud, harsh systolic ejection murmur mid to upper LSB
  - ➤ Continuous murmur of collaterals
- May have bounding pulses due to large systemic to pulmonary collaterals
- Clubbing
- Cyanosis in older children
- Abnormal facies:
  - ➤ Trisomy 21
  - ➤ DiGeorge
  - ➤ Goldenhar
  - ➤ Velocardiofacial syndrome

TESTS
- O_2 saturation
- Chest x-ray
  - ➤ Normal or smaller heart size
  - ➤ Decreased pulmonary vascular markings
  - ➤ Upturned apex with concave MPA
  - ➤ Boot-shaped heart
  - ➤ Right aortic arch: 25%
- EKG
  - ➤ Right axis deviation
  - ➤ RVH: qR, pure R, rsR', tall R, or upright T waves in V1
  - ➤ Combined ventricular hypertrophy seen in acyanotic form
- Echocardiography
  - ➤ Large malaligned ventricular septal defect w/ anterior deviation of conal septum
  - ➤ Pulmonary stenosis: valvar or subvalvar
  - ➤ Pulmonary atresia in extreme cases
  - ➤ Overriding aorta

> Right ventricular hypertrophy
> Right aortic arch (25%)
> Coronary artery abnormalities
■ CBC

DIFFERENTIAL DIAGNOSIS
■ Other cyanotic heart lesions:
> Pulmonary atresia
> TGA
> Tricuspid atresia
> TAPVR
> Truncus arteriosus
> Ebstein's
■ VSD
■ Pulmonary stenosis

MANAGEMENT
■ Assess cardiopulmonary status, need for acute intervention – depends on degree of pulmonary outflow obstruction
■ Refer to pediatric cardiologist

SPECIFIC THERAPY
Medical management
■ Prostaglandins in neonate w/ ductal dependent lesion
■ Hypoxic ("Tet") spells:
> Knee-chest position
> Oxygen
> Morphine 0.1–0.2 mg/kg IM, SC, or slow IV
> Normal saline bolus
> Propranolol 0.05 mg/kg slow IV
> Phenylephrine 0.02 mg/kg IV
> Treat acidosis: $NaHCO_3$ 1 mEq/kg IV
■ Subacute bacterial endocarditis prophylaxis
■ Oral propranolol used to prevent spells
Surgical Management
■ Palliative procedure: increase pulmonary flow
> Blalock-Taussig shunt: subclavian artery to pulmonary artery shunt if corrective repair difficult
  • Indications: prematurity, hypoplastic pulmonary arteries, hypoxic spells, severe cyanosis in pts <3 mo
■ Definitive repair: preferred management

FOLLOW-UP
- Depends on severity of disease, treatment decision

COMPLICATIONS AND PROGNOSIS
- Hypoxic spells
  - Peak incidence 2–6 mo of age
  - Often initiated by feeding, crying, stooling, increased activity
  - Features
    - Irritability
    - Hyperpnea
    - Worsening cyanosis
    - If severe: lethargy, seizures, CVA, death
- Polycythemia
- Brain abscess
- Cerebrovascular accident (CVA)
- Growth retardation
- Subacute bacterial endocarditis
- Coagulopathy
- Arrhythmia

Prognosis
- Improved with complete surgical repair
  - 90% survival to adulthood
  - Deaths occur due to arrhythmia

THALASSEMIA

SHARON SPACE, M.D., AND HALLIE KASPER, P.N.P.

HISTORY AND PHYSICAL
- Hereditary deficiency in production of alpha- or beta-globin
- Clinical presentation varies based on number of genes inherited:
  - Beta-thalassemia trait (1 beta-globin gene missing): mild microcytic anemia
  - Beta-thalassemia intermedia (1 beta-globin gene missing, low production of Hb):
    - Mild-moderate anemia
    - Possible transfusion
  - Beta-thalassemia major (Cooley's anemia, both beta-globin genes missing):
    - Presents at 6–24 mo

- Severe, transfusion-dependent anemia
- Growth retardation
- Hepatosplenomegaly
- Bone deformities

➤ Alpha-thalassemia silent carrier (1 alpha-globin gene missing): asymptomatic

➤ Alpha-thalassemia trait (2 alpha-globin genes missing): mild microcytic anemia

➤ HbH disease (3 alpha-globin genes missing):
  - Moderate-severe hemolytic anemia
  - Icterus
  - Splenomegaly

➤ Hydrops fetalis (all 4 alpha-globin genes missing; not compatible with life)

➤ Thalassemia trait (alpha or beta):
  - Hx of microcytic anemia that does not improve w/ iron therapy
  - Family Hx: anemia
  - Ethnicity: beta in Mediterranean descent; alpha in African Americans & Southeast Asians

TESTS
- CBC
- RBC indices: decreased MCV
- Hb electrophoresis (newborn screen; repeat after age 6 mo to confirm diagnosis)
- Beta trait:
  ➤ Newborn screen likely normal
  ➤ Increased HbA2: >3.5%
  ➤ Microcytic, hypochromic RBC on peripheral smear
- Alpha trait:
  ➤ Newborn screen may show Hb Bart's
  ➤ F/U Hb electrophoresis normal
  ➤ Microcytic, hypochromic RBC on peripheral smear
- HbH:
  ➤ Newborn screen shows HbH
  ➤ Hypochromia, microcytosis, RBC fragments on smear

DIFFERENTIAL DIAGNOSIS
- Iron deficiency anemia
- Thalassemia trait
- Beta-thalassemia major

- Transient erythroblastemia of childhood
- Other congenital hemolytic anemias

MANAGEMENT
- Based on severity at presentation
- Thalassemia trait:
  ➤ Draw labs to make Dx
  ➤ No need to monitor CBC
- Beta-thalassemia major:
  ➤ Treat anemia symptoms
  ➤ Chronic transfusions

SPECIFIC THERAPY
- Thalassemia trait: none
- Beta-thalassemia major:
  ➤ Hematology F/U
  ➤ Chronic PRBC transfusion q3–4 wks
  ➤ Deferoxamine/chelation therapy
- HbH:
  ➤ Folic acid
  ➤ Supportive anemia care PRN

FOLLOW-UP
- Thalassemia trait:
  ➤ Education
  ➤ Genetic counseling for pt/parents
- Beta-thalassemia major:
  ➤ Genetic counseling
  ➤ Regular hematology F/U
  ➤ Yearly eval. for iron overload

COMPLICATIONS AND PROGNOSIS
- Thalassemia trait: normal
- HbH disease: chronic hemolysis, jaundice
- Chronic transfusion:
  ➤ Iron overload
  ➤ W/o chelation therapy, death from complications of iron overload in 2nd or 3rd decade:
    • Liver disease
    • HF
    • Arrhythmia
    • Diabetes mellitus
  ➤ Consider splenectomy if chronic hypersplenism

TICS/TOURETTE SYNDROME

LAURIE DOUGLAS, M.D.

HISTORY AND PHYSICAL

- Tics: brief, sudden, purposeless, stereotyped movements or utterances
- Tourette syndrome: multiple motor tics & at least 1 vocal tic for >1 yr (may wax & wane)
- Onset: age 2–7
- Simple motor tics:
  - Eye blinking
  - Grimacing
  - Neck jerking
  - Shrugging
- Complex motor tics:
  - Touching
  - Smelling
  - Jumping
  - Pulling
  - Squeezing
- Simple vocal tics:
  - Sniffing
  - Throat clearing
  - Snorting
  - Barking
  - Coughing
- Complex vocal tics:
  - Words, phrases
  - Coprolalia
  - Palilalia (repeat own words)
  - Echolalia

History

- May be suppressed for brief periods
- Diminish w/ concentration, distraction, sleep
- Increase w/ stress, excitement, or mentioning tics in front of child
- Streptococcal infection may worsen tics
- Co-morbid conditions:
  - Obsessive-compulsive disorder
  - ADHD
- Stimulant use: tics may become more apparent

Physical signs
■ Note any stigmata consistent w/ syndromes that predispose to tics or Tourette

TESTS
■ ASO titers: helpful if rapid onset
■ EEG (seizures uncertain)

DIFFERENTIAL DIAGNOSIS
■ Stereotypies:
  ➤ Involuntary, purposeless repetitive movements (e.g., lapping, rocking, finger wiggling)
  ➤ Typically begin at age <2 yrs
  ➤ Increase w/ excitement; decrease w/ distraction
■ Chorea:
  ➤ Sudden movements, not stereotypical
  ➤ May be incorporated into voluntary movements
  ➤ Hard to suppress
  ➤ Causes:
    • Sydenham chorea
    • eurodegenerative diseases
    • Paroxysmal chorea
■ Myoclonus:
  ➤ Lightning-like jerks that can't be suppressed
  ➤ Not all myoclonus due to seizure
■ Paroxysmal dystonia:
  ➤ Co-contraction of agonist & antagonist
  ➤ Not able to suppress
  ➤ Sometimes increase w/ movement
■ Coughing & sniffing:
  ➤ Often misdiagnosed as allergy or sinus disease
  ➤ Children w/ tics will not produce mucus, have no obvious allergic trigger
■ Eye blinking: commonly misdiagnosed as ophthalmologic problem

MANAGEMENT
■ Reassure patient and family
■ Treat only if child bothered by tics

SPECIFIC THERAPY
■ Penicillin if suspect exacerbation brought about by streptococcal infection
■ Clonidine or guanfacine: mild tics

■ Neuroleptics (pimozide, fluphenazine, risperidone) for more severe tics unresponsive to clonidine or guanfacine

FOLLOW-UP
■ Those requiring medication

COMPLICATIONS AND PROGNOSIS
■ Mostly due to medications
■ Symptoms wax & wane, many remit completely
■ Few require medication

TINEA INFECTIONS

ALBERT C. YAN, M.D., F.A.A.P.

HISTORY AND PHYSICAL

History
■ Itching, flaking
■ Red areas, often annular
■ Dark- and light-colored areas of skin that don't tan well (tinea versicolor)
■ Hair loss (tinea capitis or barbae)
■ Blisters on palms or soles (bullous tinea manus or pedis)
■ Hx of diabetes or immunosuppressant therapy

Physical signs
■ Tinea capitis & barbae:
  ➤ Scaling
  ➤ Alopecia
  ➤ Lymphadenopathy (occipital & cervical)
■ Tinea faciale & corporis:
  ➤ Erythema
  ➤ Annular lesions w/ peripheral scaling
■ Tinea cruris:
  ➤ Genital erythema & maceration
  ➤ May have peripheral scaling
■ Tinea manus & pedis:
  ➤ Scaling, w/ moccasin distribution on feet
  ➤ Interdigital maceration
  ➤ Blisters
■ Tinea versicolor: hypopigmented, hyperpigmented, and salmon-colored oval macules w/ some scaling

- Tinea unguium:
  - Hyperkeratosis (thickening)
  - Onycholysis (elevation of nail off bed)
  - Subungual debris

TESTS
DIFFERENTIAL DIAGNOSIS
- Tinea corporis:
  - Nummular dermatitis
  - Atopic eczema
  - Granuloma annulare
  - Erythema annulare centrifugum
- Tinea capitis:
  - Atopic dermatitis
  - Seborrheic dermatitis
  - Psoriasis
- Tinea versicolor:
  - Seborrheic dermatitis
  - Hypopigmented mycosis fungoides
- Tinea pedis:
  - Dishydrotic eczema
  - Contact dermatitis
  - Psoriasis
- Tinea unguium:
  - Psoriasis
  - Lichen planus
  - Pachyonychia congenita
  - Dyskeratosis congenita

MANAGEMENT
- Evaluate possible fomites to prevent recurrences
- Topical antifungal agents (superficial infections)
- Oral antifungals:
  - Bullous tinea manus & pedis
  - Tinea capitis & barbae
  - Fungal nail infections

SPECIFIC THERAPY
- Triazole creams (e.g., econazole or ketoconazole) bid until clear; continue additional week
- Allylamine creams (e.g., terbinafine, naftifine, butenafine) or ciclopirox cream bid until clear; continue additional week

- Selenium sulfide shampoo:
  - Daily ×6 wk (tinea versicolor); alternative: ketoconazole shampoo
  - Biweekly ×2 wk to prevent shedding (tinea capitis)
- Systemic therapy:
  - Scalp:
    - Griseofulvin 20 mg/kg divided bid ×6–8 wk
    - Second-line therapy: terbinafine
    - Alternative for tinea capitis: fluconazole solution 5 mg/kg/d ×4 wks
  - Fingernails (>40 kg): terbinafine 250 mg po qd ×6 wks
  - Toenails (>40 kg): terbinafine 250 mg po qd ×12 wks
  - Second-line treatment of onychomycosis: itraconazole

FOLLOW-UP
- Monitor for response to therapy

COMPLICATIONS AND PROGNOSIS
- Delays in diagnosis may lead to widespread or deeper cutaneous infection
- Tinea capitis:
  - Scarring alopecia
  - Kerion
- Tinea unguium:
  - Permanent nail loss
  - Secondary bacterial infection of nail

Prognosis
- Rarely tinea corporis will resolve spontaneously
- Most respond well to treatment, with occasional recurrences or reinfection
- Treatment failures related to poor compliance or resistant organisms

TORTICOLLIS

MARISA BRETT, M.D.

HISTORY AND PHYSICAL

History
- Difficult or forceps delivery
- Head or neck trauma
- Recent otolaryngologic procedure

- Head or neck infection
- Systemic inflammatory disease
- Neurologic or ophthalmologic symptoms (posterior fossa tumor)
- Drug use, esp. antipsychotics (haloperidol), antiemetics

Physical signs
- Head and neck:
  - Tilted and rotated head
  - Sternocleidomastoid (SCM) palpation
  - SCM involvement ipsilateral or contralateral to rotation
- Meningeal signs
- Extraocular movements
- Vertebral anomalies
- Posture

TESTS
- SCM spasm: none
- Neck films (AP, lateral, open-mouth):
  - Vertebral anomalies
  - C1–C2 subluxation (eccentric odontoid in open-mouth view)
  - Soft-tissue swelling (abscess)
- CT: to confirm rotatory subluxation
- CBC, blood culture, ESR
- MRI of posterior fossa
- Reflux evaluation
- Hip films for hip dysplasia assoc. w/ congenital torticollis

DIFFERENTIAL DIAGNOSIS
- Meningitis
- Congenital (primary) torticollis:
  - Muscular torticollis: diffuse SCM swelling
  - Sternomastoid tumor: discrete SCM swelling
  - SCM involvement is opposite rotation
  - Cervical spine abnormality:
    - Hemi-vertebrae
    - Cervical scoliosis
    - Skeletal dysplasias
- Acquired (secondary) torticollis:
  - SCM spasm most common
  - Posterior fossa tumor (cranial nerve/cerebellar anomalies)
  - Rotatory atlantoaxial subluxation (most frequently traumatic):
    - Results from ligamentous laxity due to inflammation

- SCM spasm & tenderness on same side as head rotation
- eurologic deficit rare
- Other causes:
  - Cervical lymphadenitis
  - Retropharyngeal abscess
  - Neoplasm (if mass not within SCM)
  - Extraocular muscle imbalance
  - GERD (Sandifer syndrome)
  - Benign paroxysmal torticollis:
    - Pallor, vomiting
    - Onset age 2–8 mo
  - Myasthenia gravis
  - Spontaneous pneumomediastinum
  - Dystonic reaction
  - Psychogenic

MANAGEMENT
- Identify underlying cause & provide specific treatment

SPECIFIC THERAPY
- Congenital muscular torticollis:
  - Usually conservative
  - Physical therapy, massage, heat
  - Surgery needed in 5%:
    - Limitation of head rotation after age 12–15 mo
    - Facial hemihypoplasia
    - Presentation at age >1 y
- Rotatory atlantoaxial subluxation:
  - Mild: soft collar & anti-inflammatory drug
  - Severe: traction & immobilization
- SCM spasm:
  - Heat
  - Anti-inflammatory drug

FOLLOW-UP
- Full ROM of neck should return
- SCM muscle feels normal
- Resolution of scoliosis or other postural anomalies
- Treatment of underlying cause, if applicable

COMPLICATIONS AND PROGNOSIS
- Complications mitigated by therapy:

- Facial hypoplasia, plagiocephaly
- Compensatory scoliosis
- Some deformity may persist
- Surgical complications:
  - Hematoma
  - Persistent torticollis

Prognosis
- 60–80% of congenital muscular torticollis resolves spontaneously
- Good results with surgical intervention

TOXIC SHOCK SYNDROME

STEPHEN I. PELTON, M.D.

HISTORY AND PHYSICAL
- Associated with:
  - Focal infection (staphylococcal abscess) or isolation of Group A streptococci from throat or sterile body site
  - Colonization of vagina with *S. aureus* and use of tampons
  - Colonization of nose and nasal packing
- Occurs primarily in children and adolescents who lack antibody to toxin(s)
- 200 cases reported to CDC in 1994
- Requires 3 major and 3 minor criteria:
  - Major:
    - Fever $>=102°F$
    - Hypotension
    - Erythroderma with late desquamation
  - Minor:
    - Mucous membrane congestion
    - GI symptoms (diarrhea or vomiting)
    - Myalgia (increased CK)
    - Liver function abnormalities
    - Renal dysfunction
    - Thrombocytopenia

History
- Febrile illness with erythroderma (scarlet fever–like rash with Group A streptococci)

Physical signs
- Conjunctival hyperemia
- Pharyngeal inflammation
- Strawberry tongue
- Desquamation of palms and soles 7–21 d after onset (in sheets)

TESTS
- Elevated WBC count
- Elevated transaminases
- Increase in conjugated bilirubin
- Increased BUN
- Decreased platelets
- Increased CK

DIFFERENTIAL DIAGNOSIS
- Septic shock
- Scarlet fever
- Rocky Mountain spotted fever
- Viral hemorrhagic fever (ie, dengue)
- Stevens-Johnson
- Leptospirosis

MANAGEMENT
- Fluid resuscitation and ongoing replacement
- Drainage of focal infections
- Removal of tampon or nasal packing if present

SPECIFIC THERAPY
- Antistaphylococcal and streptococcal antibiotics (beta-lactamase stable)
- Some experts recommend clindamycin to inhibit synthesis of toxin
- Nonresponsive cases: consider steroids and/or IVIG

FOLLOW-UP
- ICU management
- Monitor blood pressure
- Monitor for complications

COMPLICATIONS AND PROGNOSIS
- Hypotension (most important; almost all other complications result from hypoperfusion)
- Renal failure

- Myocardial dysfunction
- ARDS (usually late in course)
- Ischemia of digits (gangrene)

Prognosis
- Depends on initial presentation

TOXIC SYNOVITIS

ERIC FLEEGLER, M.D.

HISTORY AND PHYSICAL

History
- Acute, self-limiting inflammation of synovial lining
- Pain in hip
- Males:females 2:1
- Age range: 9 mo to 18 y (most age 3–10; peak age: 5–6)
- Limp or inability to bear weight
- Referred pain to thigh or knee; 5% bilateral
- Onset:
  - ➤ Usually abrupt pain
  - ➤ Occasional Hx of recent minor trauma
- Often with antecedent or intercurrent illness (URI)

Physical signs
- Low-grade fever: <10% of children
- Nontoxic appearing
- Ipsilateral hip pain: limited motion
- Hip held in flexion, external rotation (opening hip capsule to relieve elevated intracapsular pressure)

TESTS
- Radiographs of knee, femur, hip:
  - ➤ Usually normal
  - ➤ May see displacement of obturator fat pad
- Hip U/S: 80% accuracy in diagnosing effusion
- WBC, ESR:
  - ➤ Variably elevated
  - ➤ Low sensitivity, poor specificity
- Consider hip aspiration in children w/ ESR >20 mm/h or temp >99.5°F

DIFFERENTIAL DIAGNOSIS

- Trauma (fractured proximal femur, fractured acetabulum, fractured pelvis, dislocated hip or prosthesis)
- Referred pain from knee
- Infections:
  - Septic hip
  - Osteomyelitis of proximal femur
  - Tuberculous synovitis
  - Referred pain from septic knee
  - Lyme disease
  - Osteomyelitis of distal femur or proximal tibia
- Aseptic necrosis (Legg-Calve-Perthes)
- Neoplasm (primary or secondary, leukemia)
- Hematologic condition:
  - Hemophilia
  - Sickle cell crisis
- Connective tissue:
  - Acute rheumatic fever
  - Juvenile rheumatoid arthritis
  - Henoch-Schonlein purpura
- Osteoarthritis
- Slipped capital femoral epiphysis
- Femoral hernia

MANAGEMENT

- Orthopedic consult
- Diagnosis of exclusion
- May require traction for pain

SPECIFIC THERAPY

- Analgesia (NSAIDs)
- Rest (avoid weight bearing)
- Symptoms usually resolve w/in few days but can persist for 3 wks

FOLLOW-UP

- Follow up with primary doctor or orthopedics following day

COMPLICATIONS AND PROGNOSIS

- No known permanent sequelae
- Recurrence w/in 6 mo: 4–17%
- Hip radiographs at 6 mo (3% develop Legg-Calve-Perthes)

TRANSFUSION MEDICINE

SHARON SPACE, M.D.

HISTORY AND PHYSICAL

■ Indications:
  ➤ Whole blood in severe anemia & hypovolemic shock
  ➤ Packed RBCs (PRBC) in symptomatic anemia
  ➤ Platelets: control or prevent bleeding assoc. w/ decreased platelet number or function
  ➤ Fresh-frozen plasma (FFP): control bleeding in pts lacking coagulation factors
  ➤ Cryoprecipitate: control bleeding in hemophilia A, vWD, hypofibrinogenemia, Factor XIII deficiency
  ➤ Granulocyte infusion: used rarely in neutropenic pts w/ life-threatening infection

TESTS

See Management section

DIFFERENTIAL DIAGNOSIS

■ Not applicable

MANAGEMENT

■ Ordering blood:
  ➤ Consider diagnosis: isolated or chronic transfusion
  ➤ Processing:
    • Filtration: removes WBC & platelets from PRBC
    • Significantly decreases CMV risk & risk of febrile reaction
■ Washing:
  ➤ Removes WBC & donor plasma
  ➤ Indicated for Hx of severe transfusion reaction or chronic transfusion program
■ Irradiation:
  ➤ Kills lymphocytes in cellular products, inhibits WBC proliferation
  ➤ Indicated for immunocompromised, oncology, bone marrow transplant pts

SPECIFIC THERAPY

■ PRBC:
  ➤ 1 unit = 250–350 mL

➤ Hct of unit = 60–70

➤ Volume of PRBC (mL) = [(Desired − Current Hct) × Wt (kg) × Blood Vol (80 mL/kg)]/Hct of PRBC (60%)

➤ Transfuse 3–4 mL/kg/h over 3–4 h

■ Platelets:

➤ Pooled (random donor equivalent [RDE]) vs. single-donor (apheresis) products

➤ 1 apheresis unit (equivalent to 6–10 RDE) = ~300 mL

➤ 1 RDE will increase platelet count 5–10,000 in 70-kg adult and 20,000 in 18-kg child

➤ Dose = 1 RDE/10 kg

➤ Give as rapid transfusion

➤ Transfused platelets survive 3–4 d

■ FFP:

➤ 10 mL/kg over 45–60 min

➤ 10–15 mL/kg increases all clotting factors 10–20%

■ Cryoprecipitate:

➤ $^1/_2$ pack/kg increases Factor VIII by 80–100%

➤ 15 mL/pack

➤ Give 1 pack/6 kg

➤ Given as rapid infusion

FOLLOW-UP
COMPLICATIONS AND PROGNOSIS

■ Immediate:

➤ Acute hemolytic reaction:

• Caused by ABO incompatibility

• Severe hemolysis after or during PRBC transfusion

• Shock, fever, chills, dyspnea, chest pain, hemoglobinuria

• May progress to renal failure; can be fatal

• Treatment: stop transfusion; treat shock (steroids, antihistamine); monitor for DIC

• Risk: 1:30,000, mortality up to 40%

➤ Febrile reaction:

• Temperature spike +/− chills

• Treatment: hold transfusion; give acetaminophen, antihistamine; then restart transfusion in 15–20 min

• Risk 1:200

➤ Allergic reaction:

• Fever, urticaria, wheezing, angioedema

- Decreased risk w/ products that do not contain plasma
- Treatment: stop transfusion; acetaminophen, antihistamine, steroids
- Prevent by pretreatment w/ antihistamine
- Risk: mild–moderate: 1:1,000, severe: 1:150,000
  - ➤ Circulatory overload:
    - Pulmonary edema
    - Treat w/ diuretic PRN
  - ➤ Metabolic complications:
    - Hypothermia: massive transfusion of cold blood
    - itrate toxicity/hypocalcemia: anticoagulant in blood product causes ionized calcium to form complexes; rare; seen in severe liver disease
- ◼ Delayed hemolytic transfusion reaction:
  - ➤ Unexplained decrease in Hb 4–14 d after transfusion
  - ➤ Can be assoc. w/ hyperbilirubinemia, fever, hemoglobinuria
  - ➤ Due to mild minor antigen incompatibility
  - ➤ Treat as for hemolytic anemia: observe, monitor Hb/Hct; steroids if indicated
  - ➤ Milder than acute hemolytic reaction
  - ➤ Risk 1:2,500
- ◼ Infection (estimated risk/unit):
  - ➤ Hepatitis A: 1/1,000,000
  - ➤ Hepatitis B: 1/30,000–1/250,000
  - ➤ Hepatitis C: 1/30,000–1/150,000
  - ➤ HIV: 1/200,000–1/2,000,000
  - ➤ HTLV I and II: 1/250,000–1/2,000,000
- ◼ Bacterial contamination of product:
  - ➤ Rare: 1/500,000/unit
  - ➤ Can cause fever, hypotension, septic/toxic reaction
- ◼ Alloimmunization:
  - ➤ To RBC, WBC, platelet, or protein antigen
  - ➤ No immediate symptoms
  - ➤ Future transfusions must be negative for that specific antibody
- ◼ Transfusion-associated GVHD:
  - ➤ Due to transfused T-lymphocytes w/ cellular blood components
  - ➤ Usually seen in immunocompromised pts
  - ➤ Prevented by irradiation of blood products
- ◼ Iron overload

TRANSPOSITION OF THE GREAT ARTERIES

STEVE SESLAR, M.D.
SHARON O'BRIEN, M.D.

HISTORY AND PHYSICAL

Definition: Great arteries transposed, with aorta arising anteriorly from the right ventricle and pulmonary artery arising posteriorly from the left ventricle

History
- Cyanosis
- Severity depends on degree of intracardiac [through atrial septal defects (ASD) and ventricular septal defects (VSD)] and extra-cardiac (patent ductus arteriosus, bronchial collateral circulation) mixing of deoxygenated and oxygenated blood

Physical signs
- Cyanosis
- Tachypnea
- Second heart sound: prominent, often single
- Often prominent parasternal impulse
- Harsh holosystolic murmur may be present with VSD
- Systolic ejection murmur may be present with subpulmonic stenosis
- Congestive heart failure if Dx not made in newborn period (see "Congestive heart failure" entry)

TESTS
- ABG: hypoxemia, acidosis
- Hyperoxia test. hypoxemia does not respond to oxygen
- Glucose, Ca: hypoglycemia and/or hypocalcemia, consider DiGeorge syndrome
- EKG shows right axis deviation & right ventricular hypertrophy; combined ventricular hypertrophy may be present
- CXR: may show "egg on a string" with narrow mediastinum; generally normal pulmonary markings & heart size unless VSD present
- Echocardiogram: diagnostic test

DIFFERENTIAL DIAGNOSIS
- Lung disease
- Other cyanotic congenital heart disease
- Sepsis

MANAGEMENT
■ Prostaglandin therapy: 0.025–0.1 mg/kg/min IV infusion
■ Correct acidosis, hypoglycemia, hypocalcemia
■ Oxygen for severe hypoxemia
■ Admit to ICU

SPECIFIC THERAPY
■ Cardiac catheterization: balloon atrial septostomy (i.e., Rashkind procedure)
■ Operative repair (arterial switch operation, Rastelli operation, or intra-atrial repair-i.e., Mustard or Senning); approach depends on specific anatomical features

FOLLOW-UP
■ Depends on operative intervention
■ Intra-atrial repair (Mustard or Senning procedure); follow q 6–12 mo for arrhythmias, sick-sinus syndrome, right ventricular dysfunction
■ Arterial switch operation complications less common: supravalvar pulmonary or aortic stenosis, obstruction to coronary artery flow causing myocardial ischemia & semilunar valve regurgitation

COMPLICATIONS AND PROGNOSIS
■ Apnea or hypotension from prostaglandin therapy
■ End-organ injury from hypoxemia & acidosis

Prognosis
■ Without adequate mixing, progressive hypoxemia & acidosis results in death
■ With adequate mixing (VSD, ASD, PDA) less cyanotic & acidotic but may develop CHF and pulmonary vascular obstructive disease due to excessive pulmonary blood flow

---

TRICYCLIC ANTIDEPRESSANT (TCA) INGESTION

HANAN SEDIK, M.D., F.A.A.P.

HISTORY AND PHYSICAL

History
■ History of ingestion
■ TCAs available as antidepressants and to treat headaches, chronic pain syndromes, nocturnal enuresis, school phobia, sleep disorders

- Toxic dose: 10–20 mg/kg
- Symptoms develop w/in 4–6 h, but can be delayed to 24 h

Physical signs
- Anticholinergic effects:
    - Altered mental status
    - Sinus tachycardia
    - Urine retention
    - Dilated pupils
- Adrenergic blockade: hypotension
- Quinidine-like effects:
    - PVCs
    - Ventricular tachycardia
    - Widened QRS complex
- Neurologic:
    - Lethargy
    - Disorientation
    - Ataxia
    - Myoclonus
    - Coma
    - Seizures

TESTS
- Drug screen
- ECG: toxicity predicted by:
    - QRS >0.1 sec
    - R-wave amplitude >3 mm in aVR
- TCA semiquantitative rapid serum level

DIFFERENTIAL DIAGNOSIS
- Other toxins:
    - Beta-blockers
    - Quinidine
    - Phenothiazines
    - Cocaine
    - Caffeine
    - Amphetamines
    - Anticholinergics

MANAGEMENT
- Supportive care

- Decontamination
- Enhance drug elimination
- Physostigmine contraindicated for anticholinergic toxicity in TCA ingestions

SPECIFIC THERAPY

- Decontamination:
  - ➤ Gastric lavage, even in pts presenting as late as 4–12 h after ingestion
  - ➤ Activated charcoal: multiple serial doses if bowel sounds present
  - ➤ Avoid syrup of ipecac; rapid CNS deterioration and risk of aspiration
- Enhance drug elimination:
  - ➤ Alkalinize w/ IV sodium bicarbonate (1–2 mEq/kg):
    - Keep serum pH at 7.45–7.55
    - Sodium may overcome blockade of Na/K pump
    - Indications: arrhythmias, conduction delays, seizures
    - May cause electrolyte imbalances
- Anticonvulsants for seizures

FOLLOW-UP

- Cardiac monitoring:
  - ➤ All suspected TCA ingestions for at least 4–6 h after ingestion
  - ➤ Baseline 12-lead ECG
  - ➤ Repeat ECG until normal
- Admit to ICU
- Monitor serial electrolytes and ABGs during alkalinization
- Contact local Poison Control Center

COMPLICATIONS AND PROGNOSIS

- Hypotension
- Seizures
- Cardiac arrhythmias
- Electrolyte imbalances

Prognosis

- Children more sensitive to toxic effects of TCAs; develop symptoms at relatively low doses
- Ingestion of 10–20 mg/kg: coma and cardiovascular symptoms
- Ingestion of 35–50 mg/kg: may be fatal
- Drug levels do not reliably predict severity

TUBEROUS SCLEROSIS (TS)

HOWARD BAUCHNER, M.D.

HISTORY AND PHYSICAL

- Characterized by depigmented lesions of skin, tumors of CNS, harmartomas
- Can involve virtually any organ with formation of hamartomas
- Autosomal dominant: 1/6000
- 60% spontaneous mutation other specific chromosomal abnormality

History

- Often presents as seizure disorder, particularly infantile spasms in infants
- Flank pain & hematuria
- Family history of tuberous sclerosis

Physical

- Complete neurologic & dermatologic examination
- Major criteria
  - ➤ Hypopigmented skin lesions (ash leaf)
  - ➤ Fibroadenomas (adenoma sebaceum)
  - ➤ Shagreen patch: roughened, raised lesion with orange-peel consistency in lumbrosacral region
  - ➤ Heart failure (cardiac rhabdomyoma)
- Minor criteria
  - ➤ Dental pits
  - ➤ Gingival fibromas
  - ➤ Bone cysts
  - ➤ Multiple renal cysts
  - ➤ Nonrenal hamartomas
- Diagnosis requires presence of 2 major criteria or one major & 2 minor

TESTS

- Clinical diagnosis as genetic testing not routinely available
- MRI of brain (number of tubers on MRI may correlate with severity of mental retardation or seizures)
- Echocardiogram in all newborns at risk of having inherited TS
- Imaging of kidneys
- Neurodevelopmental testing
- Other tests depend up presenting signs & symptoms

DIFFERENTIAL DIAGNOSIS
- Neurofibromatosis
- Etiology of other seizure disorders, mental retardation
- Von Hippel Lindau disease

MANAGEMENT
- Seizure control
- Referral to neurologist/geneticist, other specialists as necessary

SPECIFIC THERAPY
- Therapy directed toward specific complication

FOLLOW-UP
- Joint management with specialists
- Patients require surveillance imaging of brain, heart, & kidneys; other organs as clinically indicated based on symptoms

COMPLICATIONS AND PROGNOSIS
- Complications can occur in any organ
- Hamartomas most common in brain, eyes, heart, & kidneys
- Prognosis dependent on size & number of hamartomas

TURNER SYNDROME

JEFF MILUNSKY, M.D.

HISTORY AND PHYSICAL
- 1:2,500 females

History
- Learning disabilities common/attention deficit disorder; mental retardation rare
- Absent/abnormal menstrual periods

Physical
- Short stature
- Lack of breast development
- Transient lymphedema hands & feet
- Short webbed neck & excess nuchal skin fold
- Shield-shaped chest & wide inverted hypoplastic nipples
- High-arched palate
- Small chin
- Low-set posteriorly rotated ears
- Cubitus valgus; short 4th metacarpal/metatarsal; hyperconvex nails

- Multiple pigmented nevi
- Delayed menses

TESTS
- Chromosome analysis
  - Differentiate mosaicism, missing X chromosome, structural X chromosome abnormality
  - Check for presence of Y chromosome material (DNA testing) in Turner mosaics

DIFFERENTIAL DIAGNOSIS
- Other chromosome abnormalities
- Noonan syndrome

MANAGEMENT
- Genetics
- Echocardiogram/cardiology
- Renal ultrasound
- TFTs (serial)
- Turner syndrome growth charts
- Turner syndrome support groups
- Early intervention services

SPECIFIC THERAPY
- Estrogen replacement therapy (after 14 y)
- Growth hormone (option)
- Synthroid for hypothyroidism

FOLLOW-UP
- Anticipatory guidance for specific medical problems (see below)
- Genetics
- Endocrine

COMPLICATIONS AND PROGNOSIS
- Infertility the rule unless mosaicism present
- Cardiology
  - 50% bicuspid aortic valves
  - Monitor for dilatation aortic root
  - Periodic echo
  - ~20% coarctation of aorta
  - ~30% hypertension
- 10–30% hypothyroidism → 50% adulthood

- Frequent otitis media
- Frequent UTI when GU abnormality
- ~50% progressive sensorineural hearing loss
- 10% scoliosis
- Obesity
- GI bleeding/IBD: guaiac testing
- Keloid formation
- Glucose intolerance & insulin resistance
- Gonadoblastoma from Y chromosome material (DNA): screen in cases of mosaicism
- Mean longevity ~ 69 y

UNDESCENDED TESTICLE

STEVE MOULTON, M.D.

HISTORY AND PHYSICAL

History
- Pathologic at age 6 mo
- Empty scrotum since birth
- If retractile, testicle in scrotum during warm baths, sleeping, diaper changes
- Familial tendency
- Associated anomalies in bilateral cases:
    - Exstrophy of bladder
    - Gastroschisis
    - Prune-belly syndrome
    - Intersex anomaly

Physical signs
- More common on right
- Repeat exam in multiple positions: supine, sitting cross-legged, squatting
- Affected hemiscrotum underdeveloped
- 20% bilateral, 80% unilateral
- Determine whether testicle palpable or not in inguinal canal
- Other GU anomalies: hypospadias

TESTS
- Imaging studies not needed

- Endocrine evaluation for bilateral non-palpable testes to check for testicular tissue: LH, FSH, serum testosterone levels before & after human chorionic gonadotropin (hCG) stimulation

DIFFERENTIAL DIAGNOSIS
- Retractile testicle
- Ectopic testis: check thigh, groin, suprapubic area
- Hypoplastic testicle
- Absent testicle(s):
  - 85% unilateral
  - 15% bilateral: delayed puberty, increased FSH, LH & decreased testosterone

MANAGEMENT
- Indications for orchiopexy:
  1. Preserve fertility
  2. Risk of trauma
  3. Correct associated hernia (90%)
  4. Cosmetic
  5. Risk of testicular cancer

SPECIFIC THERAPY
- Unilateral undescended testicle:
  - Optimal age for operation: 1–2 y
  - Delay leads to interstitial fibrosis & abnormal tubular development
  - If testicle not palpable: laparoscopy to check for testicular tissue
  - If testicle palpable: inguinal incision & orchiopexy; correction limited by vessel length
  - If testicle atrophic: orchiectomy
  - If age >14 y: biopsy testicle
    - If abnormal, orchiectomy
    - If normal, orchiopexy
- Bilateral undescended palpable testicles:
  - Beta-hCG will stimulate descent in 10% of boys w/ bilateral or high scrotal testes; may adversely affect tubular development
  - Not used for unilateral; more likely an anatomic problem

FOLLOW-UP
- Routine post-op and 3 mo post-op

COMPLICATIONS AND PROGNOSIS
- Vascular injury <5% secondary to compression, twisting, tension

Prognosis
- Fertility:
  - Uncorrected unilateral: 40–65%
  - Corrected unilateral <6 y: 92%
  - Corrected bilateral <6 y: 50%
- Malignancy:
  - 12% of testicular tumors
  - 40× increased risk
  - 200× increased risk if testicle atrophic or intra-abdominal
  - Average age at detection: 26 y
  - Lower risk of malignancy if orchiopexy age <5 y versus >10 y

UPPER GI BLEEDING

MARISA BRETT, M.D.

HISTORY AND PHYSICAL

History
- Amount of bleeding
- Bright-red blood vs. coffee ground emesis
- History of forceful vomiting
- Ingestion of foreign body
- Ingestion of caustic agents
- Medications: NSAID/aspirin
- History of bleeding disorder
- Jaundice or chronic liver disease
- Reflux history
- History of breastfeeding (cracked nipples; swallowed maternal blood)
- History of nosebleeds

Physical signs
- Hemodynamic status
- Skin exam:
  - Eczema
  - Cutaneous lesions
  - Telangiectasias
  - Rash
- Nasopharynx to identify bleeding
- Evidence of acute abdominal process
- Liver disease/portal hypertension

TESTS
- Gastroccult to verify subtle bleed
- Nasogastric lavage
- CBC, PT/PTT
- Liver function tests
- Coagulation studies
- Apt test:
  - Mix blood from aspirate with 1% NaOH
  - Adult (maternal) Hgb turns brown, fetal Hgb stays pink
- KUB (foreign body)
- Doppler ultrasound:
  - Liver disease
  - Portal hypertension
  - Vascular anomalies
- Consider upper GI study or endoscopy

DIFFERENTIAL DIAGNOSIS
- Artifact (i.e., food coloring, beets)
- Swallowed maternal blood/nosebleeds
- Foreign body ingestion
- Mallory-Weiss tear
- Esophagitis
- Gastroduodenal ulcer/gastritis
- Varices
- GI obstructive lesion
- Coagulopathy
- Vascular anomaly
- Hemophilia
- Trauma or Munchausen by proxy

MANAGEMENT
What to do first
- ABCs, including access, fluid resuscitation

General measures
- Type and crossmatch blood
- Correct coagulopathy
- Empiric acid-blockers or surface gut protection
- Hospitalization for most because rate of re-bleed variable, can be catastrophic

SPECIFIC THERAPY

- Endoscopy with sclerotherapy/ligation for varices; may consider trial of octreotide
- Angiography/embolization for life-threatening bleeds
- Coagulopathy: vitamin K, fresh-frozen plasma if severe/recalcitrant
- Portal hypertension: may need portosystemic shunt

FOLLOW-UP

- Follow hemodynamic status
- Repeat gastric irrigation in ongoing upper GI bleed
- Small upper GI bleeds from mucosal lesions improve w/ conservative management; require workup for underlying cause

COMPLICATIONS AND PROGNOSIS

- Mortality rare in children
- Therapy effective for most etiologies, incl. anatomic lesions
- Complications related to underlying disorders

URINARY TRACT INFECTION

JOSHUA NAGLER, M.D.

HISTORY AND PHYSICAL

History

- Symptoms vary depending on age
- Infants:
  - Nonspecific symptoms
  - Fever
  - Irritability
  - Poor feeding
  - Poor weight gain
  - Lethargy
  - Vomiting, diarrhea
  - Abdominal pain
  - Jaundice
  - Sepsis
- Older infants & toddlers:
  - Frequency
  - Dysuria
  - Malodorous urine

- School age & older:
  - Suprapubic pain
  - Dysuria
  - Urgency
  - Frequency
  - Hesitancy
  - Enuresis
  - May have flank pain, fever, vomiting w/ upper UTI
- Risk factors:
  - Uncircumcised male (tenfold increased incidence)
  - VUR
  - Toilet training
  - Wiping incorrectly
  - Bubble baths
  - Tight clothing
  - Constipation
  - Anatomic abnormality (e.g., labial adhesions)
  - Incomplete bladder emptying
  - Sexual activity

Physical signs
- Flank pain/masses, suprapubic tenderness
- Evidence of fecal impaction
- GU exam for labial adhesions, meatal stenosis

TESTS
- Urine culture: gold standard
- Catheterization: infants & young children unable to void into specimen container
- Suprapubic aspiration if unable to obtain catheter specimen
- Clean voided catch, midstream sample (CVS) for older children & adol.
- Bag specimens should **not** be sent for culture
- Positive culture:
  - Catheter specimen: $>50 \times 10^3$ CFU/mL
  - CVS: $>10^5$ CFU/mL
- Urinalysis interpreted in setting of clinical suspicion
- >5 WBC/hpf, (+) nitrites, or (+) leukocyte esterase may suggest UTI
- More than one finding on U/A: increases sensitivity & specificity
- Bacteriuria: unreliable for diagnosis

- Urine Gram stain:
  - Not done routinely
  - 1 organism/hpf = at least 10^5 colonies/mL
- Lab work: CBC & blood culture for complicated UTI or suspected pyelonephritis or sepsis only

Imaging
- Indications: any child age <5, & older females w/ recurrent or febrile UTI
- Renal US: R/O anatomic abnormality, hydronephrosis, obstruction, abscess
- VCUG: evaluate for VUR
- RNC in place of VCUG (1/100th radiation exposure); cannot grade reflux or see urethral anatomy
  - Imaging done once antimicrobial therapy has been initiated; no need for 2–6-wk delay

DIFFERENTIAL DIAGNOSIS
- Gastroenteritis
- Vaginitis, urethritis
- Foreign body
- Cervicitis/PID
- Appendicitis
- Nephrolithiasis

MANAGEMENT
- Antibiotics
- Fever control
- Encourage fluids: IV for vomiting, dehydration
- Radiologic imaging

SPECIFIC THERAPY
- Mild symptoms or doubtful diagnosis: delay treatment until culture results known
- Severe symptoms: treat empirically after urine specimen collection
- Inpatient treatment:
  - Age <3 mo
  - Vomiting/rigors
  - Ill appearing
  - Fever >102°F
  - Flank/abdominal pain
  - Abnormal BUN/Cr

- ➤ WBC >25,000
- ➤ Urologic abnormality
- ■ Simple cystitis
  - ➤ Treat promptly to prevent progression to pyelonephritis & possible scarring
  - ➤ First line:
    - Co-trimoxazole
    - Amoxicillin
    - Cefixime
  - ➤ Alternatives:
    - Nitrofurantoin
    - Fluoroquinolones once growth plates fused
  - ➤ Duration: 7–10 d; 3–5 d may be sufficient in school age & older
- ■ Pyelonephritis:
  - ➤ Neonates & young infants w/ febrile UTIs: assumed to have pyelonephritis
  - ➤ Broad-spectrum parenteral coverage awaiting cultures
  - ➤ First-line:
    - Ampicillin + gentamicin
    - Ampicillin + cefotaxime/ceftriaxone
  - ➤ Some advocate IM/IV dose followed by outpatient oral dosing
- ■ Prophylaxis:
  - ➤ Continue on qd prophylactic oral antibiotics after treatment course, until VCUG excludes VUR
  - ➤ Frequent UTIs, VUR, neurogenic bladder, or known urologic obstruction: daily prophylaxis
  - ➤ Daily prophylaxis recommended for 6 mo after pyelonephritis for younger children (risk of recurrence)

FOLLOW-UP
- ■ Repeat culture if no clinical improvement in 48 h on appropriate therapy
- ■ Repeat culture recommended after completion of antimicrobial therapy to document sterility; may be done at time of VCUG
- ■ VUR:
  - ➤ Serial VCUG or RNC
  - ➤ Serial ultrasound to evaluate renal size/growth
- ■ Urologic referral for obstructive lesions, or grade 4 or 5 VUR

COMPLICATIONS AND PROGNOSIS
- ■ Renal scarring from pyelonephritis, esp. in infants & young children

- Risk of progression to chronic renal insufficiency: low even w/ pyelonephritis
- Hypertension: from recurrent pyelonephritis

URTICARIA

ANDREW MACGINNITE, M.D., PH.D.

HISTORY AND PHYSICAL
- Intensely pruritic
- Called "hives" by pt, parents
- Often no obvious antecedent exposure
- Common identifiable causes:
  - Infection
  - Food (nuts, chocolate, seafood, eggs)
  - Drugs
  - Skin contact
  - Insect stings
- Physical urticarias:
  - Dermographism: hives with pressure
  - Cholinergic urticaria: hives with overheating
  - Cold urticaria
- Erythematous, raised lesions w/ irregular borders; blanch w/ pressure
- Chronic urticaria: as >6 wk
- Hypotension & wheezing (symptoms of anaphylaxis; see "Anaphylaxis" entry)

TESTS
- Generally not indicated

DIFFERENTIAL DIAGNOSIS
- Angioedema: occurs deeper in dermis w/ less well-demarcated lesions and less pruritus
- Anaphylaxis: urticaria w/ hypotension, wheezing, other systemic manifestations
- Viral exanthem, other rashes

MANAGEMENT
- Assess for respiratory compromise
- Remove offending antigen, if possible

■ Oxygen therapy
■ May need IV line
■ Pharmacologic management

SPECIFIC THERAPY
■ Antihistamines: diphenhydramine available over the counter; effective but sedating
■ Newer, nonsedating antihistamines: effective w/ fewer side effects
■ 2nd-line therapy w/ steroids (rarely needed)
■ May need subq epinephrine or nebulized beta agonists for patients with wheezing

FOLLOW-UP
■ Generally benign, self-limited
■ Chronic urticaria (>6 wks): careful search for environmental exposures & underlying systemic illness (mastocytosis, parasitic infection, collagen vascular disease)
■ Evaluation of chronic urticaria guided by Hx, physical
■ Majority of cases remain idiopathic

COMPLICATIONS AND PROGNOSIS
■ Self-limited w/o long-term complications
■ Chronic urticaria

Prognosis
■ Generally excellent

VAGINAL BLEEDING

ELSIE TAVERAS, M.D.

HISTORY AND PHYSICAL
■ Approach based on age

History
■ Prepubertal:
  ➤ Recent trauma
  ➤ Foreign body
  ➤ Sexual abuse
  ➤ Signs of precocious puberty
  ➤ Symptoms of vaginitis

> Dysuria or pain occurring with cough or straining
> Vaginal or anal pruritus

- Pubertal:
  > Last menstrual period
  > Usual length of menses
  > Irregular, heavy menses
  > Pregnancy
  > Sexual activity
  > Use of contraception
  > Previous STDs
  > Vaginal discharge
  > Easy bruising, family history of bleeding or clotting disorder

Physical signs

- Prepubertal:
  > Signs of hormonal stimulation (breast development, pubic hair growth)
  > Evidence of trauma, incl. ecchymoses in vulva & periclitoral folds suggesting a saddle injury, or lacerations of labia or tear in hymen from penetrating injuries
  > Intravaginal foreign bodies
  > Vulvar inflammation & erythema (vulvovaginitis)
  > Excoriations of anal & perineal area (pinworm infestation)
  > Vulvar & perianal hypopigmentation (lichen sclerosus)
  > Friable red-blue (doughnut-like) annular mass (urethral prolapse)

- Pubertal:
  > Genital warts
  > Speculum exam: note any vaginal vault lacerations, foreign bodies, or discharge
  > Punctate cervical hemorrhages (strawberry cervix): trichomonal vaginitis
  > Cervical bleeding after swabbing & mucopurulent discharge (common w/ *Chlamydia trachomatis*)
  > Uterine mass: intrauterine pregnancy; adnexal mass for possible ectopic
  > Note active bleeding from open cervical os (spontaneous abortion)

TESTS

- Qualitative pregnancy test

- Cervical specimen for GC and chlamydia
- CBC: Hct, platelets
- KOH prep
- Urinalysis & stool guaiac
- "Scotch tape" test

DIFFERENTIAL DIAGNOSIS
- Prepubertal:
  - Trauma
  - Vulvovaginitis
  - Foreign body
  - Urethral prolapse
  - Precocious puberty
  - Lichen sclerosus
- Pubertal:
  - Dysfunctional uterine bleeding
  - Disorders of pregnancy: threatened, incomplete, ectopic
  - PID
  - Bleeding disorders: von Willebrand disease
  - Breakthrough bleeding (OCPs)
  - Endometriosis

MANAGEMENT
- Identification & treatment of shock, acute hemorrhage, & trauma
- Hct
- Pregnancy test

SPECIFIC THERAPY
- Please see entries for most disorders
- Urethral prolapse:
  - Usually resolves w/ nonsurgical treatment
  - Sitz baths
  - Topical estrogen cream
  - Prolapse w/ dark, necrosing tissue requires surgical excision
- Lichen sclerosus:
  - Mild–moderate:
    - Eliminate local irritants
    - Protective ointments (e.g., A and D Ointment)
  - Moderate: 1–3-mo course of low-potency topical steroid cream or ointment
  - Moderate–severe: topical testosterone cream applied nightly for several months

- Ectopic pregnancy:
  - ➤ Quantitative beta-hCG determination
  - ➤ Transvaginal or transabdominal ultrasonography
  - ➤ Obstetric consult

FOLLOW-UP
- After bleeding controlled, follow-up depends on diagnosis

COMPLICATIONS AND PROGNOSIS
- Depends on specific diagnosis

VAGINAL DISCHARGE

ELSIE TAVERAS, M.D.

HISTORY AND PHYSICAL
- Approach based on age

History
- Vaginal irritation, itching, dysuria
- Color, consistency, quantity, odor of vaginal discharge
- Other illnesses (i.e., diabetes)
- Recent medications (i.e., broad-spectrum antibiotics)
- Recent sexual activity

Physical signs
- Prepubertal children:
  - ➤ Examine external genitalia with child in frog-leg position
  - ➤ Collect vaginal secretions w/ moistened cotton-tipped swab

TESTS
- Standard speculum & bimanual pelvic exam
- pH, saline prep, KOH prep, endocervical culture for GC & endocervical DNA probe for Chlamydia, qualitative pregnancy test
- High index of suspicion for PID: CBC with differential, ESR, RPR
- Consider urine dipstick, urine culture

DIFFERENTIAL DIAGNOSIS
- Prepubertal:
  - ➤ Physiologic leukorrhea
  - ➤ Infections (consider sexual abuse):
    - • Gonococcal infection
    - • Shigella & group A beta-hemolytic streptococcal vaginitis

- Trichomonal vaginitis (age <6 mo)
- Chlamydia
➤ Foreign body
➤ Ectopic ureter
■ Pubertal:
   ➤ Physiologic leukorrhea
   ➤ Candida vaginitis
   ➤ Trichomoniasis
   ➤ Bacterial vaginosis
   ➤ Gonorrhea
   ➤ Chlamydia
   ➤ Foreign body
   ➤ Allergic vaginitis

MANAGEMENT
■ Prompt characterization of discharge, microscopy, & Gram stain

SPECIFIC THERAPY
■ Physiologic leukorrhea:
   ➤ Whitish, mucoid discharge; normal estrogen effect
   ➤ May be copious & watery midmenstrual cycle, stickier & scantier during second half of cycle w/ rising progesterone levels
   ➤ Wet mount: epithelial cells w/ no leukocytes or pathogens, pH <4.5
   ➤ Reassurance & explanation
■ Shigella and group A beta-hemolytic vaginitis:
   ➤ White to yellow discharge; may be bloody
   ➤ Erythema, inflammation, or ulceration of vulva
   ➤ Definitive Dx: culture of vaginal discharge; important to R/O STD
   ➤ Oral antibiotics:
      - Based on sensitivity testing
      - Penicillin (drug of choice for Group A strep)
■ Candida vaginitis:
   ➤ Curdlike, white clumped, odorless discharge
   ➤ Intense burning & pruritus
   ➤ Predisposing factors: diabetes mellitus, pregnancy, antibiotic use, obesity
   ➤ pH <4.5, KOH: budding yeast & pseudohyphae, leukocytes
   ➤ Fluconazole, miconazole, or clotrimazole suppositories
   ➤ Partner: treat w/ topical preparation if recurrent infections

- Bacterial vaginosis:
  - Malodorous, yellow or gray discharge adherent to vaginal walls
  - Mild or no pruritus
  - pH >4.5, positive "whiff" test w/ KOH prep, presence of clue cells on wet mount
  - Gram stain: gram-negative rods
  - Nonpregnant pts: metronidazole
  - Pregnant pts: clindamycin or amoxicillin/clavulanate
  - Partner: treat if pt has recurrent infections
- Gonorrhea:
  - Often asymptomatic; may cause purulent, gray-white vaginal discharge from cervicitis in symptomatic patients
  - Endocervical culture on Thayer-Martin media
  - Gram stain: gram-negative, intracellular diplococci
  - Ceftriaxone + doxycycline
  - Always treat for presumptive Chlamydia co-infection
  - Partner: evaluate & treat w/in 60 d of contact
- Chlamydia:
  - Mucopurulent, yellow cervical discharge; may be asymptomatic
  - Endocervical DNA probe or culture for Chlamydia
  - Azithromycin, doxycycline, or tetracycline
  - Test of cure 3–6 wk after treatment
  - Partner: evaluate & treat w/in 60 d of contact
- Trichomonas:
  - Frothy, malodorous yellow-green discharge that may cause itching, dysuria, postcoital bleeding, or dyspareunia
  - Vulvar erythema & excoriations
  - Cervical punctate hemorrhages & swollen papillae (strawberry cervix)
  - Wet mount: flagellated, motile organisms; pH >5
  - Metronidazole
  - Partner: treat; refrain from intercourse until completion of treatment

FOLLOW-UP
- Observe patient for response to therapy and resolution of symptoms

COMPLICATIONS AND PROGNOSIS
- Treatment of failures and re-infections
- Depend on specific diagnosis

VARICELLA ZOSTER VIRUS (VZV): CHICKENPOX AND SHINGLES

ELLEN COOPER, M.D.

HISTORY AND PHYSICAL

Chickenpox
- Season: winter/spring (temperate climates)
- Airborne spread
- Incubation: 10–21 d (varicella zoster immune globulin [VZIG] may prolong to 30 d)
- Usually mild during childhood, may be severe in adolescent; severe or fatal if immunocompromised
- Highly contagious: 80–90% attack rate after household exposure
- Contagion: 2 d before rash until lesions are crusted

Physical signs
- Fever & pruritic papulovesicular rash involving skin & mucous membranes
- Rash appears first on head; centripetal distribution
- Begins as macules & papules
- Quickly progresses (in hours) to vesicles, pustules, and then to crusts (persist 1–2 wks)
- Lesions appear in crops (3 to 5 crops at ~24-h intervals)
- Different lesion stages present at same time
- Shingles
- Always preceded by chickenpox (often >10 yrs before)
- Infectious: as chickenpox
- Normal hosts: usually self-limited in young
- May be presentation of AIDS in younger individuals; more common in adults
- The more immunocompromised, the greater the likelihood

History
- Precipitating factors:
  - X-ray
  - Trauma
  - Malignancy
  - Sun exposure
  - Stress

Physical signs
- Localized unilateral vesicular skin eruption involving 1–3 dermatomes (lesions resemble varicella, but tend more toward confluence, are more likely to be painful)

Tests
- Labs (usually unnecessary)
- Skin lesions :
  - Culture
  - PCR
  - Immunofluorescence
  - In situ hybridization
- Tzanck smear: not specific but suggestive; can focus differential Dx

DIFFERENTIAL DIAGNOSIS
- HSV
- Scabies
- Stevens-Johnson
- Rickettsial pox
- Coxsackie A

MANAGEMENT
- Adequate hydration (esp. difficult if lesions in mouth)
- Supportive care

SPECIFIC THERAPY

Prevention
- VZIG w/in 3 d:
  - Intimate exposure & high-risk susceptible pts:
    - Immunocompromised on steroids
    - HIV
    - Malignancy
    - Premature
    - Neonate of mother w/ varicella
  - If varicella develops after VZIG, usually ameliorated course
- Varicella vaccine:
  - "Live" attenuated vaccine
  - 90% protection
  - Adolescents & adults: 2 doses 4–8 wks apart, children 1 dose
  - Contraindications:
    - Pregnancy

- Severe immunocompromise
- Allergy
- Treatment – Acyclovir:
  - Immunocompromised pts, primary pneumonia
  - Orally to children w/ chickenpox: shortens course by 1 d, but drug has poor GI absorption
  - Other antivirals: if resistant virus develops
- Treatment for shingles
  - Similar considerations
  - Acyclovir, other antivirals
  - No VZIG

FOLLOW-UP
- None necessary in uncomplicated cases
- F/U complicated cases or abnormal host w/in 24–48 hrs

COMPLICATIONS AND PROGNOSIS
- Chickenpox:
  - Hepatitis: elevated hepatic enzymes
  - Streptococcal/staphylococcal superinfection (cellulitis, fasciitis, osteomyelitis)
  - Pneumonia (more common in adults)
  - Cerebellar ataxia, encephalitis
  - Rare: myocarditis, acute glomerulonephritis
  - Immunocompromised:
    - DIC
    - Shock
    - Primary viral pneumonia
    - Death
- Congenital varicella syndrome (2%):
  - Scarred rash
  - Hypoplastic limbs
  - Eye, CNS damage
  - Early zoster
- Shingles:
  - Postherpetic neuralgia after healing of rash (25–50% of people age >50 yrs)
  - Disseminated zoster:
    - Crossing dermatones; often past midline of body and assoc. w/ severe disease
    - Usually requires IV acyclovir therapy

VENTRICULAR SEPTAL DEFECTS

SHARON E. O'BRIEN, M.D.

HISTORY AND PHYSICAL

History
- Family Hx of CHD
- Varies depends on size/location
- May be asymptomatic
- Tachypnea, dyspnea, orthopnea
- Cyanosis
- Feeding intolerance
- Vomiting
- Diaphoresis w/ feeds
- Failure to thrive
- Easy fatigability

Physical signs
- Heart rate, weight, height
- Associated syndromes (e.g., trisomy 21)
- Active precordium
- Asymmetric chest wall
- Palpation for thrill or RV heave
- Loud and possibly single S2 with large defects and pulmonary hypertension
- Systolic murmurs vary on defect size
  - Trivial: high-pitched, well localized, short systolic
  - Small: high-pitched, holosystolic
  - Moderate: medium-pitched, harsh, holosystolic
  - Large: short, systolic, crescendo-decrescendo
- Diastolic murmur may represent:
  - Relative mitral stenosis 2° to LA/LV volume overload
  - Pulmonary insufficiency with high pulmonary diastolic pressures
  - Aortic insufficiency 2° to prolapse of aortic cusp into defect
- Arterial pulses may be normal, brisk, or diminished depending on defect size

TESTS
- ECG: tachycardia, left atrial enlargement, right or left ventricular hypertrophy

- CXR: variable; normal, pulmonary overcirculation, cardiomegaly
- O_2 saturation
- Echocardiogram

DIFFERENTIAL DIAGNOSIS
- Innocent murmur
- Other cardiac defect:
  - AV valve regurgitation
  - Pulmonary stenosis
  - Subaortic membrane
  - Aortic stenosis
  - IHSS

MANAGEMENT
- Optimize weight gain
- Treat CHF
- Prevent subacute bacterial endocarditis
- Prevent damage to lungs, aortic valve

SPECIFIC THERAPY

Treatment
- Anticongestive medication: Lasix, digoxin, captopril
- Enhanced caloric density
- SBE prophylaxis (See "Endocarditis" entry)
- Transcatheter closure
- Surgery

FOLLOW-UP
- Varies depending on defect size, complications
- More frequent in very young with large defects or in complicated pts
- Older patients w/ small or moderate defects & no complications: yearly evaluation
- Auscultate for changing murmur, esp. onset of new diastolic murmur
- Evaluate prolonged febrile illness, weight loss, change in murmur, positive blood cultures, esp. with *S. viridans* for endocarditis

COMPLICATIONS AND PROGNOSIS

Complications
- CHF
- Pulmonary hypertension
- Eisenmenger's syndrome

- SBE
- Destruction of aortic valve

Prognosis
- 85% small muscular VSD spontaneously close by age 1 y
- Uncomplicated small VSD: excellent prognosis
- Large VSD w/ irreversible pulmonary hypertension and/or Eisenmenger's: poor prognosis
- Increased morbidity/mortality if complicated by CHF, aortic regurgitation, SBE

VERTIGO

ROBERT VINCI, M.D.

HISTORY AND PHYSICAL

History
- Room spinning
- Onset during sudden upright posture
- Ringing in the ears
- Vomiting, unsteady gait, or loss of balance
- Recent head trauma
- Hearing loss
- Weakness, diplopia, or dysarthria
- Acuity:
  - ➤ Central lesion: usually acute
  - ➤ Peripheral lesion: usually insidious onset

Physical signs
- Orthostatic vital signs
- Nystagmus:
  - ➤ Horizontal with rotary component (peripheral lesion)
  - ➤ Vertical or changing position of nystagmus (central lesion)
- Examine tympanic membrane for cerumen or middle ear effusion
- Neurologic exam with bedside hearing test and cerebellar test

TESTS
- Nylen Barany test:
  - ➤ Pt head 45° to one side; move patient from sitting to supine position, keeping head turned & hanging over bed

- Observe for nystagmus & symptoms of vertigo
- Central lesion: immediate, mild nystagmus
- Peripheral lesion: delayed intense nystagmus
- Hearing test
- Head CT (trauma/acute bleed)
- MRI (suspected CNS lesion)

DIFFERENTIAL DIAGNOSIS

- Nystagmus of peripheral origin:
    - Cerumen or foreign body in ear canal
    - Otitis media/labyrinthitis
    - Cholesteatoma
    - Head trauma
    - Perilymphatic fistula
    - Benign paroxysmal vertigo:
        - Usually age <4 yr
        - Intense nausea, vertigo, flushing
        - All motor activity stops
        - Attacks last from seconds to minutes
- Nystagmus of central origin:
    - Seizures
    - Basilar artery migraine
    - CNS lesions
    - Demyelinating disorders (e.g., multiple sclerosis)

MANAGEMENT

What to do first

- Protect from falls & self-injury

General measures

- Bed rest or decrease physical activity
- IV fluids
- Antiemetics
- Vestibular suppressants

SPECIFIC THERAPY

- Treat underlying cause
- Vertigo may be managed with:
    - Dimenhydrinate 1–1.5 mg/kg IM
    - Meclizine (for children <12 yr)
    - Valium (sedation)

FOLLOW-UP
- Follow response to therapy

COMPLICATIONS AND PROGNOSIS
- Depends on underlying disorder
- Benign positional vertigo: spontaneous resolution
- Benign paroxysmal vertigo: migraine headaches in adult life

VESICOURETERAL REFLUX (VUR)

MICHAEL J.G. SOMERS, M.D.

HISTORY AND PHYSICAL

History
- Culture-proven UTI in age <7 y
- Older child: repeated UTIs
- Recurrent unexplained fevers
- Family history
  - VUR (parent/sibling)
  - Renal failure, dialysis, transplantation

Physical signs
- Often asymptomatic
- Vital signs, esp. BP
- Abdominal mass
- Palpable bladder
- Flank pain
- External genitalia
- Neuro exam (lower extremities)

TESTS
- Urinalysis, urine culture
- Urine protein/Cr ratio if proteinuria
- Serum BUN, Cr

Imaging
- Renal US:
  - Kidney size, position, & parenchyma
  - Detects hydronephrosis or ureter/bladder anomaly
  - Not diagnostic
- Voiding cystourethrogram (VCUG):
  - Diagnostic

- Graded for severity:
  - Grade 1: reflux into ureter only
  - Grade 2: ureter & collecting system involved; no dilatation
  - Grade 3: mild calyceal blunting
  - Grade 4: >50% calyces blunted; ureter tortuous
  - Grade 5: all calyces blunted; papillar impressions lost; ureter tortuous

DIFFERENTIAL DIAGNOSIS

- Primary reflux:
  - Congenital
  - Not assoc w/ neuromuscular deficit or urinary tract obstruction
  - Tendency to be inherited
  - Suboptimal insertion of ureter into bladder
  - Often outgrown
- Secondary reflux:
  - Causes:
    - Obstruction
    - Neuromuscular deficit
    - Voiding anomaly
  - High intravesical pressures overwhelm physiologic antireflux mechanisms
  - Must treat underlying cause

MANAGEMENT

- Medical:
  - Prophylactic daily oral antibiotic
  - Await spontaneous resolution
- Surgery:
  - Ureteral reimplantation
  - Indications:
    - Grades 4–5
    - Medical failure
    - Secondary causes
- Siblings of index case:
  - Up to 35% have VUR
  - Consider radionuclide cystogram (RNC) as screen

SPECIFIC THERAPY

- Antibiotic prophylaxis (low-dose qd):
  - Co-trimoxazole/trimethoprim (2 mg/kg) or nitrofurantoin (2 mg/kg):
    - Effective

- • Fewer GI effects
- ➤ Amoxicillin (15 mg/kg) or cephalosporins: more GI effects
- ➤ Complications:
  - • Noncompliance
  - • Breakthrough UTIs
  - • Side effects
- ■ Surgical repair:
  - ➤ Open repair
  - ➤ Endoscopic repair w/ Teflon paste less effective (VUR may recur)
  - ➤ Few complications, but no long-term advantage over medical Rx for Grades 1–4

FOLLOW-UP
- ■ Monitor urine cultures q3–4 mo
- ■ Yearly imaging:
  - ➤ RNC or VCUG: document presence & grade
  - ➤ Renal US: document kidney growth & assess parenchyma for scarring

COMPLICATIONS AND PROGNOSIS
- ■ Recurrent UTIs: up to 35% despite therapy
- ■ Renal scars:
  - ➤ 25–60% of children w/ febrile UTI & VUR
  - ➤ Most due to pyelonephritis
  - ➤ More common in younger children & higher grades
- ■ Hypertension:
  - ➤ Sequela of renal scarring
  - ➤ Up to 25% of cases
  - ➤ May take years to manifest
  - ➤ Toxemia in pregnancy possibly more common
- ■ Renal insufficiency:
  - ➤ Up to 10% progress to renal failure & dialysis/transplant
  - ➤ Generally preceded by hypertension & proteinuria

VIRAL HEPATITIS

MAUREEN M. JONAS, M.D.

HISTORY AND PHYSICAL

History
Hepatitis A (HAV)
- ■ Exposure: infected individual or common source during outbreak
- ■ Fecal-oral spread: contaminated food or water

- Incubation: 30 d
- Risk: day-care or household contact
- Infants/young children:
  - Asymptomatic or gastroenteritis-like syndrome
  - Rarely jaundice
- Older children:
  - Prodrome:
    - Fever
    - Headache
    - Malaise
  - Acute:
    - Jaundice ± pruritus
    - Nausea
    - Abdominal pain
    - Vomiting
    - Anorexia
- Symptoms resolve: 2–3 wks
- Jaundice resolves: 4 wks
- Atypical HAV:
  - Cholestatic hepatitis:
    - Jaundice >12 wks
    - Severe pruritus
  - Biphasic/relapsing:
    - 2nd or 3rd episode
    - Recurrence of jaundice
    - High aminotransferases

Hepatitis B (HBV)
- Parenteral, sexual, or perinatal transmission
- Risk:
  - IV drug use
  - Male homosexual activity
  - STD
- Incubation: 90 d
- Symptoms:
  - As in older children w/ HAV
  - 1–3% fulminant hepatitis

Hepatitis C (HCV)
- Parenteral, perinatal transmission
- Risk:
  - IV or intranasal drug use
  - Tattoo or body piercing

➤ Blood product transfusion <1992
➤ Infected mother
- Incubation: 35–45 d
- 25% acute hepatitis
- Fulminant hepatitis rare

Physical signs
- Jaundice
- Tender hepatomegaly
- Dehydration if nausea/vomiting
- Fulminant:
    ➤ Asterixis
    ➤ Mental status changes

TESTS
- ALT (20–100× normal), PT, bilirubin
- Electrolytes if dehydrated
- HAV:
    ➤ Anti-HAV IgM
    ➤ First total anti-HAV then IgM if +
- HBV:
    ➤ HBsAg & anti-HBc (core antibody)
    ➤ IgM diagnostic
- HCV:
    ➤ ± Anti-HCV with + PCR diagnostic
    ➤ Does not confirm acute infection (ie, disease superimposed on chronic HCV)

DIFFERENTIAL DIAGNOSIS
- Infants:
    ➤ Metabolic liver disease
    ➤ Enteroviral infections
    ➤ TORCH infections
- Older children/teens:
    ➤ Human herpesvirus 6
    ➤ Parvovirus B19
- Acute hepatitis D in chronic HBV
- EBV hepatitis
- Hepatitis E: recent immigrant from endemic area
- Drug hepatotoxicity
- Wilson disease
- Autoimmune hepatitis

MANAGEMENT

General measures
- Hospitalize:
  - Vomiting/dehydration
  - Prolonged PT
  - Altered mental status
- Correct fluid/electrolyte

SPECIFIC THERAPY
- Supportive Rx
- HAV: contact precautions for diapered/incontinent pts for first week
- HCV: interferon/ribavirin to decrease chronic infection
- Prophylaxis for contacts
- HAV:
  - Immune serum globulin (IM gamma globulin) 0.02 mL/kg
  - Household contacts w/in 2 wks
  - Vaccinate age >2 y
  - Community outbreak: vaccinate to decrease # of cases
- HBV:
  - Hepatitis B immune globulin 0.06 mL/kg
  - Vaccinate nonimmune sexual/parenteral contacts, needlestick exposures
- HCV: no immunoprophylaxis

FOLLOW-UP
- Monitor for resolution:
  - ALT, bilirubin
  - HBsAg & HBsAb after 4–6 wks, resolution, or development of chronic HBV
  - HCV RNA by PCR after 6 mo to determine chronic HCV
- Monitor for fulminant hepatitis:
  - PT
  - Mental status

COMPLICATIONS AND PROGNOSIS
- HAV: no chronic disease
- HBV: 5–10% of older children chronic variable course & prognosis
- HCV:
  - Untreated: >75% rate of chronic HCV
  - Complications of chronic liver disease over several decades
- Fulminant hepatitis: with HAV or HBV (<5%):
  - Mortality high
  - Liver transplant possible

VON WILLEBRAND'S DISEASE (VWD)

SHARON SPACE, M.D., AND HALLIE KASPER, P.N.P.

HISTORY AND PHYSICAL
- Characterized by abnormal quantity or structure of von Willebrand's factor (vWF)
- VWF is important in clotting:
  - Mediates adhesion of platelets to subendothelium to form platelet plug
  - Forms complex with Factor VIII
- Type 1:
  - Most common (80%)
  - Decreased quantity of vWF
- Types 2 and 3:
  - Less common
  - Abnormal structure or function of vWF

History
- Easy bruising
- Mucous membrane bleeding (epistaxis, gums, menorrhagia)
- Petechiae
- Bleeding with surgery or tooth extraction
- Family history of bleeding (autosomal dominant)

Physical signs
- Bruising or petechiae on exam
- May see signs/symptoms of anemia secondary to blood loss

TESTS
- CBC and platelets (normal platelet count)
- PT (normal)
- PTT (prolonged or normal)
- Factor VIII level
- Factor VIII-related antigen (measures vWF)
- Ristocetin cofactor (measures vWF activity)
- vWF multimers (determines type)
- May need to repeat workup to make diagnosis

DIFFERENTIAL DIAGNOSIS
- ITP
- Hemophilia
- Dysfunctional uterine bleeding of other etiology

MANAGEMENT
- Control acute bleeding
- Confirm diagnosis and classification
- Develop treatment plan for bleeding, surgery

SPECIFIC THERAPY
- DDAVP:
  - Vasopressin analog
  - Stimulates release of endogenous vWF from endothelial stores
  - Nasal spray or IV (IV dose, 3 mcg/kg)
  - Give qd for 2–3 d; not effective after because stores are depleted and must be restored
  - Indications:
    - Before surgery or tooth extraction
    - To stop/control bleeding in acute setting (nosebleed)
    - At start of menses to control menorrhagia
  - Type 1 responds but Types 2 and 3 may not
  - Consider DDAVP trial (measure labs before and 30 minutes after dose to determine response)
- Cryoprecipitate:
  - Contains large amounts of Factor VIII, vWF, fibrinogen, fibronectin (1 bag = ~100 units vWF)
  - Use in acute setting to control bleeding (trauma, surgery)
  - Dose: 1 bag/6 kg q12 h
  - Human-derived Factor VIII concentrate contains large amount of vWF: use in acute setting to control bleeding
- If severe anemia secondary to prolonged bleeding: iron therapy

FOLLOW-UP
- Follow females with severe menorrhagia closely: monitor Hct and response to DDAVP

COMPLICATIONS AND PROGNOSIS
- Good
- Not at risk for spontaneous bleeding

WARTS

ALBERT C. YAN, M.D., F.A.A.P.

HISTORY AND PHYSICAL

History
- Verrucous papules and plaques

- Common forms:
  - Common
  - Plantar
  - Genital
  - Flat
- Widespread lesions: in patients w/ renal insufficiency or immune deficiency
- Lesions may produce pain, distortion of anatomic structures (nail plate), and can be cosmetically disfiguring
- If genital lesions present, obligatory to R/O sexual abuse

Physical signs
- Black pepper spots (thrombosed capillaries) on individual lesions
- Face, extremities, genitals

TESTS
- Usually clinical diagnosis
- Biopsy:
  - Of chronic, persistent lesions (esp. on feet and under nails) to R/O verrucous carcinoma
  - Of persistent lesions in genital area to R/O transformation to squamous cell carcinoma

DIFFERENTIAL DIAGNOSIS
- Molluscum contagiosum
- Nevus sebaceous
- Epidermal nevus
- Lichen striatus

MANAGEMENT
- Most resolve spontaneously over months to years

SPECIFIC THERAPY
- Topical salicylic acid (17%):
  - Soak affected areas in hot water for 5 min, apply salicylic acid, and cover with occlusive tape overnight; repeat nightly until warts resolve
  - Plantar warts: additional use of salicylic acid plasters at higher concentrations (40%)
- Imiquimod cream: primarily for genital warts
- Tretinoin or tazarotene gel:
  - To debride warts
  - Particularly useful against flat warts and molluscum
- Cimetidine (possible therapeutic effect in children)

- Cantharidin (with or without added podophyllin and salicylic acid): applied in office, left on under tape occlusion x 4–6 h, then washed off
- Cryotherapy
- Surgical curettage or excision: not generally recommended because of resulting scar
- Dermatology referral for refractory warts

FOLLOW-UP
- Treated warts re-evaluated and retreated q 2–3 wks until resolved to minimize risk of recurrence
- Prolonging interval between treatments associated with slower response to therapy and lower cure rate

COMPLICATIONS AND PROGNOSIS
- Post-therapy pain and discomfort
- Hypopigmentation or hyperpigmentation after treatment
- Scarring
- Risk of malignant transformation (large, chronic lesions or genital lesions)

Prognosis
- Most resolve spontaneously in immunocompetent hosts
- More aggressive therapy for immunodeficient patients

WILMS TUMOR

SUZANNE SHUSTERMAN, M.D.

HISTORY AND PHYSICAL
- Asymptomatic abdominal mass: most common
- Abdominal pain
- Hematuria
- Fever
- Hypertension (25%)
- Subcapsular hemorrhage:
  - Rapid abdominal enlargement
  - Pain
  - Anemia
- Median age:
  - 44 mo: unilateral tumor
  - 30 mo: bilateral tumor

- Associated syndromes, genetics:
  - WAGR syndrome (<u>W</u>ilms, <u>A</u>niridia, <u>G</u>U anomalies, mental <u>R</u> etardation)
  - Denys-Drash
  - Beckwith-Wiedemann (hemihypertrophy, macroglossia, omphalocele, visceromegaly)
  - Isolated hemihypertrophy, other overgrowth syndromes
  - Inactivation of tumor suppressor gene WT1 (11p13)
- Prevalence 1:10,000
- 5–6% of all childhood cancers

Physical signs
- Abdominal mass
- Hypertension
- Aniridia
- Hemihypertrophy
- Hypospadias, cryptorchidism

TESTS

Basic tests
- CBC, electrolytes
- Renal & liver function tests
- PT, PTT (rare association with von Willebrand disease)
- Urinalysis (hematuria)

Specific diagnostic tests
Local disease
- Abdominal CT w/ contrast:
  - Nature, extent of mass
  - Lymph node, liver involvement
  - Contralateral kidney
  - Ultrasound w/ Doppler: Identify renal mass
  - IVC involvement
Metastatic disease
- Chest x-ray +/− chest CT
- Bone scan & skeletal survey (clear cell sarcoma)
- Head CT or MRI (clear cell sarcoma or rhabdoid tumor)
- Pathology:
  - Tissue for definitive diagnosis
  - Classically triphasic histology: blastemal, stromal, epithelial elements
  - Anaplasia (focal or diffuse)

DIFFERENTIAL DIAGNOSIS
- Neuroblastoma
- Other intra-abdominal tumor
- Other intrarenal neoplasm:
  - Clear cell sarcoma
  - Rhabdoid tumor
- Nonmalignant renal:
  - Polycystic kidney disease
  - Hydronephrosis

MANAGEMENT

What to do first
- Surgical excision if safe, then chemo +/- radiation therapy

General measures
- Determine tumor stage:
  - Stage I: localized disease, completely excised
  - Stage II: local extension beyond kidney, completely excised
  - Stage III: residual intra-abdominal tumor postop
  - Stage IV: hematogenous spread; most common: lungs
  - Stage V: bilateral renal disease

SPECIFIC THERAPY
- Surgery:
  - Remove primary tumor & involved kidney
  - Assess local tumor spread
  - Inspect contralateral kidney
  - Very large tumors:
    - Biopsy initially
    - Excision after tumor reduction w/ chemo
- Bilateral disease:
  - Biopsy both kidneys
  - Renal-sparing surgery after tumor reduction w/ chemo
- Chemotherapy
  - Cerapy Stage I & II: vincristine + actinomycin
  - Stage III & IV: add doxorubicin
  - Anaplastic, Stage II, III, IV: add cyclophosphamide
- Radiation for primary tumor:
  - Stage I & II: none
  - Stage III & anaplastic stage II: 1080 cGy to tumor bed; whole abdomen if tumor spillage
  - Pulmonary metastasis: whole lung radiation 1,200 cGy

FOLLOW-UP
- Off therapy: chest x-ray, US at regular intervals for first 5 y

COMPLICATIONS AND PROGNOSIS
- Acute treatment-related toxicity:
  - Hair loss
  - Nausea, vomiting
  - Bone marrow suppression
  - Peripheral neuropathy (vincristine)
  - Hemorrhagic cystitis (cyclophosphamide)
- Late treatment-related toxicity:
  - Cardiomyopathy (doxorubicin):
  - Second malignant neoplasms in irradiated areas

Prognosis
- Overall: >90% survival
- Stage IV: 70–80% survival

WISKOTT-ALDRICH SYNDROME

ANDREW KOH, M.D.

HISTORY AND PHYSICAL
- X-linked recessive syndrome with:
  - Atopic dermatitis
  - Thrombocytopenia
  - Recurrent infections

History
- Thrombocytopenia:
  - Prolonged bleeding from circumcision
  - Bloody diarrhea during infancy
  - Cerebral hemorrhage
- Eczema
- Encapsulated bacterial infections (eg, pneumococci):
  - Otitis media
  - Pneumonia
  - Meningitis
  - Sepsis

TESTS
- CBC/bone marrow: few and small defective platelets with normal-appearing megakaryocytes

- Immunoglobulin levels:
  - ➤ Low IgM
  - ➤ Elevated IgA and IgE
  - ➤ Normal or slightly low IgG
- Reduced antibody response to polysaccharides
- Lymphocytes: reduced CD3, CD4, CD8+ subsets
- Deletion of WASP gene at X11p

Differential diagnosis
- Primary immunodeficiency diseases
- Chronic granulomatous disease
- Common variable immunodeficiency
- Severe combined immunodeficiency
- X-linked agammaglobulinemia
- Leukocyte adhesion deficiency

MANAGEMENT
What to do first
- Obtain tests & genetic confirmation

General measures
- Treat infections
- Supportive care for eczema
- Refer to pediatric hematologist

SPECIFIC THERAPY
- Bone marrow transplantation w/ matched sibling marrow: best chance for survival & correction of underlying defect
- Splenectomy improves thrombocytopenia but need antibiotic prophylaxis for increased risk of encapsulated bacterial infection

FOLLOW-UP
- Monitor platelet counts, Ig levels
- Watch for infections

COMPLICATIONS AND PROGNOSIS
- Infection:
  - ➤ Encapsulated bacteria (*S. pneumoniae*, *H. influenzae*, *Salmonella sp.*, *Neisseria sp.*)
  - ➤ Otitis media, pneumonia, meningitis, sepsis
  - ➤ *Pneumocystis carinii*
  - ➤ Herpesviruses

- Bleeding:
  - ➤ Bloody diarrhea
  - ➤ Cerebral hemorrhage
- Malignancy (eg, lymphoma)

Prognosis
- Survival beyond teens rare
  - ➤ Major causes of death: infection, bleeding
  - ➤ Fatal malignancies less common
- Partial syndromes seen occasionally in adults

YERSINIA INFECTIONS

EILEEN A. KENECK, M.D.

HISTORY AND PHYSICAL
- *Yersinia enterocolitica*, *Y. pestis*, and *Y. pseudotuberculosis* : Gram-negative bacilli
- Most commonly cause enteritis
- Incubation period: 4–6 d
- Period of communicability unknown, probably ~6 wk after diagnosis

History
- Usually transmitted by ingestion of contaminated food (water, unpasteurized milk, raw pork)
- *Y. enterocolitica* most often causes acute gastroenteritis, often w/ blood & mucus, especially in younger children
- *Y. pseudotuberculosis*:
  - ➤ Triad of fever, rash, & abdominal symptoms
  - ➤ Abdominal symptoms from mesenteric adenitis, terminal ileitis, or appendicitis

Physical signs
- Mesenteric adenitis, fever, RLQ tenderness, leukocytosis (pseudoappendicitis syndrome), more common in older children
- May also cause pharyngitis, osteomyelitis, meningitis, pneumonia
- May also have diarrhea, septicemia, sterile pleural or joint effusions
- Postinfection: erythema nodosum or arthritis, esp. in adults
- Rash usually scarlatiniform

TESTS
- Often positive stool leukocytes
- Stool culture (must tell lab of *Yersinia* suspicion): usually positive during 1st 2 wks
- Antibody test (usually goes to reference lab)
- Culture from other body fluids (urine, bile, CSF), from throat swabs, or blood

DIFFERENTIAL DIAGNOSIS
- Enteritis from other pathogens:
  - *Shigella*
  - *Salmonella*
  - *Campylobacter*
  - Invasive *E. coli*
- Appendicitis
- Kawasaki (*Y. pseudotuberculosis*)

MANAGEMENT
- Supportive: fluid replacement and fever control
- Antibiotics (controversial)

SPECIFIC THERAPY
- Antibiotics:
  - Uncertain benefit if only GI symptoms
  - Useful if infection at other sites or immunocompromised pt
- Aminoglycosides, third-generation cephalosporins, tetracycline (if age >8), chloramphenicol, co-trimoxazole, possibly fluoroquinolones

FOLLOW-UP
- Continue to monitor fluid and electrolyte balance
- Admit patients with infections at sites requiring antibiotics

COMPLICATIONS AND PROGNOSIS
Complications
- Rare
- Septicemia more likely in immunocompromised pts & those with iron overload

Prognosis
- Generally self-limited; most recover in 2–3 wks
- 50% mortality if pt has septicemia, even with antibiotics